THIRD EDITION

RESEARCH METHODS

Principles, Practice, and Theory for Nursing

Catherine H. C. Seaman, R.N., Ph.D.
Professor and Chair
Department of Anthropology and Sociology
Sweet Briar College
Sweet Briar, Virginia

Formerly Coordinator of Undergraduate Research
University of Virginia
School of Nursing
Charlottesville, Virginia

D1417646

**Appleton
&Lange**
Norwalk, Connecticut/Los Altos, California

This edition is dedicated to the memory of my mother, Bertha Davis Hughes; my father, William Irby Coleman; my brother, Pvt. William Irby Coleman, Jr.; and my former colleague, Phyllis Verhonick.

0-8385-8275-3

Notice: The author(s) and publisher of this volume have taken care that the information and recommendations contained herein are accurate and compatible with the standards generally accepted at the time of publication.

87 88 89 90 91 / 10 9 8 7 6 5 4 3 2 1

Prentice-Hall of Australia, Pty. Ltd., Sydney
Prentice-Hall Canada, Inc.
Prentice-Hall Hispanoamericana, S.A., Mexico
Prentice-Hall of India Private Limited, New Delhi
Prentice-Hall International (UK) Limited, London
Prentice-Hall of Japan, Inc., Tokyo
Prentice-Hall of Southeast Asia (Pte.) Ltd., Singapore
Whitehall Books Ltd., Wellington, New Zealand
Editora Prentice-Hall do Brasil Ltda., Rio de Janeiro

Library of Congress Cataloging-in-Publication Data

Seaman, Catherine H. C.
  Research methods.

  Rev. ed. of: Research methods for undergraduate students in nursing. 2nd ed. c1982.
  Bibliography: p.
  Includes index.
  1. Nursing—Research—Methodology. 2. Nursing—
Research. I. Seaman, Catherine H. C. Research methods for undergraduate students in nursing. II. Title.
  [DNLM: 1. Education, Nursing, Baccalaurate. 2. Research—
methods. WY 20.5 S438r]
  RT81.5.S4 1987   610.73'072   86-28667
  ISBN 0-8385-8275-3

Design: M. Chandler Martylewski

Contents

Preface to the Third Edition

It has been a pleasure to write the third edition of *Research Methods*. It was a challenge to meet the expanding interest of nurses in research, theory, and published research reports. A primary goal of this edition, therefore, was to bring these interests together in a way that would be helpful to undergraduate and graduate students and to practicing nurses.

This new edition gives increased attention to examples from actual nursing research, which enables the student or practicing nurse to identify the problems that nurse-researchers select for study, how they study the problems, and what they find. In addition, each chapter of the book concludes with a synopsis of an actual research report that illustrates the major points made in the chapter. An additional chapter examines the theories that nurse-researchers most often use to explain and summarize what they have observed. An expanded section on research designs includes separate chapters on each of the major designs used in nursing research, including new information on qualitative research designs. Chapters on data analysis include additional ways to analyze research data that examine more than one variable.

Like the second edition, the third edition organizes the research process into a simple framework that provides a step-by-step introduction to the construction of research projects. It answers questions such as: What makes nursing research scientific and ethical? How are nursing observations, concepts, and theory interrelated? What are the steps necessary to plan and execute a research project? What are the various designs and methods used? How does the nurse-researcher obtain study subjects? Collect and analyze data? How does a nurse read a research report critically? Use the new microcomputer?

My thanks go to those of my nursing colleagues who read and commented on the book as it was being revised; to Charlie Bollinger, who suggested the third edition; and to the several editors at Appleton-Century-Crofts who subsequently worked on the revision, especially Janice E. Yaeger, who guided the revision to completion. I am also grateful to Sweet Briar College, which provided financial assistance for the purchase of a word processor that greatly assisted the task of revision.

Catherine Seaman

Preface to the Second Edition

The second edition of this book endeavors to meet the expanding interest of nurses in research. The primary goal is to organize the research process into a simple framework that not only provides a step-by-step introduction to the construction of research projects but that answers questions such as: What makes nursing research scientific? How does scientific reasoning enter into research? How are nursing observations and theory related? What are the various designs and methods used in nursing research? How does the student obtain study subjects? Collect and measure the data? Summarize the findings?

The book is written both for the undergraduate nurse and for the graduate student who has not had an undergraduate research course. The aim of the book is to assist the student to understand the research process well enough to read the publications in nursing research with a critical perspective, propose and carry out a circumscribed research project, and integrate the reasoning and observations that make nursing research scientific.

Because of the growth of nursing research, the revision of the book has been a sweeping one. Every chapter has been rewritten, although occasional portions of the first edition remain. Every page was written with the image of Phyllis Verhonick in mind. Consultation with her was sorely missed.

My thanks go to my colleagues who read and commented on the book as it was being revised, and to Charles Bollinger, who encouraged and stimulated the publication.

PART I

Introduction to the Research Process

1

Scientific Research in Nursing

Scientific research is a process in which observable, verifiable data are systematically collected from the empirical world—the world we know through our senses—in order to describe, explain, or predict events. Scientific research differs from nonscientific research undertaken by scholars such as theologians, whose work may be careful and systematic but concerned with unseen phenomena such as supernatural spirits. In contrast, scientific research deals only with what can be observed by one scientist and verified by another. The objectives of scientific research are to answer questions, to discover or revise facts or theories, or to solve problems. Scientific research, as Notter (1963, p. 49) notes, is every nurse's business.

Upon completion of this chapter, the student will be able to: (1) define basic and applied research; (2) state the purposes of research in nursing; (3) trace the rise of scientific research in the ancient art of nursing; (4) describe the place of research in the emergent profession of nursing; and (5) identify trends in the future of nursing research.

APPLIED AND BASIC RESEARCH IN NURSING

Applied research is a process whereby the researcher collects nursing data to be used—that is, *applied*—in the clinical, administrative, or instructional areas. Applied research is designed to: (1) find solutions to nursing problems; (2) evaluate nursing practices or curricula; (3) assess needs; or (4) make decisions to change or continue various aspects of nursing. The research of Kalisch et al. (1985), Chapman (1977), Hain and Chen (1976), and McGillicuddy (1977) includes applied aspects.

For example, Kalisch et al. (1985) developed a news-based forecasting

3

model to predict what the image of nursing would be in order to *aid policy-making* in nursing and *assist in* the *promotion* of an effective image of nursing. A review of newspaper articles from 1978 to 1981, combined with a model constructed to show the effects of key nursing issues on the image of nursing, enabled the researchers to forecast the image of nursing for 1982 to 1984.

Chapman (1977) conducted a clinical study to determine whether measures of patient stress and welfare differed when various approaches to nursing care—individualized, informative, and routine—were used in the perioperative period. She found that both the individualized and the informative approaches to nursing care were more effective than routine nursing care to reduce both the patient's requirement for postoperative analgesics and the length of hospitalization. Her findings suggest solutions to nursing problems concerned with the use of postoperative analgesics and with length of hospital stay. The study also provides data upon which to base decisions to change the approach to nursing care.

Another example of applied research is that of Hain and Chen (1976), who assessed the health needs of elderly persons living in high-rise apartments. After identifying various health problems, the researchers recommended a number of solutions, including screening for windows and employment of health personnel.

McGillicuddy's research (1977) on the relationship between mothers rooming-in with their children during a child's hospitalization and change in the child's behavior enabled her to recommend both administrative changes, such as changes in visiting regulations, and changes in nursing education to allow experience for the nursing student in caring for a family.

Each of these studies centers upon the practical application of research, clearly relating research to problem solving, evaluation, assessment, and intervention.

In contrast, basic research aims to advance scientific knowledge, whether or not this knowledge is immediately usable in nursing. One example of basic research by nurse scientists is that of Parsons et al. (1981), who examined the extent of nerve fiber degeneration in rats' brains following a single cerebral concussion. Since such experimental research is impossible using human subjects, findings from lower mammals may cast some light upon the effects of concussion in general. Similar research is that of Raff (1977), who studied the relationship between prenatal exercise and postnatal growth and development in the offspring of albino rats. However, using the research findings in nursing practice is not the immediate objective of such basic research. Basic research adds to the pool of scientific knowledge, but the implementation of this knowledge in nursing is left to others.

Many nursing studies contain elements of both basic and applied research. Often the distinction between the two has more to do with administrative decisions about financial support than with study content. In this sense, "basic research" may only imply that the researcher was free to work in the area of choice without justifying the work by immediate practical advantage.

THE PURPOSES OF NURSING RESEARCH

The purposes of nursing research may be summarized as follows: to observe in order to know; to know in order to predict; to predict in order to control; and to control in order to practice and prescribe in a professional manner. Each of these purposes will be briefly examined.

To observe in order to know is the aim of all nursing research. The nurse who observes, verifies, and documents observations works at a crucial level of research. These studies are often called *descriptive* or *exploratory*. They begin when the nurse asks the question "What?" For example, Verhonick (1961) asks, "What are bedsores? What are the objective criteria to use to measure bedsores? What causes skin to break down in the first place?" Williams (1972) asks, "What factors contribute to skin breakdown?" Once the factors are discovered and named, the nurse can then explore how they are related to one another. For example, are the factors of age, skin thickness, and diagnosis interrelated to the occurrence of bedsores? Thus, descriptive studies are closely oriented to observation. Yet the very perception of nursing data is often structured by the scientist's background and education. That is, the nurse observes, or "sees," data from a viewpoint that differs from that of a psychologist or geneticist. For example, the nurse–midwife wants to describe, or "know," the physiological, psychological, social, and cultural factors associated with maternal and child care. She wants to know how the procedures are alike for all patients and how they differ for some, such as rural or urban women, lower-class or middle-class women, and women of various ethnic origins. However, all scientists ultimately use their observations to try to explain how concepts are interrelated. Such explanations lead to the second purpose of nursing research—to predict.

To predict, the nurse begins with an explanation, predicts what should be found on observation, and tests these predictions in nursing research. The researcher may predict causality or may predict that correlations will be found between specified factors. Causality means that one variable, such as germ X, causes a change in another variable, such as the state of health. Causality is established if the events under specific conditions may be related in such a way that event Y (such as syphilis) will always be observed to follow event X (exposure to the spirochete). However, because many complex factors influence human health and welfare, it is not always possible to establish causality as neatly as the germ theory allows. For example, scientists cannot yet say exactly what causes lung cancer. However, they can say that lung cancer increases as pollution of the inhaled air increases. Predictions can be made that certain factors appear to be associated with a rise in lung cancer. As evidence increases, stronger statements can be made, such as that of the Surgeon General concerning cigarette smoking as a health hazard.

Correlations, or concomitant variations and associations, as these are also called, state that a change in the amount of one variable is related to a change in the amount of another. Correlations may be either positive or negative: as one increases, the other also increases; or, as one increases, the other decreases.

Once such interrelations are made, the nurse can predict that certain populations are at risk to develop lung cancer; for example, those who smoke. Predictions such as these can be tested further in research; if the research findings support the predictions, steps can be taken to control harmful factors.

To control is a major purpose of applied nursing research. It means that the nurse has the ability to check, regulate, and exercise directing power over factors that influence the health and comfort of patients or clients. To control pain, discomfort, sickness, anxiety, or fear is an objective of patient care; to control ignorance and superstition is an objective of nursing teaching; and to control the proper flow of information and communication is a goal of nursing administration. A revolutionary approach in nursing is to return control of the patient's body and mind to the patient, with as little recourse to drugs and dependence upon health personnel as possible.

When nursing is able to describe, understand, and explain nursing phenomena; when we can predict what will happen each time we intervene; and if our ability to predict allows us to control the harmful factors and promote the positive; then nursing research can fulfill the final purpose—to prescribe.

To prescribe requires a deep involvement in research and practice. In addition, it involves a conception of what is good and desirable—the values of the profession and society. A prescription is based on the fact that the goal to be achieved is a desirable one and that the way to achieve the goal is to follow the prescription. To bring about and maintain good health, the prescription states, one must comply with the prescribed regimen of treatment, diet, or medication.

Nurses have long practiced and prescribed intuitively. Experience has often told them to do one thing rather than another. However, the research process helps nurses to put experience and intuition into a statement that summarizes or predicts relationships among concepts and variables. It helps them to test the statement in research and then to share the findings with the profession as a whole. In this way, research adds to the accumulating body of nursing science and enables nurses to solve problems and recommend changes.

THE RISE OF SCIENTIFIC RESEARCH
IN THE ART OF NURSING

Long before nursing was a science, it was an art. Many aspects of contemporary nursing are rooted in the thousands of years during which nurses attempted to care for and cure the sick with tender, loving care rather than with science. Nursing helped others to do what they could not do for themselves—deliver a baby, feed the wounded, or bathe the helpless.

Scanty evidence exists from the archeological record to indicate who were the nurses of antiquity. The work of Solecki (1971) in an ancient cave in Iraq suggests that, about 60,000 years ago, women, children, and occasionally an old man remained close to the hearth fires of home. Perhaps they were the first nurses. Evidence from ancient bones found near the hearth suggests that early patients were the handicapped and the injured. The cave dwellers of Shanidar, called the *flower people* by Solecki because they placed clusters of flowers in the graves of their dead, may have utilized local plants as poultices or herbal remedies. Elsewhere in the ancient world, Marshack (1972) found finely made figurines that, he suggests, may have been used in magical rites to assist women in childbirth.

Nursing care moved out of the home when priests established a causal link in the minds of their followers between evil spirits and sickness. For example, in Greece, by 1200 B.C., the sick were being treated in temples, where the priests prescribed rest, diet, and bathing.

Among early Christians, both women and men cared for the sick and aged; this practice continued as the Church gained control over society. However, the dirty and unpleasant work associated with the art of nursing was often left to the lower levels of nurses, who performed disagreeable tasks in hope of a later reward in heaven. The well-to-do and educated tended to supervise rather than deliver direct care. During the Crusades, men and women of high status served as nurses. In fact, the association of nursing with war and the military left its mark on the character of nurses' training, as well as on the military-like stratification that has long been a part of nursing practice. In the West, nursing tended to become a task performed by women, while research tended to be exclusively in the hands of men.

Following the Protestant Reformation, the status of nursing, now based on wage labor supported by taxes, declined. Low wages, lack of education, and the servant-like status of women who were nurses soon brought nursing to a position of disrespect and contempt. The art of nursing fell to untrained, uneducated women, some of whom were inmates of workhouses or penal institutions. However, humanitarian reform arose in reaction to the Industrial Revolution, with its accompanying exploitation of the poor and the sick. In Germany, Pastor Fliedner established a five-year program to train nurses. Among those who examined the functioning of the school was Florence Nightingale, who (in 1860) founded a school of nursing at St. Thomas's Hospital in England. Nightingale approached nursing primarily as an art but was also the first nurse-scientist. Her *Notes on Nursing* (1859) not only stresses the use of observation but also contains a wealth of material inviting research.

The most important practical lesson that can be given to nurses, Nightingale writes (p. 65), is to teach them how and what to observe. In Nightingale's view, devotion is useless without ready and correct observations. While statistics inform us what percentage of the population may die, she writes, observation tells us which ones will die.

Nightingale was a firm believer in applied research, noting that observations are made for the sake of saving lives and increasing comfort rather than for piling up miscellaneous information or curious facts (p. 70).

Nightingale's approach to nurses' training assisted in the rise of the modern hospital, which came into being along with the improvement of bedside nursing, hospital management, the science of bacteriology, and the introduction of aseptic surgery. At that time, nurses' training included the mastery of scientific techniques and procedures, if not scientific theory. Nonetheless, the rise of science and research in nursing was underway.

The Development of Nursing Research

Following Nightingale's era, research in nursing practice declined for nearly a century. It was replaced in the United States by research in nursing education and administration, such as that conducted by Nutting (1907), and by research on the function of nurses, such as that reported by Hughes et al. (1958).

During the decade of the 1950s, more and more nurses entered the universities to complete undergraduate or graduate education. Research was required to complete the graduate degree. In the universities, many nurses began to form intellectual alliances with those in the social and behavioral sciences (Benne and Bennis, 1959), with several consequences. First, nurses became researchers in the domains of the social and behavioral sciences neglected by many physicians. Second, the profession of nursing began to integrate a holistic approach to patients, family, and community, which supplemented the former "organ" or "disease" orientation. Third, the conceptual and theoretical frameworks of the social and behavioral sciences began to make their way into nursing to supplement the theory of the natural sciences. For example, the integrated approach enabled nurses to treat mental illness, rapidly becoming the most prevalent disease in the Western world, with a considerable level of sophistication. Moreover, the appearance of the journal *Nursing Research* also provided nurses during the 1950s with both a forum and a stimulus for research.

During the 1960s, research concerned with patient care and nursing practice began to appear in the literature once more. *Patient-Centered Approaches to Nursing*, by Abdellah et al. (1960), ushered in the new era. Orlando's *The Dynamic Nurse–Patient Relationship* (1961) focused attention on interaction between nurse and patient. Brown's *Newer Dimensions of Patient Care* (1961–1962) integrated the scientific approaches of anthropology and nursing. *Better Patient Care Through Nursing Research*, by Abdellah and Levine (1965), exemplified the rise of the importance of research in nursing.

From this time forward, publications that dealt with nursing research began to accelerate. The National Commission for the Study of Nursing and Nursing Education reinforced the importance of science and research in nursing in its 1970 report, *An Abstract for Action*, which established research as one of the four priorities in the future of nursing. In *Research in Nursing: Toward a Science of Health Care* (1976), the American Nurses' Association reported contemporary trends in nursing research and suggested that nursing was moving toward becoming the science of health care. During the 1970s, edited studies in nursing research appeared, including the series *Communicating Nursing Research*, edited by Marjorie V. Batey (1968–1978, 11 vol.); Verhonick (1975; 1977); and Downs and Fleming (1979).

During that time, publications concerned with theory in nursing also began to appear: Rogers (1970); Murphy (1971); Hardy (1973); Hardy and Conway (1978); and Stevens (1979). The decade of the 1980s has brought more, including both revisions of old works and new publications, such as those by Kim (1983), Chinn (1983), and Walker (1983).

Basic and applied clinical nursing research has shown a similar growth. At first, clinical studies centered upon particular diseases, such as tuberculosis; then studies focused on maternal and child care. Recent clinical research includes a wide variety of topics and designs, such as Cleland's (1971) concern with the prevention of bacteriuria in female patients with indwelling catheters, and Jacox's (1973 and 1977) work on pain. Diers (1979) combined research in the clinical area with a theoretical orientation developed by Dickoff and James (1968).

The Importance of Research to the Nursing Profession

Research is of vital importance to nursing today, more so than it has ever been in the past. The rapid advance of knowledge in the fields of health maintenance, health promotion, and disease prevention, together with the public's demand for the quality of life that good physical and mental health bring, have moved nursing quickly forward. To meet new challenges, investigate unsolved problems, and scrutinize the changes underway in nursing, the individual nurse must actively seek to understand and apply the basic principles of research.

Likewise, research provides the abstract knowledge that is the foundation for establishing nursing as a profession. According to Carr-Saunders and Wilson (1933), the distinguishing mark of a profession is the combination of knowledge and technique. Caplow (1971), a more recent work, includes a knowledge base, autonomy and monopoly in practice, and serious consequences of practice to society. A code of ethics is another distinguishing feature of the professional. Each of these five criteria will be examined briefly, in order to assess the place of research in the rising profession of nursing.

1. *The possession of a large body of abstract knowledge is directly related to research and theory.* From what pool of abstract knowledge does nursing draw to make decisions? What theory explains the reasoning behind a decision to intervene in practice, change a curriculum, or reverse an administrative decision? Writing over 25 years ago, Johnson (1959, p. 292) suggests that professional nursing draws its knowledge from the basic sciences. Nurses then apply this knowledge in practice to achieve carefully defined goals. Research findings useful to nursing include those of physics, chemistry, microbiology, physiology, psychology, anthropology, sociology, law, and economics. In her view, nursing research should be designed to test the findings from these disciplines so as to expand nursing's body of knowledge.

2. *The achievement of autonomy in nursing is underway.* Bullough (1975) notes the autonomy of the clinical specialists, while Foster and Anderson (1978, p. 199) relate the autonomy gained by nurse-practitioners to their willingness to assume major responsibilities. However, further research is needed to establish the nature and permanence of autonomy in nursing. Is nursing autonomy related to the supply of doctors? Will nurses achieve true autonomy only in ghettos or sparsely populated areas where medical doctors do not choose to practice? Does federal funding of the health care of the poor enable nurses to be autonomous? How will the curtailment of federal funds to health and welfare, currently underway, affect nursing? Answers to such questions are crucial to the establishment and survival of autonomy in nursing.

3. *Monopoly of nursing practice is a legal question, contingent upon both a definition of nursing and support at the legislative level.* As Hinsvark (1974) notes, only a few states, such as Washington, have laws that give nurses the right to expanded practice. Research is needed, not only to keep abreast of legal questions, but also to determine the most effective way to promote the profession and protect the image of nursing.

4. *The social consequences that follow autonomy and monopoly of nursing practice are serious.* This is evident in the report of the

National Commission for the Study of Nursing and Nursing Education (1970, p. 163):

> We have become intimately acquainted with the history and the disappointments, as well as the great joys of nursing. Out of this has come the recognition that nursing is not only important, but critical to the future of health care in America.

The social consequences that would follow if all nurses withdrew from hospitals, clinics, nursing homes, and public health agencies indicate the seriousness of nursing practice.

5. *The nursing code of ethics is concerned with moral and ethical questions for which the nurse is responsible.* The nursing profession must continually review its code to reflect both the changing status of nursing and societal demands. A comparison of the Florence Nightingale Code with the current American Nurses' Association Code (1976), for example, reveals changes in the relationship between nursing and medicine.

There are virtually no formal teaching structures for nursing ethics, in either schools of nursing or other schools for health professions, Gortner notes (1979, p. 193). Greater attention must be given to ethics, she suggests, in both research and practice.

Future Directions of Nursing Research

Nowhere is the importance of research in the future of nursing better demonstrated than in the statement of The National League for Nursing (1978), which includes research as one of the ten characteristics of baccalaureate education in nursing. Emphasis upon research in the undergraduate curriculum assures that a new generation of nurses will possess research skills.

What areas of research will nurses pursue in the future? Lindeman (1975) reports the findings of a nationwide survey of nurses, the Delphi survey, which identified the most important areas needing research (Table 1–1). Evaluation, nursing practice, nursing interventions, and nursing roles were considered to be important areas for research. Fleming (1979) suggests that research in the future should focus on preventive health measures, nursing care, and persistent nursing problems (Table 1–2). In Fleming's view, nursing researchers must find ways to incorporate research findings into nursing practice. Yet Stetler and Marram (1976) warn that research findings must first be evaluated before they are applied to nursing problems. Nurses should be able to predict and assess outcomes of applied research findings. Loomis (1985), in a study designed to document the emerging content in nursing, undertook to analyze and classify the content of dissertations from 25 nursing doctoral programs between

TABLE 1–1. FUTURE DIRECTIONS OF NURSING RESEARCH SUGGESTED BY LINDEMAN'S 1975 SURVEY

Research *to determine:*
1. How to use research in practice
2. Valid and reliable indicators of quality nursing care
3. Interventions by nurses most effective in reducing patients' psychological stress
4. Valid and reliable methods for staffing that reflect patients' needs and contain costs
5. Effective means of communicating and implementing change in practice
6. The nursing behavior and setting most likely to produce positive effects in a crisis

Research *to evaluate:*
1. Effects of nurses' expanding role in patient care
2. Functions and clinical parameters of nurse-practitioners
3. Processes used to provide nursing care in terms of patient outcomes
4. Nurses' role in preventive health service in terms of patient outcomes
5. Effectiveness of various approaches to peer review
6. Nurses' interventions that are most effective in reducing the psychological stress of patients
7. Change in nursing practice

Research *to establish* the relationship between clinical nursing research and quality care.

Research *to develop* a set of physical and psychological procedures to assess and improve patient care and nursing intervention.

Research *to explore* means of enhancing nurses' ability to cope with stress.

Research *to clarify* concepts, such as the expanding role of the nurse.

Research *to delimit* the functions and clinical parameters of nurse-practitioners.

Research *to assess* the relationship between quality of nursing leadership and quality of nursing practice in institutions.

1976 and 1982. She divided the content into two categories: clinical nursing and social issues. She found that 78.4 percent of the dissertations pertained to clinical nursing, while 21.6 percent studied social issues in nursing.

The American Nurses' Association Commission of Nursing Research has identified a number of questions that it hopes will be answered in future nursing research (A.N.A., 1976): (1) How are individuals persuaded to use available measures to prevent illness? (2) How are individuals helped to maintain health? (3) How are people helped to cope with illness? (4) How are complications reduced among those hospitalized or chronically ill? (5) How is illness prevented for those subject to health risks, such as the premature and the elderly? Each question represents a fruitful area to explore in research. Forthcoming answers will not only prevent suffering but will save countless time and money and will reduce the investment of energy.

In Leininger's view (1976), future research in doctoral programs will focus on four areas: the identification of cultural influences on health practices and values; definition of ways to achieve new levels of health

TABLE 1–2. RESEARCH NEEDS IDENTIFIED BY FLEMING (1979)

Preventive Health

Research to understand behaviors detrimental to health:
1. Excess use of alcohol and mood-altering drugs
2. Cigarette smoking
3. Poor nutritional practices
4. Carelessness that results in accidental injury
5. Sedentary life styles and improper exercise
6. Improper care and supervision of children
7. Lack of knowledge to carry out the parenting role

Research to understand preventive health problems for age groups:
1. Health care of the young
2. Lack of immunization among children
3. Quality of life for city children
4. Child neglect and child abuse
5. Psychosocial disability from poor bonding between mother and infant
6. Extent to which a disabling condition can be decreased
7. Rate and consequences of teenage pregnancies
8. Preventive mental health services to families and youth
9. Health education to improve access to comprehensive care
10. The economics of maintaining and caring for the aged
11. Aspects of leisure time, retirement, coping abilities, and health status of the elderly
12. Demand for health care and hospitalization of the aged

Types of Care

Research related to primary health care:
1. Clarification of the role of the nurse who is practicing primary care
2. Changes in the delivery system of primary care
3. Planning, delivery, assessment, and monitoring of primary care for all ages and socioeconomic statuses

Research related to long-term health care:
1. Identification and resolution for long-term care of chronic conditions such as: diabetes, urological conditions, arthritis, cardiac conditions, glaucoma, cataracts, cancer, cerebral vascular accidents, and mental aberrations

Current Conditions Likely to be Prevalent in the Future

Research related to:
1. Drug abuse: narcotics; alcohol; cigarette smoking; effect on user and, in case of women, on the fetus
2. Stress: identifying, assessing, measuring, and implementing intervention plans to alter loneliness, pain, fear, and adjustment problems
3. Venereal disease; cancer; nutrition problems; and cultural diversity

Problems Identified by Nurses

Research to reduce complications of hospitalization and surgery; to improve outlook for high-risk parents and infants; to improve health care of the elderly; to study life-threatening situations; to study adaptation to chronic illness; to study self-care systems; to study new technological development.*

*See Priorities for Research in Nursing. Kansas City: ANA Commission on Nursing Research, 1975.

care; invention of systems to classify nursing phenomena; and the formulation of systems to evaluate major components of health care.

In the views of Abdellah (1971), Gortner (1975), and Barnard and Neal (1977), the profession will direct future attention to theory development, conceptual clarification, and research, a practice already underway.

SUMMARY

Scientific research is a process in which observable data are systematically collected from the empirical world by one scientist and verified by another. Research is commonly divided into two types, basic and applied. *Basic research* advances scientific knowledge, regardless of whether the knowledge is immediately usable or not. *Applied research* is used in nursing practice, teaching, or administration. Most research projects contain elements of both types of research.

The purpose of research is to observe in order to know; to know in order to predict; to predict in order to control; and to control in order to practice and prescribe in a professional manner. Descriptive or exploratory studies help the nurse know what the subject matter of nursing is and what should be studied. Prediction allows the nurse to identify associated factors in order to control other factors, such as pain. Once nursing attains the knowledge necessary to understand and predict, it will be more able to control harmful elements, and nurses will move into practice and prescription with greater assurance.

The art of nursing—helping others to do what they cannot do for themselves—is an ancient tradition rooted first in the home and then in religious institutions. The decline of nursing as a service to God put nursing practice in a low-status, wage-earning position. Nightingale, scientist and scholar, raised the status of nursing and stressed that observation should be applied for the sake of saving lives and increasing the comfort of the sick. Following Nightingale's era, nearly a century elapsed before research focused on the patient rather than on the nurse or nursing. In the universities, alliances between nursing and the social and behavioral sciences influenced the direction of nursing research.

In order to provide a body of knowledge that allows the nurse discretion and autonomy in practice, research is crucial to the emergent profession of nursing. Research is becoming the focus of many teachers, and the behavioral sciences have influenced the direction of nursing research.

EXAMPLE FROM NURSING RESEARCH

Julia S. Brown, Christine A. Tanner, Daren P. Padrik (1984): Nursing's search for scientific knowledge. Nursing Research, 33, 26–32.

In this article, the authors examine four characteristics found in the literature that are presumed to be essential for the development of a scientific base in nursing. These include the following: (1) research should be conducted by members of the nursing discipline; (2) research should be concerned with clinical problems; (3) scientific research should be anchored in a theoretical framework that is continuously refined and extended through replication of research studies; and (4) methods of research should be sound.

To examine whether these characteristics of research have changed since 1952, the authors selected a sample of 137 research articles published in four journals—*Nursing Research*; *The International Journal of Nursing Studies*; *Research in Nursing and Health*; and the *Western Journal of Nursing Research*. Years selected for study include 1952, when the journal *Nursing Research* appeared, and each decade year thereafter: 1960, 1970, and 1980. Selections included all studies in *Nursing Research* in 1952–1953 and 1960, as well as a random sample of the 63 studies published in the 1970 and the 95 articles published in the 1980 issues of the journals.

To summarize and discuss the results of the study, the authors asked four questions: To what extent have nurses responded to the call to conduct research? Has the focus of research shifted toward clinical practice? Has nursing research become more theoretically oriented? What methods were used in nursing research, and how have the methods changed over the past decades? Each question was answered in turn.

1. *To what extent have nurses responded to the call to conduct research?* Nursing research has increased: the number of journals concentrating on research has increased from 1 to 4, while the number of articles published increased from 17 in 1952–1953 to 136 in 1980. In addition, by 1980, nurses comprised 78 percent of the senior authors; 48 percent of these had doctoral degrees.

2. *Has the focus of nursing research shifted toward issues of clinical practice?* To answer this question, four categories were devised: nursing education, nurse characteristics, administration, and clinical practice. It was found that the focus of research has shifted to clinical problems.

3. *Has nursing research become more theoretically oriented?* The authors found that the answer to this was yes. The proportion of studies with no theoretical framework, explicit or implicit, has declined. However, the theoretical perspective most frequently employed was psychological and social–psychological in nature.

4. *What methods have been employed in nursing research? How have they changed over the past three decades?* To answer these questions, the authors examined aspects of the research design, data collection techniques, measurements, sampling, and analysis of data. They found that research designs, classified according to purpose, were methodological, descriptive, or explanatory. The most frequently used design was the explanatory (36 cases, or 57 percent of the total, in 1980), with correlational designs (and ex-post-facto) accounting for most of these. Use of descriptive designs declined sharply over the years, while use of the methodological design remained quite small. The cross-sectional study was the most frequently used time frame-

work, with only 4 percent of the studies using a longitudinal approach that examines trends, processes, and dynamics of change.

The major method of data collection was that of asking questions by interview and questionnaires, while measurement tools included previously published tools, mostly from psychology, with about equal use of tools created by the researcher. By 1980, nearly half of the researchers specified the reliability of their measurement tools, and one third the validity. This is an improvement over 1952–1953, when it was rare to report either.

Sampling was almost always a nonprobability sample, usually a convenience sample, while median sample size decreased from 84 in 1952 to 60 in 1980. Study units were nearly always persons—the students, nurses, and patients found in hospitals, clinics, and schools of nursing.

Analysis of data changed from equal stress on both qualitative and quantitative research to emphasis on quantitative, with bivariate analysis being the most frequently used type.

The authors included the following recommendations. Nursing should: (1) direct efforts toward the development of instruments to measure phenomena of interest to nursing; (2) use a wider variety of data sources including records, archives, observational techniques, unobtrusive measures, and qualitative materials; (3) use more longitudinal designs to study change; (4) replicate studies; (5) use multivariate analyses where appropriate; (6) link research to prior work to refine, extend, or refute theoretical formulations; and (7) relate all hypotheses to theory, in order that research findings can be tied into past work.

STUDY QUESTIONS

1. Define the kind of research that has application in the clinical area. Can you propose such a research project?
2. State the four purposes of nursing research.
3. Describe a descriptive or exploratory project that you would like to conduct and identify which of the four purposes of nursing research it would fulfill.
4. Write a statement that predicts a causal relationship between germs and disease.
5. Can you use any knowledge gained in nursing to make a prediction about nursing care?
6. Describe some of the factors in patient care that you have tried to control, and describe the factors that enabled you to achieve or maintain control.
7. Write a nursing prescription. How is it similar to nursing intervention?
8. Write a nursing prescription that the patient can use to intervene in a process that is not good for his or her health.

9. Which purpose of nursing research did Nightingale stress? Explain whether or not it is relevant today.
10. At times, nurses give patients backrubs. Is this an art or a science? Why?
11. To what do you attribute the rise of research in nursing?
12. What trends can you identify in future nursing research?
13. Examine Tables 1–1 and 1–2. Which of these research needs most interests you? Which would you like to study or examine in research?
14. Read the preceding example from *Nursing Research*, "Nursing's search for scientific knowledge." Which of the recommendations do you find most important or attractive?

REFERENCES AND SUGGESTED READINGS

Abdellah, F. (1971): Foreword. In Murphy, F. (ed.), Theoretical Issues in Professional Nursing. New York: Appleton-Century-Crofts, pp. xi–xii.

Abdellah, F. et al. (1960): Patient-Centered Approaches to Nursing. New York: Macmillan. *Abdellah et al. change the focus of research from nurses to patients.*

Abdellah, F. and Levine, E. (1979): Better Patient Care Through Nursing Research (2nd ed.). New York: Macmillan. *The second edition of a comprehensive book that integrates research with patient care. Part 4 looks at contemporary status of nursing research.*

American Nurses' Association (1976): Research in Nursing: Toward a Science of Health Care. Kansas City: The American Nurses' Association. Preparation of Nurses for Participation in Research. Code No. D-54 2500. Kansas City: The American Nurses' Association. Priorities for Research in Nursing. Kansas City: The American Nurses' Association. *Publications of the association that reflect the rising emphasis on research.*

Batey, M. (ed.) (1968–1978): Communicating Nursing Research. Boulder: Western Interstate Commission on Higher Education (WICHE). *Eleven volumes of report papers delivered in a conference on research held yearly since 1968. Each research paper is followed by a critique from another nurse-scientist.*

Barnard, K. and Neal, M. (1977): Maternal-child nursing research: Review of the past and strategies for the future. Nursing Research, 26, 193–200. *The authors call for the development of classificatory systems of concepts used in practice.*

Benne, D. and Bennis, W. (1959): The role of the professional nurse. American Journal of Nursing, May, 837–882. *The authors discuss the problems of the drive for professionalism in nursing and note the alliances formed in universities between nursing and the social and behavioral sciences.*

Brown, E. (1948): Nursing for the Future. New York: Russell Sage. (1961): Newer Dimensions of Patient Care I. New York: Russell Sage. (1962): Newer Dimensions of Patient Care II. New York: Russell Sage. *An anthropologist interested in nursing published the three books above that provided insight into the nursing profession.*

Brown, J. et al. (1984): Nursing's search for scientific knowledge. Nursing Research, 33, 26–32.

Bullough, B. (1975): Factors contributing to role expansion for registered nurses. In Bullough, B. (ed.), The Law and the Expanding Nursing Role. New York: Appleton-Century-Crofts, pp. 53–61.

Bullough, B. (ed.) (1980): The Law and the Expanding Nursing Role (2nd ed.). New York: Appleton-Century-Crofts. *A collection of papers that examine the use of law, perspectives on the expanding role of nurses, and other topics.*

Caplow, T. (1971): Elementary Sociology. Englewood Cliffs, N. J.: Prentice-Hall. *Chapter VIII contains discussion on professions and occupations.*

Carr-Saunders, A. and Wilson, P. (1933): Professions. In Seligman, E. (ed.), Encyclopaedia of the Social Sciences. New York: Macmillan. *Nearly 50 years old, this article still provides insight and understanding.*

Chapman, J. (1977): Effects of different approaches upon selected postoperative responses of male herniorraphy patients. In Downs, F. and Newman, M., A Sourcebook of Nursing Research. Philadelphia: F. A. Davis, pp. 15–23.

Chinn, P. (ed.) (1983): Advances in Nursing Theory Development. Rockville, Md.: Aspen.

Cleland, V. (1977): Investigations in the clinical setting. In Verhonick, P. (ed.), Nursing Research II. Boston: Little, Brown, pp. 33–75. *Discusses two studies: the effect of situational stressors on the cognitive performance of general nurses, and a study to assess the relative effectiveness of different types of perineal care in preventing bacteriuria in female patients with indwelling catheters.*

Cleland, V. et al. (1971): Prevention of bacteriuria in female patients with indwelling catheters. Nursing Research, 20, 309–318.

Diers, D. (1979): Research in Nursing Practice. Philadelphia: J. B. Lippincott. *Uses ideas generated by Dickoff and James and others to develop chapters on clinical judgment, and studies of factor-searching, relation-searching, association and causal hypotheses testing, and prescription testing.*

Dickoff, J. and James, P. (1968): Theory in a practice discipline. Practice oriented theory (Part I). Practice oriented research (Part II). Nursing Research, 17, 415–435; 545–554. *Develops theory related to practice.*

Downs, F. and Fleming, J. (eds.) (1979): Issues in Nursing Research. New York: Appleton-Century-Crofts. *Seven articles cover particular problem areas in research.*

Downs, F. and Newman, M. (eds.) (1977): A Source Book of Nursing Research (2nd ed.). Philadelphia: F. A. Davis. *Sixteen articles deal with research in nursing.*

Fleming, J. (1979): The future of nursing research. In Downs, F. and Fleming, J. (eds.), Issues in Nursing Research. New York: Appleton-Century-Crofts. *Reports on the acceptance and scope of research in nursing, research needs, and other issues.*

Foster, F. and Anderson, B. (1978): Medical Anthropology. New York: Wiley. *Chapter 11 deals with "Professionals in Medicine, Nursing."*

Gortner, S. (1975): Research for a practice profession. Nursing Research, 24, 193–197. *Notes a trend in nursing to integrate theory and research to provide knowledge base.*

Hain, M. and Chen, S. (1976): Health needs of the elderly. Nursing Research, 25, 433–439. *A study of the elderly living in high-rise apartments.*

Hall, V. (1975): Statutory Regulation of the Scope of Nursing Practice—A Critical Survey. Chicago: National Joint Practice Commission. *Author comments on various definitions found in Nurse Practice Act.*

Hardy, M. (ed.) (1973): Theoretical Foundations for Nursing. New York: MSS Information Corp. *Editor brings together a number of articles contributing to theory.*

Hardy, M. and Conway, M. (1978): Role Theory: Perspectives for Health Professionals. New York: Appleton-Century-Crofts. *Twelve articles deal with role.*

Henderson, V., Nite, G. et al. (1978): Principles and Practices of Nursing (6th ed.). New York: Macmillan. *Part I: Place of nursing in health services.*

Hinsvark, I. (1974): Implications for action in the expanded role of the nurse. Nursing Clinics of North America, *9*, 411–423. *Effect of nursing and medical practice acts on work activity of nurses.*

Hughes, E. et al. (1958): Twenty Thousand Nurses Tell Their Story. Philadelphia: J. B. Lippincott. *Five-year study on nurses initiated by the A.N.A.*

Jacox, A. and Steward, M. (1973): Psychosocial Contingencies of the Pain Experience. Iowa City, Iowa: University of Iowa College of Nursing. *A study of pain as a biopsychosocial phenomenon.*

Jacox, A. (ed.) (1977): Pain: A Sourcebook for Nurses and Other Health Professionals Boston: Little, Brown. *Overview of pain.*

Johnson, D. (1959): The nature of a science of nursing. Nursing Outlook, *7*, 291–294. *The emergence of nursing as a science.*

Kalisch, B., Kalisch, P., and Belcher, B. (1985): Forecasting for nursing policy: A news-based image approach. Nursing Research, *34*, 44–49.

Kim, H. (1983): The Nature of Theoretical Thinking in Nursing. Norwalk, Conn.: Appleton-Century-Crofts.

King, I. (1971): Toward a Theory for Nursing. New York: Wiley.

Leininger, M. (1976): Doctoral program for nurses: Trends, questions, and projected plans. Nursing Research, *24*, 434–441. *Ideas of cultural influences on health.*

Lindeman, C. and Van Aernam, V. (1971): Nursing intervention with the presurgical patient—the effects of structured and unstructured preoperative teaching. Nursing Research, *20*, 196–209. *Authors examine effect of preoperative teaching on postoperative behavior.*

Lindeman, C. (1975): Delphi survey of priorities in clinical nursing research. Nursing Research, *24*, 434–441. *Priorities for nursing research.*

Marshack, A. (1972): The Roots of Civilization. New York: McGraw-Hill. *An examination of the prehistory of people.*

McGillicuddy, M. (1977): A study of the relationship between mothers' rooming in during their children's hospitalization and changes in selected areas of children's behavior. In Downs, F. and Newman, M. (eds.), A Sourcebook of Nursing Research. Philadelphia: F. A. Davis, pp. 64–77. *Author recommends changes in practice area from research findings.*

Murphy, F. (1971): Theoretical Issues in Professional Nursing. New York: Appleton-Century-Crofts. *Collection of articles dealing with theories useful in nursing.*

National Commission for the Study of Nursing and Nursing Education (1970): An Abstract for Action. New York: McGraw-Hill. *A national study of nursing.*

National League for Nursing (1978): Characteristics of Baccalaureate Education in Nursing. *A revision of the 1974 statement.*

Nightingale, F. (1859): Notes on Nursing (1970 ed.). London: Gerald Duckworth. *A small book everyone interested in nursing should read.*

Notter, L. (1963): Nursing research in every nurse's business. Nursing Outlook, *11*, 49–51. *Notter's view of research.*

Nutting, M. (1907): The Educational and Professional Position of Nurses. U.S. Gov. Printing. *An early study of nurses in the United States.*

Orlando, I. (1961): The Dynamic Nurse–Patient Relationship. New York: G. P. Putnam's Sons. *Communication between nurse–patient.*

Parsons, C. et al. (1981): Nerve fiber degeneration following a single experimental cerebral concussion in the rat. Neuroscience Letter, *24*, 199–204.

Raff, B. (1977): The relationship of planned prenatal exercise to postnatal growth and development in the offspring of albino rats. In Downs, F. and Newman, M. (eds.), A Sourcebook of Nursing Research (2nd ed.). Philadelphia: F. A. Davis. pp. 78–85. *Example of basic research.*

Rogers, M. (1970): Introduction to the Theoretical Basis of Nursing. Philadelphia: F. A. Davis. *Uses principle of reciprocity to relate man to environment.*

Seligman, E. (ed.) (1933): Encyclopedia of the Social Sciences. New York: Macmillan. *Old, but still relevant.*

Solecki, R. (1971): Shanidar: The First Flower People. New York: Knopf. *Excavations in Iraq reveal prehistoric health conditions.*

Stetler, C. and Marram, G. (1976): Evaluating research findings for applicability in practice. Nursing Outlook, *24*, 559–563.

Stevens, B. (1979): Nursing Theory. Boston: Little, Brown. *An analysis and evaluation of nursing theory in its present state.*

Verhonick, P. (ed.) (1975): Nursing Research I. Boston: Little, Brown. (1977): Nursing Research II. Boston: Little, Brown.

Verhonick, P. (1961): Decubitus ulcer observations measured objectively. Nursing Research, *10*, 211–214. *Use of observation to answer "what" questions.*

Walker, L. and Avant, K. (1983): Strategies for Theory Construction in Nursing. Norwalk, Conn.: Appleton-Century-Crofts.

Williams, A. (1972): Study of factors contributing to skin breakdown. Nursing Research, *21*, 238–243.

2

Ethical Issues
in Nursing Research

A good research problem conforms to moral, ethical, and legal standards
of scientific inquiry. A researcher should have deep concern for human
welfare and sensitivity for the rights of research subjects. Any research
that may be harmful violates the ethical code of nursing and may be
illegal.

This chapter is designed to help the student become aware of the
issues related to the use of human subjects in research. Upon completion
of this chapter, the student should be able to: (1) describe the relationship
between values and ethics; (2) state the rights of human subjects; (3)
identify subjects who are vulnerable and need to have their rights protected; (4) describe problems concerned with the researcher's withholding
information or with fully disclosing research plans to subjects; (5) identify
the steps to take to secure informed consent; and (6) discuss the nurse's
role in research.

VALUES AND ETHICS

Values are the ideas that members of a society share about what is important, worthwhile, good, and bad. Values underlie standards and are
the criteria by which means and ends are judged. *Ethics* refers to the
study and evaluation of human conduct. *Applied ethics* examines actual
human conduct in real situations. Research involves both values and
ethics. For example, it is a basic scientific value that it is better to know
than not to know. The behavior associated with this value is to seek
knowledge through research. This applied ethic may come into conflict
with the right of human beings to determine for themselves what will be

done to them. A tension exists, therefore, between human rights that restrict the freedom of inquiry and the injunction to seek knowledge, which promotes research.

The need to protect human rights is amply demonstrated by research in which potentially harmful experiments were performed on elderly patients, children, and sick persons. Aged and infirm hospital patients were injected with live cancer cells without being informed that cancer was in any way involved (Langer, 1966). Mentally retarded children were deliberately exposed to infectious hepatitis, which could have resulted in considerable physical harm to them (Capron, 1973).

When the research designs of these experiments became public, the resulting outcry led to the development of guidelines to protect human subjects at both governmental and professional levels. For example, the federal government, through the Department of Health, Education, and Welfare, developed policies that mandated informed consent (1974) and privacy (1976). The American Nurses' Association developed *Human Rights Guidelines for Nurses in Clinical and Other Research*, which were first adopted in 1967 and updated in 1975.

THE RIGHTS OF HUMAN SUBJECTS

The first right of human subjects is not to be harmed physically, psychologically, or emotionally. Other rights include self-determination, privacy, confidentiality, the right to maintain self-respect, the right to refuse to participate in research or to withdraw from participation without any penalty, and the right for services. Each of these will be examined.

1. *The right not to be harmed has received little consideration in the past.* It is reported that Edward Jenner deliberately exposed an 8-year-old child to cowpox in order to try a new vaccine (Hayter, 1979). The good that Jenner did is remembered, while the possibility that the child may have been harmed has been forgotten. Unforgotten in the Western world, however, are the Nazi experiments that were conducted by highly qualified scholars with a flagrant disregard for the well-being of their captive human subjects.

   The best-known example of psychologically harmful research is that of Milgram's (1963) study of obedience to authority. The test was designed to determine how many persons would continue to obey the commands of an authority figure, even when they thought they were endangering the life of another. The procedure required that the subjects give what they thought were increasingly powerful electric shocks to another person (who was actually a stooge). Of the 40 subjects, 65 percent continued to give shocks to the end of the series, even though there was a question of harming what they thought was a powerless person. Urged on by the researcher to continue giving the shocks, the subjects were clearly anguished and tense: sweating, stuttering, and trembling. One subject had a violently convulsive seizure. The right of the subject not to be harmed had been brought into serious question.

2. *The right of self-determination includes informed voluntary consent.* Subjects who give *voluntary consent* are free from constraint and coercion of any kind. *Informed consent* means that the subjects have full knowledge and understanding about the research project in which they are being asked to participate. Volunteers should be free to decide to participate or not after they have been fully informed about the research. Informed consent includes providing subjects with a full description of:

   1. the purpose of the project and its general value;
   2. all procedures used in the research and why;
   3. the subject's part in the research, including the amount of time and energy that the research will take;
   4. any possible pain, discomfort, stress, or loss of autonomy or dignity;
   5. how privacy, confidentiality, and anonymity will be guarded;
   6. the manner in which data will be used.

   Informed consent implies that promises will be kept, no deception will be practiced, the self-respect of subjects will be protected, and ethical guidelines will be carefully followed. The manner in which data will be used should be explained, and the subject should give permission for such use. To allow the data to be put to any other use, or to fail to describe all of its uses, is unethical.

3. *The right to privacy in our society is a tradition of considerable importance.* In some cases, the idea of being watched is illegal— the "peeping Tom" is liable for prosecution. Any intimation that "Big Brother" is watching in the privacy of the home or that anyone else is observing private behavior is repugnant. Privacy enables a person to behave and think without interference or the possibility that private behavior or thoughts may be used to embarrass or demean the person later. Therefore, research methods that observe or question may invade privacy.

   Participant observation is a method of collecting data in the field, or "natural" setting, by direct observation. This method may invade the privacy of individuals who do not realize they are being studied. Degrees of the researcher's participation range from total participation by living and working with the research subjects to nonparticipating observation by merely observing. The degree of disclosure to subjects also varies—from no disclosure, to partial concealment, to full disclosure. Participant observation is considered a powerful method for exploratory research, but there is a serious question of an invasion of the subject's privacy. Since the research setting is a part of everyday activity, little effort is made by the subject to conceal behavior. In particular, disguised participant observation is viewed as unethical.

The Privacy Act of 1974 (NIH Guide, 1974) raises questions concerning data collection techniques that use drugs, tests, or other processes that may invade privacy. Tests such as the "F scale" (fascistic scale) may reveal aspects of a person's personality, such as antidemocratic or authoritarian characteristics, that could prove embarrassing. The use of instruments such as tape recorders, cameras, or one-way mirrors to collect data without a subject's knowledge or permission is an invasion of privacy. Questioning sedated persons or giving mind-altering drugs without the full knowledge of the subject is unethical and may be illegal.

Personal activities, opinions, attitudes, beliefs, letters, diaries, and records are private property and are not subject to study without permission. The researcher must ascertain the extent to which each subject is willing to share privacy. Even if the researcher promises to maintain privacy of research data, data may fall into other hands if records are stored. The records may be subpoenaed or stolen, or crucial material may be copied by someone with temporary access to the records.

Data stored in computers are a potential threat to privacy, since individuals often do not know what is stored or even if the material stored is accurate. The use of such data is not only unethical; it may mislead the research. Use of records of patients to which the nurse has full access in practice requires the patient's permission.

4. *Confidentiality and anonymity are two processes that protect the subject best. Confidentiality* is the researcher's ability to keep data sources protected. *Anonymity* is the researcher's ability to keep subjects nameless. Anonymity is potentially handicapping to the researcher, because it prevents the researcher from contacting subjects in a survey who do not return questionnaires. Rather than sending reminders to the few who do not respond, the entire sample would have to be sent reminders, sometimes a rather expensive undertaking. Anonymity also prevents any longitudinal or follow-up studies. Confidentiality may be the best means of protecting subjects without damaging the research. To maintain confidentiality, the data are coded with numbers instead of names,

and the records that note which names go with which numbers are kept under lock and key. Names and code numbers are kept in different locations entirely. The data may then be kept for further study long after the names are needed and have been destroyed. If a loss of confidentiality is threatened, all records should be destroyed. Subjects should be informed of all measures used to maintain confidentiality and anonymity.

To maintain confidentiality and anonymity in published reports, pseudonyms are useful for subjects, agencies, and geographical settings. The keys to the pseudonyms, like the names associated with the numbers, are kept locked and in different locations. Any other information that can reveal the identity of persons or places is carefully handled, being burned or shredded, rather than thrown into wastebaskets (from which retrieval is possible).

5. *The right to maintain self-respect and dignity is associated with the right not to be harmed in any way.* This includes the right not to be deceived or led into doing things that may later distress or cause injury to the subject's self-concept. The Milgram experiments are a good example of the use of deceit. The use of "stooges" and the experimenter's prestige and power to urge the subject to do things caused distress during the experiment and later. *Debriefing* is a process of disclosing to the subject all information previously withheld and explaining why the information was withheld. This is an attempt to undo any harm that was done, either by withholding information or by deceit. Debriefing is more effective if the subject is told in advance of the research that it is not possible to reveal every aspect of the research ahead of time, but that the subject will be fully informed later. This information allows the subject to consider this aspect of the research before giving consent. The subject should be informed of all that was withheld and should decide whether or not the data should be published.

6. *The right to refuse to participate or to withdraw from participation without fear of recrimination is the subject's right, even though withdrawal may damage the research project.* The researcher must make the subject aware of this right and allay any fears that the subject may have that refusal to participate or withdrawal from the project will in some way hurt him or her. Patients have been known to believe that health care would be withdrawn if they either refused to participate or wished to withdraw. Any promises of reward, such as money, free nursing care, or better nursing care, should not be used, since these may be coercive. The cooperation of patients or subjects is better achieved by explaining

what the research is about and the importance that the findings may have. Either altruistic motives or the possibility of making a contribution to scientific knowledge is often enough to encourage participation. Should the subject decide to stop participating, the researcher must be prepared to accept the decision.

7. *The right for services is a concern of the researcher, if the patient who comes for service is involved in research at the same time.* Some patients may be denied services or may be exposed to an approach that is experimental rather than traditional (Walizer and Wiener, 1978, p. 159). The solution to this problem is to let everyone get both the experimental and the traditional forms of treatment, but at different times. However, this is not always possible. A patient dying of cancer may insist upon the new experimental drug and is not likely to have the time for both the traditional and the experimental treatments. To evaluate traditional services and to provide the best possible service requires research and sometimes experimentation. However, the rights of the subjects as persons require that they exercise informed consent and be allowed to volunteer in an experiment.

VULNERABLE SUBJECTS WHO NEED SPECIAL PROTECTION

Vulnerable subjects either are unable to give informed consent or are captive subjects. The less able a person is to protect him- or herself, the more vigilant the researcher must be. Vulnerable subjects include children, the mentally ill or retarded, the aged, captive persons, the poor, the dying, and the sedated or unconscious.

1. *Children are believed to be incapable of weighing the risks and benefits of a research project and should not even be asked to give informed consent.* However, the question arises of the definition of a *child*. At what age does a person leave childhood and become capable of making a decision regarding research? Various criteria are applied: marriage, military service, economic independence by working, living away from home, graduating from high school, or being of a certain age, such as 18 or 21. Minors have been allowed to make a number of crucial decisions by court order. One judge allowed a 14-year-old to make the decision to be a kidney donor. In the past, parents were able to give consent for their children, but this is now being questioned. Hayter (1979, pp. 125–126) cites a number of studies that deal with this issue. Certain circumstances, such as being chronically ill, emotionally disturbed, or alienated from the family, tend to increase the child's risk of being harmed by participation in research. Children may also be dam-

aged by being put in a position of informing on parents or conditions in the home.

2. *The mentally ill or mentally retarded are vulnerable subjects because they may be unable to comprehend the implications of the research.* In such instances, informed consent may have to come from both the subject and a relative or guardian. Some agencies appoint responsible persons as patients' advocates to assess the risk-benefit ratio.

3. *The aged need special consideration.* Some cannot comprehend and, in this way, resemble children or the mentally incompetent. Others comprehend well, but feel a pressure to comply, especially if they are not in a good position to make all their own choices. The dependent, those in nursing homes, or the incapacitated may feel that they should please those in authority. This requires the researcher to exercise special care.

4. *Captive persons, such as prisoners, men and women in the armed forces, students, the dependent poor, friends and family of researchers, and employees are all vulnerable* (Hayter, 1979). In the past, prisoners have been used for research and are vulnerable to promises of early parole, money, special privileges, or prestige. Soldiers, sailors, and others in the armed services are trained to obey superior officers and, in that sense, may be rather helpless. Students, too, are under the authority of professors or are subject to peer pressure. Without being fully aware of the pressure, the researcher may ask family and friends to participate in a study. The love and trust of friends and family may override their concern. This puts the burden on the researcher to be aware of the dangers and risks.

5. *The poor, who are dependent on certain facilities for health care, may believe that they must comply with a request for research.* At times, money is forthcoming to study an aspect of health care in a poverty-stricken area. However, money may not be available to maintain services once the research is complete. The ethical issues involved in these cases must be carefully weighed by the researcher, who must be concerned about the rights of human subjects.

6. *The dying, sedated, or unconscious person is vulnerable.* At best, the dying are under stress and may be incapable of dealing with research issues. At the same time, however, some may gain satisfaction from the help they are able to provide others. Each case is unique, requiring the researcher to deal with it differently. The sedated person is seldom able to handle implications of the research. For example, a student who wishes to study the various

methods of childbirth should obtain informed consent before the time of labor. The unconscious or anesthetized should only be subjects of research if they have given informed consent when totally conscious.

The key to research on vulnerable subjects who need special protection is to eliminate all subjects who cannot give informed consent freely and with understanding. The less able a subject is to protect him- or herself, the greater is the burden on the researcher to protect the subject.

WITHHOLDING INFORMATION

A major problem with informed consent is that disclosure of the details of a study may change the nature of the subject's response. Some researchers believe that informed consent may be avoided or that misleading explanations may be given if there is a very low risk to the subjects. The "cover story," for example, satisfies the curiosity of the participants without revealing the true nature of the research. In such cases, the subjects' right of free choice has been sharply diminished, thereby raising ethical questions. Deception, the willful use of false information, is unethical, even if the subjects are later apprised of the deception. The Milgram study described earlier is a classic case of deception: the subjects were deceived about the true nature of the experiment and about the fact that stooges were being used. Debriefing, a complete disclosure of all information previously withheld, does not always reverse the harm that is done. If information will be withheld, the subject should be advised of this before he or she gives informed consent.

STEPS TO TAKE TO SECURE INFORMED CONSENT

The first step is to locate or construct a proper informed consent form (Fig. 2–1). The form must include all of the information that the subject needs in order to make an informed decision to participate in the research or not. The following information should be included:

1. An invitation to participate in the study, with times, dates, and purpose of the study clearly stated.
2. An explanation of why the subject was selected.
3. A statement describing all procedures that will be used, the purpose and frequency of each procedure, and how long each will take.
4. An explanation of the subject's part in the procedures, including the amount of time and energy necessary.
5. Any possible discomfort, stress, inconvenience, or loss of dignity and autonomy that may be experienced.

Purpose of the study: _____.
Invitation to participate: _____.
Why subject was selected: _____.
Procedures, purpose, length of time needed, frequency of procedure: _____.
Discomforts, inconveniences expected: _____.
Risks, if any: _____.
Benefits, if any: _____.
Withholding standard treatment, if any: _____.
Time, energy required of subject: _____.
How confidentiality, anonymity, privacy will be maintained: _____.
Compensation to be expected, if any: _____.
Right of subject to refuse to participate or withdraw: _____.
Assurances that researcher will answer all questions: _____.
Concluding statement: "I have read all the information above and have made a
    decision whether or not to participate. My signature indicates that I have been
    informed and have decided to participate."

_____   _____
Date   Signature of subject

_____   _____
Time   Signature of subject advocate, if
                                       necessary; note relationship

_____   _____
Signature of witness   Signature of researcher

Figure 2–1. Informed consent guidelines.

6. The risk/benefit ratio that may be expected.
7. A description of any standard treatment being withheld.
8. A statement explaining the ways in which confidentiality and anonymity will be maintained.
9. Any compensation to be expected, whether monetary or otherwise.
10. The right of the subject to refuse to participate or to withdraw from participation without fear of recrimination.
11. Assurance that the researcher will answer all questions.
12. A statement noting that the researcher has explained all elements of the study to the subject, and that the subject indicates by signature that he or she has read the information provided and has decided to participate.

Below the informational portion of the form, space must be allowed for the signature of the subject, the researcher, and a witness, along with the time and date of the signatures.

Once the consent form is constructed and pretested, the student is ready to secure the approval of the appropriate human rights committees.

Many universities that receive federal funding require research to be approved by various supervising committees. Schools of nursing often form their own committees to preview the students' research proposals and to review consent forms. A committee may be both regulator and resource to the student. In the process of review, committee members may advise the student of proper steps to take to improve the research approach.

After the consent form and the proposed research have been approved, the student must identify subjects and agencies and must approach them for consent. For example, a study of hospital nurses may require the student to obtain permission from the director of nurses before contacting the individual nurses. If patients are the subjects of research, the task may be more difficult. Most hospitals have human investigation committees that review all research in which patients are involved. The student must present the proposal to the committee and must defend it. Before contact with patients is made, suggested revisions must be incorporated into the study.

THE ROLE OF THE NURSE IN RESEARCH

The nurse may be the investigator, participant, or subject of research. As in other applied sciences, the nurse is also a consumer of research, interested in findings that may point the way to more efficient practice. As an investigator, the nurse must understand the scientific principles associated with empirical research. As a participant in others' research, the nurse has the right and responsibility to be informed and to consent to the role that he or she is designated to play. As the subject of research, the nurse has the right of informed consent and self-determination.

SUMMARY

Ethics is the study and evaluation of human conduct. *Applied ethics* examines actual human conduct in real situations. *Values* are the ideas that members of society share about what is important, worthwhile, good, and bad. Research involves both ethics and values. However, the value held by scientists—that it is better to know than not to know—may come in conflict with the rights of human subjects for self-determination.

Rights of human subjects include the right not to be harmed, the right of self-determination, the right to privacy, and the right to obtain services. Each of these is related to other rights, such as the rights to maintain self-respect and dignity, to remain anonymous, and to have confidential material remain confidential.

Vulnerable subjects who need to have their rights protected are of special concern to the researcher. These subjects include children; the mentally ill or retarded; the aged; the poor; the dying or unconscious; and captive persons, such as prisoners, those in the armed forces, students, and friends and families of researchers.

A major problem with informed consent is the effect that disclosure may have on the research. Deception is unethical, but the researcher may inform subjects that full disclosure will follow the research. Debriefing informs the subject of all elements of the research after the research but before publication. This allows a subject who has given permission for delayed disclosure to refuse to have the information that concerns him or her published.

A number of steps must be taken to secure consent from study subjects. The researcher must describe all procedures that will be used, including the amount of time and energy that subjects will be required to expend. Any discomfort that subjects may experience, as well as the risk/benefit ratio, must be described. The subjects must be informed of the manner in which data will be used and why the collection of such data is valuable. The subjects must understand that they may refuse to participate in the study or may withdraw without fear of recrimination. The researcher must state how confidentiality and anonymity will be maintained and must assure subjects that all questions will be answered. The informed-consent statement must be dated and signed by the researcher, the subject, and at least one witness.

The nurse may be a researcher, a participant, a subject, or a consumer of research. In all cases, the nurse must be alert to all possible ethical questions and speak out against any unethical practice that becomes known.

EXAMPLES FROM NURSING RESEARCH

Subjects who are employees, studied at the place of work. Jordan-Marsh (1985) studied the development of a tool for diagnosing changes in concern about exercise. The subjects were employees of a Southern California industry that sponsored a comprehensive health promotion program provided through a major university consulting center. The researcher recruited subjects from persons standing in the waiting line during the blood pressure screening program. Jordan-Marsh asked subjects to fill out a questionnaire and background data sheet, informing the subjects of the following: (1) the questionnaire was not required for the blood pressure reading; (2) names would not be included in study reports; and (3) the questionnaires would not be available to either the employer or the health care program staff. In addition, the researcher provided a box for the return of all questionnaires so that employees were able to return blank or incomplete forms without revealing their refusal to participate. Jordan-Marsh considered that consent to participate in the study was implied when subjects filled out the questionnaire.

Alexy (1985) compared the effectiveness of three methods of setting goals that were designed to reduce health-risking behavior. The subjects were employees at three different places of work. The researcher obtained a convenience sample from persons eligible for periodic health examination at the place of employment who agreed to participate in the study. The researcher assured subjects that confidentiality would be maintained and that they could withdraw from the study at any time.

Subjects who are patients in the hospital, studied in their home after discharge. Hilbert (1985), studying the relationship between spouse support and compliance of myocardial infarction patients, obtained data from a sample of 60 couples. The researcher interviewed the patient in his home and asked his wife to fill out a questionnaire. Hilbert drew the sample of study subjects from a group of consenting couples, conducting an informed-consent procedure prior to home interviews.

Study subjects who were veterans studied in their homes. Robb (1985), studying urinary incontinence verification in elderly men who were also veterans, does not report how she identified the subjects, other than to say that they were veterans over 60 years of age, residing at home within 25 miles of the Veterans Administration Medical Center, who volunteered to be included in the study. Robb solicited potential subjects to ask them to volunteer to undergo an assessment of their urinary incontinence problem including a history, physical examination, and tests to measure urine loss, all to be conducted in the veteran's home. Subjects were free to refuse participation in any of the components.

Adult hospital patients from medical-surgical units in three community hospitals. Samples et al. (1985), studying circadian rhythms as a basis for screening for fever, purposed to determine if the peak of the circadian thermal rhythm is the optimal time to screen and the necessary frequency for measurement. The researchers utilized ethical procedures in the study to: (1) gain approval for the study from the institutional review board of the medical center by submitting a proposal for the research; (2) gain permission to participate in research from directors of nursing in the participating hospitals; (3) review when possible with the head nurse of each ward under study to determine whether contraindications for including selected study subjects existed. Following these procedures, a member of the research team met with study subjects to instruct each on the purpose and plan of the study and to obtain verbal consent for participation in the study. Subjects were informed that they could withdraw from the study at any time during the period of data collection.

Study subjects from county health department maternity clinics. DiIorio (1985), studying first-trimester nausea in pregnant teenagers, drew her sample from patients attending three county health department maternity clinics. The researcher guaranteed confidentiality and asked each subject who agreed to participate to sign an informed-consent form prior to completing a questionnaire.

Children who are in school. Lamontagne, Mason, and Hepworth (1985) studied the effects of relaxation on anxiety in children in order to identify implications for coping with stress. The sample was comprised of 46 second-grade children in two classrooms who volunteered for the study upon receiving parental consent. Apparently, the researchers had also worked with the administration and with teachers in the school, since teachers used an audiocassette tape provided by Gillis to record items.

STUDY QUESTIONS

1. What is the relationship between values and ethics in nursing?
2. You are the chief nurse in a privately supported children's rehabilitation center. A research team has been given permission to conduct research in the clinic. What are the rights of the patients? What are your responsibilities?
3. As a nurse, which persons must you be particularly concerned about when they are potential subjects in research? Why?
4. Discuss how you would feel if you had been a subject in Milgram's experiment and the researcher fully "debriefed" you.
5. You are planning a research project on pain. The project has been approved and the adult subjects have been selected. To give full information about the project—special nursing care and a placebo versus routine nursing care and medication—would damage the validity of the findings. What should you do?
6. You are planning to conduct a study to determine by questionnaire the attitudes of nursing students toward abortion. Write a brief form that is usable for informed consent.
7. What is the role of a nurse who reads a research project that seems to be unethical?

REFERENCES AND SUGGESTED READINGS

Abdellah, F. (1967): Approaches to protecting the rights of human subjects. Nursing Research, *16*, 316–320. *Ethical values in nursing research.*

Alexy, B. (1985): Goal setting and health risk reduction. Nursing Research, *34*, 283–288. *Includes use of ethics in research, confidentiality, right to withdraw.*

American Nurses' Association (1968): The nurse in research. ANA Guidelines on Ethical Values. Nursing Research, *17*, 104–107. (1975): Human Rights Guidelines for Nurses in Clinical and Other Research. Kansas City, Mo.: The American Nurses' Association. *Guidelines in nursing research.*

Annas, G. et al. (1977): The Subject's Dilemma. Cambridge, Mass.: Ballinger. *Includes research with children, prisoners, fetus. Describes efforts of legal system to deal with laws of informed consent.*

Arminger, B. (1977): Ethics of nursing research: Profile, principles, perspective. Nursing Research, *26*, 330–336. *Research situations.*

Besch, L. (1979): Informed consent: A patient's right. Nursing Outlook, *27*, 32–35.

Capron, A. (1973): Legal considerations affecting clinical pharmacological studies in children. Clinical Research, *21*, 141–150. *Exposure of children to infectious hepatitis.*

Cortin, L. and Flaherty, M. (1982): Nursing Ethics: Theories and Pragmatics. Bowie, Md.: Robert J. Brady Co.

Davis, A. (1985): Informed consent: How much information is enough? Nursing Outlook, *33*, 40–42.

Davis, A. (1979): Ethics rounds with intensive care nurses. Nursing Clinics of North America, *14*, 45–55.

Davis, A. and Aroskar, M. (1978): Ethical Dilemmas and Nursing Practice. New York: Appleton-Century-Crofts.

Diers, D. (1979): Research in Nursing Practice. Philadelphia: J. B. Lippincott. Chap. 11.

Dilorio, C. (1985): First trimester nausea in pregnant teenagers: Incidence, characteristics, intervention. Nursing Research, *34*, 372–374.

Downs, F. (1967): Ethical inquiry in nursing research. Nursing Forum, *6*, 12–20.

Gortner, S. (1982): Ethics issues: The boundaries between practice and research. CNR Newsletter *10*, 2. Published by the Council of Nurse Researchers.

Gortner, S., Hudes, M., and Zyzanski, S. (1984): Appraisal of values in the choice of treatment. Nursing Research, *33*, 319–324. *Includes the research protocol.*

Gray, B. (1976): An assessment of institutional review committees in human experimentation. Nursing Digest, *4*. *The place of the institutional review committee.*

Hayter, J. (1979): Issues related to human subjects. In Down, F. and Fleming, J. (eds.), Issues in Nursing Research. New York: Appleton-Century-Crofts, pp. 107–147. *Examination of informed consent and other ethical issues.*

Hilbert, G. (1985): Spouse support and myocardial infarction. Nursing Research, *34*, 218–220.

Jacobson, S. (1973): Ethical issues in experimentation with human subjects. Nursing Forum, *12*, 58–71. *Ethics in experimental research.*

Jordan-Marsh, M. (1985): Development of a tool for diagnosing changes in concern about exercise: A means of enhancing compliance. Nursing Research, *34*, 103–106.

Kelly, K. and McClelland, E. (1979): Signed consent: Protection or constraint. Nursing Outlook, *27*, 40–42.

Lamontagne, L. et al. (1985): Effects of relaxation on anxiety in children: Implications for coping with stress. Nursing Research, *34*, 289–292.

Langer, E. (1966): Human experimentation: New York verdict affirms human rights. Science, *151*, 663–666. *Experiment on elderly patients.*

May, K. (1979): The nurse as researcher: Impediment to informed consent. Nursing Outlook, *27*, 36–39.

Milgram, S. (1963): Behavioral study of obedience. Journal of Abnormal and Social Psychology, *67*, 371–378. *Experiment with human subjects.*

National Institute of Health Guide 3 (1974): Research projects involving human subjects. *Guides for Ethical Research; HEW policies.*

Phillips, L. and Rempusheski, V. (1985): A decision-making model for diagnosing and intervening in elder abuse and neglect. Nursing Research *34*, 134–139.

Robb, S. (1985): Urinary incontinence verification in elderly men. Nursing Research, *34*, 278–280.

Samples, J. et al. (1985): Circadian rhythms: Basis for screening for fever. Nursing Research, *34*, 377–379. *Includes series of steps taken to obtain permission and informed consent for research.*

Swider, S., McElmurry, B., and Yarling, R. (1985): Ethical decision making in a bureaucratic context by senior nursing students. Nursing Research, *34*, 108–112.

Veatch, R. and Bransom, R. (eds.): Ethics and Health Policy. Cambridge, Mass.: Ballinger. *Examination of ethics, including informed-consent bibliography.*

Watson, A. (1982): Informed consent of special subject. Nursing Research, *31,* 43–47.

Walizer, M. and Wiener, P. (1978): Research Methods and Analysis. New York, Harper & Row. *Chapter 6 examines the ethics of research on human subjects.*

3

Elements of the Scientific Research Process

The central element of the scientific research process is observation. However, scientific observation is intimately related to theory, which is a general statement that explains the interrelationships among observed facts and propositions. Theory without scientific observation is untested "armchair speculation," while observation without theory is confined to limited statements about what has been observed. Therefore, the student needs to utilize both observation and theory, and needs to relate each to the other. To relate theory and observation, the student uses her or his mind to reason, either beginning with a theory and then moving to observation to test theory, or beginning with observation and then moving to theory to formulate theory. The type of logical reasoning that begins with theory is called deductive reasoning, while the kind of logical reasoning that begins with observation is called inductive reasoning. The student needs to understand how logical reasoning and research observations function together in nursing research.

To achieve this understanding, the student needs a scientific vocabulary that includes such basic terms as *observation, concept, variable, hypothesis, empirical generalization, theory,* and *logical reasoning.* Such expressions are a part of the language of science—those words whose meaning is shared by members of the scientific community. Each nurse must learn the language of science, not only to be able to read and understand publications in nursing and allied sciences, but to be able to think, observe, and write in such terms. However, scientific language often includes words without exact meaning that are used in everyday conversation. The use of such terms in research requires not only that students define each one precisely, but that they understand how each term functions in the research process.

Upon completion of this chapter, the student should be able to: (1) depict the relationships among observation, proposition, logical reasoning, and theory; (2) identify and define basic terms used in nursing research; (3) state how scientific observation and logical reasoning function to test theories, and (4) formulate, reformulate, and clarify theories used in nursing research.

A MODEL OF THE BASIC ELEMENTS AND METHODS OF RESEARCH

The scientific process in nursing is built upon dual foundations: logical thought (or theorizing), and scientific observation (or empirical research). Figure 3–1 brings these dual foundations together and depicts the interrelationships among theorizing and empirical research. The model can be examined from two viewpoints. It can be divided horizontally in order to study separately what is meant by theorizing and by empirical research. In addition, it can be divided into a right side and a left side in order to study separately how theory and research observations are integrated from two perspectives: either that which begins with a theory and then moves, by deductive reasoning, toward observation to test a theory, or that which begins with observations and moves, by inductive reasoning, to construct a theory. Each of these will be discussed in turn.

Theorizing and Empirical Research

Theorizing involves thinking about observations—either what the researcher will find upon observation or what has been found by observation. Theorizing is depicted on the top half of Figure 3–1, and empirical research is depicted on the bottom half. *Empirical research* involves conducting the observation, as well as summarizing what has been observed. Theorizing and empirical research mutually share the hypothesis and empirical generalization.

Theorizing includes thinking by both deductive and inductive reasoning. *Deductive reasoning* involves thinking about a particular theory and then predicting what will be found when the researcher makes observations. From a theory, the researcher creates a proposition—an *hypothesis*—a statement that predicts the relationship that will be found between variables upon observation. Deductive reasoning is used to test a known theory utilized in nursing research, such as learning theory; theories of development, adaptation, and stress; systems theory; and social and cultural theories. In contrast, *inductive reasoning* involves thinking about observations after they have been made. The researcher thinks about the facts observed, utilizes concepts to stand for related observations, and creates a proposition—*an empirical generalization*—that states the relationship observed between two facts or concepts.

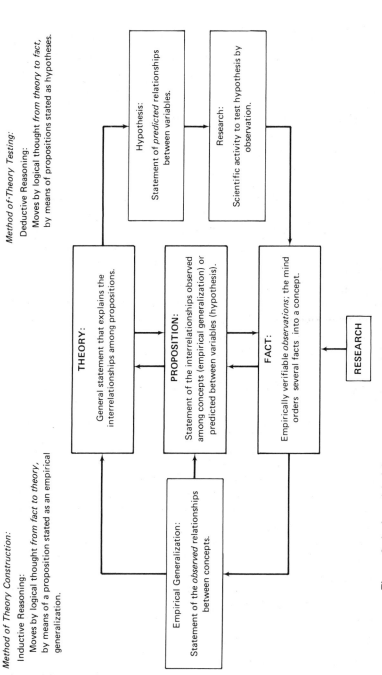

Figure 3–1. A model of theory construction and theory testing, using elements and methods of the scientific research process.

Method of Theory Construction:

Inductive Reasoning:

Moves by logical thought *from fact to theory,* by means of a proposition stated as an empirical generalization.

Method of Theory Testing:

Deductive Reasoning:

Moves by logical thought *from theory to fact,* by means of propositions stated as hypotheses.

THEORY:

General statement that explains the interrelationships among propositions.

PROPOSITION:

Statement of the interrelationships observed among concepts (empirical generalization) or predicted between variables (hypothesis).

FACT:

Empirically verifiable *observations*; the mind orders several facts into a concept.

Hypothesis:

Statement of *predicted* relationships between variables.

Research:

Scientific activity to test hypothesis by observation.

Empirical Generalization:

Statement of the *observed* relationships between concepts.

RESEARCH

The empirical generalization is a specific, isolated, and limited statement that the researcher formulates directly from observation. It is the starting point for inventing a theory. It should be kept in mind that the empirical generalization retains a meaning independent of the theory invented to explain it, because the empirical generalization is based on observational evidence and therefore will survive even when the theory invented to explain it may have to be reformulated or discarded.

Empirical research is the process of systematically collecting observable, verifiable data. It includes both observation and the activity that goes on before and after observation. Before observation, the researcher must identify from the hypothesis what is to be observed, then plan how observations are to be made and how hypotheses are to be tested. If the research begins with observations, the researcher must summarize what has been observed and must create an empirical generalization to summarize relationships between two facts or concepts that have been observed.

Scientific observation involves either directly watching and recording what goes on in the selected research area, or asking people by interview or questionnaire what they have observed or experienced. The means by which the researcher observes depends on what is to be observed. As we saw, the researcher who begins with a theory next creates an hypothesis that states what is to be observed. The hypothesis must now be linked with observation if it is to be useful in research. Therefore, the researcher spends considerable time choosing a sample to observe and identifying or creating instruments to assist with observation. *Instrumentation* refers to all processes that aid observation, including paper-and-pencil aids (operational definitions, observation checklists, survey schedules, scales); machines that measure data; or laboratory tests that analyze data. Following observations, the researcher summarizes data, tests hypotheses, or creates empirical generalizations.

The researcher who begins with observation is partly dependent on other elements in the scientific process, but is partly independent, as well. That is, the researcher often begins with observation when studying new material that has not been described previously. Therefore, it may not be clear how to prepare for observation until the researcher goes into the field. At the same time, the researcher does not go naively into observation but brings all past education and experiences to bear, both on making plans for observation and on executing these plans. The researcher may begin with particular objectives in mind or may formulate a working hypothesis based on knowledge and experience rather than on a theory. The researcher then plans to use as many instruments as are available to assist with making observations. Following a careful documentation of what has been observed, systematic patterns in the observations are sought. Research data (facts) are put into categories and are analyzed for a pattern of relationships. If no name (concept) exists to describe the patterns of observation found, the researcher must invent one. Where relationships are found between two facts and concepts, the researcher states these in a proposition—the empirical generalization.

Testing a Theory: Bringing Theorizing and Observation Together

To integrate theorizing and the observation used to test a theory, the researcher begins with the theory and moves to observation—the process depicted on the right side of Figure 3–1. The researcher first conducts a review of the literature in order to study existing theories and past research associated with the theory. Next, the researcher either finds an appropriate hypothesis in the literature, or reasons from the theory in order to create an hypothesis—to predict what will be found on observation. Then the researcher commonly takes some or all of the following steps to prepare for observation: first, each concept in the hypothesis is defined to transform it into a variable—i.e., make each concept observable and measurable. Next the researcher selects a research design, a research method, a method of selecting a sample of objects or persons to study, and the instruments to use in research. Following observations, the data are summarized, and the hypotheses tested. The researcher then makes a judgment as to whether the observations support the hypothesis and thus contribute to the theory from which the hypothesis was drawn.

Formulating a Theory: Bringing Together Observation and Theorizing

To integrate observation and theorizing, the researcher begins with observations and then reasons inductively in order to summarize what has been observed—the processes depicted on the left side of Figure 3–1. The first step after observation is usually to describe in detail what has been observed. This step is especially important if no other accounts of such observation exist. Next the researcher summarizes the observations by placing similar observations into categories; he or she then locates a concept in the literature that names the categories or invents names if none are found. Next, the researcher creates a proposition, an empirical generalization that states a relationship between concepts. Finally, from the empirical generalization, the researcher theorizes by means of inductive reasoning to relate the new empirical generalization to other empirical generalizations found in the literature. Or, the researcher may invent higher-level, more abstract, and unobservable concepts that are more generally applicable. From these, the researcher formulates a theory—a general statement that explains the relationship among the propositions (the empirical generalizations) or among the more generalized concepts.

BASIC TERMS OF RESEARCH

A number of the basic terms utilized in research have been examined briefly above. *Observation* is a method of collecting research data in which the researcher scientifically watches and records pertinent information. A *fact* is an empirically verifiable observation, which the mind orders into a *concept*, the word or symbol that stands for the mental image that the researcher forms from observation.

Concepts are the building blocks of propositions such as hypotheses or empirical generalizations, both of which are intimately related to theory. A *theory* is a general statement that explains the relationships among facts, concepts, or propositions. The relationship among fact, concept, and theory is well illustrated by the following example, which Charter (1975, p. 2) draws from a specific nursing situation:

> The nurse caring for a patient admitted to the hospital following an automobile accident would obtain certain factual information from the patient and family. The recording of facts might include: 40-year-old male, conscious, no external bleeding; vital signs—blood pressure, 90/40; pulse, 100; respiratory rate, 20. She immediately thinks of shock (*concept*) as she studies the relationship between blood pressure and pulse (*facts*). She knows that gravity will return the blood to the heart and aid circulation (principle), and she is prepared to elevate the foot of the bed . . . Thus, the principle used for nursing care is also supported by theories from physiology and physics.

The nurse described here went through a very swift process of logical thought and scientific research. First, drawing on her education and experience, she implicitly *began with a theory* derived from physiology and physics, one that explained the relationship between gravity and the circulation of blood. Then, by rapid *deductive reasoning* (from the theory to a created hypothesis, to the collection of facts), she formed a *working hypothesis*—a proposition that predicted what would be found upon observation. Her hypothesis predicted the following: *If* a person has been in a car accident, and has lowered blood pressure and elevated pulse, *then* he is at risk to be in shock. Shock is a *concept*, a word that, in this case, had already been invented to stand for a complex idea or a constellation of facts. To test the hypothesis, the nurse made observations, watching and recording the following pertinent information: bleeding, if any; state of consciousness; and measurements of blood pressure and pulse rate. After collecting these data, the nurse made a judgment that her hypothesis was supported by the observed facts, and prepared to elevate the foot of the bed.

Concepts and Variables: the Building Blocks of Propositions

The basic units of scientific research, logical thinking, and propositions are concepts and variables. *Concepts* are the abstract words or symbols that stand for the mental images we form from reality, while *variables* are concepts that have been defined in a manner that makes them observable and measurable. For example, the concept "shock" is not observable until it is defined in a way to make it observable and measurable: we measure blood pressure, count the pulse, take the temperature, look for bleeding and the amount (if any), and look for state of consciousness and for sweating.

Scientific concepts get their precise meanings from the formal definitions that scholars and scientists assign to each word or symbol. Unfortunately, the definitions may differ among scientists, and meanings may change over time. For example, it has been suggested that the concept "burnout" was originally invented to stand for a space-age phenomenon —the spent fuel tank that burned out and dropped back to earth as the rocket sped into space. The term passed into literature and found its way into nursing. Dailey (1985) became interested in the concept and describes the symptoms reported by nurses who respond positively to a "burnout" test. These include reports of feelings such as fatigue, depression, and hopelessness; feelings of being "stretched too thin," of failure at work, and of low morale; attitudes toward patients such as insensitivity, seeing patients as subhuman, or feeling physically distanced from patients; and behaviors including spending less time with patients, increased absenteeism, hiding in paperwork, and escaping patients by moving on to higher education.

The concept of burnout has thus changed from one that was close to observation—the spent fuel tank falling to earth—to an abstract concept that is not directly observable and that is itself comprised of other abstract terms. Such concepts, composed of several other concepts, are called *constructs*. Only time will tell whether "burnout" will remain in the scientific nursing literature. Not all concepts or constructs survive the passage of time. For example, "shell-shocked," a term coined during World War I, has dropped out of the literature.

When disparities in the definitions of concepts are found, the researcher must be careful to clarify precisely how to define each concept used in research, noting the scholarly sources. Examples of concepts in nursing include "nursing care," one of the oldest nursing concepts (used since the time of Nightingale); "patient-centered care," suggested by Abdellah and Levine (1965, p. 84) two decades ago; "self-care," used by Orem (1971); and, more recently, a number of concepts subsumed under "nursing diagnosis." Concepts deal with varying levels of abstraction. They may be close to observations, such as "crying," or highly abstract and unobservable, such as "grieving."

Chagrine.

To transform an abstract, unobservable concept into a measurable, observable variable, an operational definition is used. An *operational definition* is a step-by-step set of directions that specify what the researcher must do in order to observe and measure the concept under study. For example, Jacobson et al. (1985) were interested in whether there was a relationship between handwashing, ring-wearing, and the number of microorganisms found before and after handwashing. Although handwashing is a concept that is close to observation, there are many ways to wash hands. Therefore, in order to ensure that all researchers are observing the same kind of handwashing, and to clarify the different kinds of handwashing that were being studied in the experiment, several types of handwashing were defined by operational definitions, as follows: (1) a timed 60-second rinse of both hands using friction only; (2) a timed two-minute scrub and rinse of the hands to above the wrists using liquid Ivory soap, a sterilized surgical scrub brush, and cold, running tap water; and (3) scrubbing with soap for one minute, followed by a one-minute rinse.

Variables are classified in several ways: independent variables; dependent variables; extraneous variables; and attribute variables. The *independent variable*, also called the experimental, causal, stimulus, or treatment variable, is manipulated by the researcher to study its effect upon the dependent variable. *Manipulation* refers to the fact that the researcher does something with the independent variable. If the independent variable is a nursing treatment, the researcher manipulates it by giving the treatment to some study subjects and withholding it from others. The purpose of the manipulation is to see if the treatment made a difference. The *dependent variable*, also called the effect, the response, or the criterion measure, is the behavior or outcome that the researcher wishes to predict and explain. The change in the dependent variable is presumed to be caused by, or associated with, the independent variable. For example, Jacobson et al. wanted to examine whether different types of handwashing, the independent variable, affected the number of microorganisms (the dependent variable) found after washing. Lindeman and Van Aernam (1971) were interested in the effect of preoperative teaching (the independent variable) on the length of stay and the need for analgesics in the postoperative patient (the dependent variables). They wanted to predict what caused one patient to need fewer analgesics and to stay in the hospital fewer days. Did the preoperative instruction make a difference? Their research was structured to answer this question.

Extraneous variables are those variables present in large numbers in the research environment that may interfere with the research findings by acting as unwanted independent variables that confuse the results of the research. For example, race may be utilized as an independent variable to see how it is associated with hypertension. However, race becomes an extraneous variable when another factor, such as a drug, is being studied to determine *its* effect on high blood pressure. Then, the race of the person may be a factor that acts upon the blood pressure and confuses whether the drug actually caused the observed effect.

Attribute variables are preexisting characteristics of the study subjects, such as education, occupation, income, age, weight, medical diagnosis, or any other characteristic that varies from one individual to another. Such characteristics themselves may be studied as independent variables.

Concepts and variables are the components of hypotheses that the researcher creates to predict what will be found upon observation. Brown et al. (1984) report an increase in efforts of nursing researchers to establish relationships between variables—i.e., to test hypotheses. However, they found a need for nurse-researchers to state hypotheses more explicitly. Therefore, in planning research or reading research reports, it is important for the student to know what an hypothesis is, the source of hypotheses, how to state an hypothesis, and how to test it.

Hypotheses: Statements Constructed for Prediction and Testing

Hypotheses are statements that predict a relationship between two or more variables. Hypotheses are forward-looking, guiding the researcher in collecting and analyzing data. Sources of hypotheses include theory, assumptions, observations, work experiences, and the literature. The formulation of hypotheses and the definitions of their variables come early in the planning phase. Formulation requires painstaking work. Testing hypotheses requires a judgment: Do the data warrant the support of the hypotheses? The sources of hypotheses, and the formulation and testing of each hypothesis, are now examined.

1. *Sources of hypotheses include: (1) theory; (2) assumptions; (3) observations; (4) working experiences; and (5) the literature.* To derive hypotheses from theory, we proceed in the classic manner by means of a formal deductive system. However, such systems appear more frequently in the older sciences, which have had a longer period of development than nursing. But nursing can use these systems to develop hypotheses related to nursing. For example, behavior modification proposes that behavior is a direct function of the environment. Using such a proposition, the student may predict a relationship between rewards and punishments and a change in behavior detrimental to health, such as drug use, cigarette smoking, or poor eating habits. Rottkamp (1981) developed the hypothesis that "spinal cord-injured patients with impairment in body-positioning behaviors who receive an intervention that incorporates behavior-modification techniques . . . will improve in their body-positioning performance to a measurable degree. . . ."

To derive hypotheses from *assumptions*, statements whose accuracy is taken for granted, the researcher first states the assumption and then predicts what will be found in research. For example, Robischon (1971) became interested in pica, the habitual ingestion of nonedible substances, because she was concerned over the poisoning of children from eating lead paint. She believed that hand-to-mouth behavior associated with eating in general was related to development. Her assumptions included the following: child development proceeds as an integrated system in interaction with the environment; and development proceeds in orderly, patterned, identifiable, and measurable sequences. Based on these assumptions, Robischon created the following hypothesis: children who practice pica will have a lower developmental level than children who do not exhibit these behaviors.

To derive hypotheses from observation, the researcher makes a statement about the relationships between the observed regularities (that is, the facts or concepts), called the *empirical generalization*. From this statement, then, the researcher may deduce an hypothesis. For example, Alderson (1974) observed that patients who had high fevers seemed to experience time differently, and thought that a possible relationship existed between the concepts *high fever* and *perception of time*. To predict a relationship, Alderson derived the following hypothesis: if body temperature rises a specified number of degrees above normal, then the patient will experience time differently.

Hypotheses that arise during the experiences and observations of everyday life are called *working hypotheses*, predictions that lie close to observed data (Conant, 1947, p. 137). As the nurse encounters certain facts or observations in the course of nursing practice, the nurse thinks of alternative explanations, which she or he then tests. For example, if a nurse sees a patient with hypertension collapse on the floor, some explanations flash through the nurse's mind: the patient has had a cerebral accident; the patient has had a heart attack. To test these working hypotheses, the nurse observes signs and, if possible, questions the patient. If the first hypothesis seems wrong, the nurse may test others in rapid succession. A *nursing diagnosis* is defined as a statement of the probable relationships between an identified negative health behavior and the factors contributing to its occurrence (Brill and Kilts, 1980, p. 154). It is a predictive statement that refers to a possible relationship between factors. Such working hypotheses must be tested in research.

To derive hypotheses from the literature, the student may begin with any of the points above: the theory stated in research reports, the assumptions, or the documented observations and working experiences.

2. *Formulation of hypotheses requires the student first to identify what relationship she or he is predicting.* For example, a nurse familiar with Alderson's (1974) work on the relationship between high fever and the perception of the passage of time may wonder if homebound patients with fevers who take their own medication can accurately perceive the passage of time in order to take medication on schedule. To state the relationship, the nurse must link the abstract idea of perception to the actual fact of taking medications on time. In addition, the nurse must predict what he or she expects to find in research and must define the variables in such a manner that each is observable and measurable: if a patient's temperature rises three degrees above normal, then the patient will take medications off-schedule. Once the initial statement is written, the student must ask the following questions to judge the statement's usefulness: Is the statement concise and unambiguous? Are the concepts and variables stated in a clear and specific manner? Do the variables refer to data that are observable and measurable? Do instruments exist to measure the variables, or can the variables be easily developed and tested? Are the sources from which the hypothesis was formulated clearly identified and stated? Careful work, self-criticism, and assistance from experts are essential in the development of the art and science of hypothesis formulation.

3. *In many ways, testing hypotheses is similar to a trial by a jury.* The jury is comprised of ourselves and our fellow scientists, who examine all aspects of the research, beginning with the research hypothesis and including a scrutiny of research design, sampling methods, research methods, and data analysis. In cases where the hypothesis and findings can be expressed and analyzed in quantitative form, statistical tests are likewise helpful.

The research hypothesis is formulated to test either for association or causality. Establishing causality is a difficult task when the research involves the complex behavior of persons, because causal factors are often multiplex rather than single. Associations, or correlations, indicate how specified factors occur or vary together: as one increases the other may increase (positive correlation), or as one increases the other may decrease (negative correlation). For example, Olgas (1974) was interested in the association between the health status of parents and the way that their children perceived their own bodies. She sought to predict whether children of handicapped parents have a body image that is different from that held by children of nonhandicapped parents: is there an association between the body image of the child and the health status of the parent, whether handicapped or not? In such cases, the difficulty of establishing causality is obvious—

many factors contribute to the body image of a child. But, if it can be demonstrated that the body image of a child is associated with the handicap of the parent, nursing intervention may be considered on the basis of this information.

Causal hypotheses state that cause X must occur in time before effect Y. An experiment that includes before and after tests, as well as an experimental and a control group, is the most effective method for establishing a cause–effect relationship. For example, Van Ort and Gerber (1976) hypothesized that the topical application of insulin (the cause) would cause decubitus ulcers to heal faster (the effect). However, to test this hypothesis, two groups of patients who are alike in every way (sex, age, race, diagnosis, kind of decubitus ulcer) would have to be tested. One group would receive topical applications of insulin, while one would not. If the experimental group who received the insulin healed faster than the group who did not receive the insulin, the insulin may be said to have "caused" faster healing. However, other variables may have intervened. For example, genetic factors may have influenced the results, or undetected factors may have been responsible.

Nursing research publications over the last three decades indicate increased efforts to establish relationships between variables and to test hypotheses (Brown et al., 1984). However, hypotheses are likely to remain implicit rather than explicit and are rarely grounded in theory (in terms of stating interrelated propositions deduced from theory).

Yet, the relationship between hypotheses and theory is an intimate one. The researcher who incorporates theory into research is making a more general contribution to nursing knowledge—one that leads to an understanding of the interrelationship among observed facts.

Theory: Scientific Explanations of Relationships Among Propositions

Theory is a scientific explanation for the interrelationships among facts, concepts, and propositions. The key words are *explanation* and *interrelationships*. An explanation for interrelated phenomena is a goal of all science, but the practicing professions (such as medicine, nursing, law, applied anthropology, clinical sociology, and engineering) go one step beyond explanation to application. One of their goals is to use theory in practice to control, to prescribe or, as Diers (1979, p. 33) notes, to change the world for the better. However, care must be taken to recognize that not everyone may agree on what constitutes "better." The values of one segment of society may not always coincide with all segments.

Nonetheless, people tend to agree that it is better to be well than to be sick. Theories that explain health and sickness are sought everywhere, in order to control sickness and to prescribe measures to recover and maintain good health. For example, the germ theory explains why and how germs and disease are interrelated. The explanation allows practitioners to control disease caused by germs by prescribing vaccination or medication. Few would argue that such change is not for the better.

Theories abound in human cultures, but not all of these theories are scientific. For example, in the past, philosophy and religion provided explanations of events in this world and the next. The medieval view that the world was flat arose from the theory that angels held up the four corners of the earth. Proceeding from this premise, or theory, deductive reasoning led to predictions that, if one sailed toward the horizon, one would eventually fall off the edge of the earth. No provision was made for testing such hypotheses, because religious explanations were considered to be eternal truths. Those with inquisitive minds were hampered in testing alternative hypotheses by a lack of instruments and by convention, which frowned upon such ventures. Armchair philosophers of the time believed general principles to be self-evident and in no need of empirical testing and observation.

In contrast, scientific theory deals with the empirical world that we know directly, through our senses or through inventions that extend our senses, such as the sphygmomanometer or the microscope. Scientific theory is the symbolic dimension of our experiences and observations, a mental invention that systematically orders the things that we observe. If the theory is a fruitful one, we can derive statements (propositions, hypotheses) that predict from the theory, and we can then test the predictions in research. However, the theory itself cannot be proven. All theories are tentative: they tentatively explain what we *have* observed in research, and these explanations can be used to predict what we *will* observe in research. Thus, research, observation, and theory are intimately related to one another.

Nursing Theory and Theory in Nursing. There are several views about the construction and use of theory in nursing. One view is that of Mathwig (1970), who believes that theoretical knowledge of nursing must evolve from nursing and nursing alone. She seems to reject the idea of using theory developed in other disciplines. The problem with this approach is that knowledge unique to nursing and nursing alone may be difficult to find and that, should such a unique body of knowledge develop, nursing may find it difficult to communicate its meaning to other health disciplines (Stevens, 1979, p. 63).

Johnson (1968), Henderson (1978, p. 22), and others suggest that it is hazardous to attempt to differentiate between borrowed and unique theory, because knowledge does not belong innately to any one field of science; thus, definitions of what is borrowed and what is unique have no permanence or real meaning.

A view that integrates both of these views in some measure is that of Wald and Leonard (1964), most recently adopted by Diers (1979). This view suggests that the development of *nursing practice theory* is distinct from the theory of practice in any other health field. However, theory and research from other disciplines are readily used, although Diers (p. 65) suggests that a careful evaluation is necessary to fit theory to the problems at hand. Relying on the ideas generated by philosophers Dickoff and James (1968), Diers defines a *theory* as a mental invention whose purpose is to describe, explain, predict, or prescribe (Diers, 1979, p. 69). She examines four levels of theoretical inquiry: (1) naming theory; (2) theory that suggests the connection among concepts; (3) theory that explains and predicts; and (4) theory that both states the goals to be achieved in nursing practice and prescribes activities to achieve those goals (Diers, chap. 2).

The construction of nursing theories often begins with observations and inductive reasoning, while the testing of theories begins with theory or assumptions and deduces hypotheses to be tested. Induction and deduction alternate in the development and testing of theory. Each of these will be examined.

Inductive Reasoning: Constructing Nursing Theory from Observation. Inductive reasoning is the means by which we explain the things that we have observed. It begins with specific observations and moves to construct a general explanation or theory. The first step in the inductive process is to collect data that are significant to the nursing problem under investigation. The second step is to summarize the collected data, using scales, measurements, graphs, and tables. The third step is to synthesize the summarized data into a single statement or observation—the empirical generalization—that states a proposed relationship between concepts. The fourth step is to use the relationships expressed to initiate, reformulate, or clarify theory.

The proposed steps are fluid rather than fixed: the researcher tends to move back and forth between inductive and deductive reasoning, testing and probing as necessary, seldom moving in a straight line. The inductive process may be illustrated with an example that will help clarify the steps usually taken.

As nurses in practice, we may have observed that a number of persons in the local area are committing suicide. Therefore, we wish to observe and study the phenomenon scientifically in order to arrive at an explanation of suicide that will enable us to intervene in the process. We may begin by reading the literature, paying particular attention to a classic 19-century European study of suicide from which we take the definition of *suicide* as "cases of death resulting directly or indirectly from a positive or negative act of the victim himself, which he knows will produce this result" (Durkheim, trans. 1951, p. 44).

Next, we must decide which data about suicide we should collect—work data, personal data, family data, or other. And we must decide how to collect the data. We decide to collect data about the characteristics of the persons who commit suicide—their sex, religion, occupation, and marital status—using a broad review of all of the official documents available.

Once we collect the data, we summarize the observations. We count the frequency of suicide by category, such as sex and religion, summarizing the data in tables or graphs. In analyzing the summaries, we find that certain categories of persons in the population—males of the Protestant faith—are committing suicide with greater frequency than others. We can now make a statement, the empirical generalization, that summarizes the uniformities between two or more variables: Protestant males commit suicide more frequently than others in the population; that is, suicide varies by sex and religion. From such an empirical generalization, inductively reached, we may now use deduction (reasoning from a *premise* rather than from observations) to formulate a working hypothesis that predicts future findings: if one is a Protestant male, then he is in a population at risk for suicide. Induction and deduction alternate in the process of rational thought. Once we state the hypothesis, we may collect further data to test the hypothesis or to develop another empirical generalization.

Yet, we still cannot explain why male Protestants kill themselves more often than others in the population. At this point, the creative ability of the mind enters the process. Drawing on material in the literature, we may attempt a biological explanation; it is the genetic endowment of the individual that explains suicide; that is, males are more susceptible to suicide because of a genetic disposition toward depression that leads to suicide. Or we may develop a psychological explanation: males committing suicide have a death wish. However, these explanations do not account for the variable of religion. Why are Protestants committing suicide more frequently than Catholics or Jews? To deal with all of the variables, we need a social explanation that relates the value system of Protestantism, internalized by males of the faith, with a later vulnerability to commit suicide. Reared to be self-reliant and independent of his family and other primary groups, the Protestant male cannot depend upon the group to sustain him during periods of deep, unrelieved anxiety and distress. Therefore, he is at risk to commit suicide because of his individualistic approach to life. We invent a new concept, "individualism," or "egoism," to stand for the constellation of observations and ideas that arise. Personal disorganization in individuals who are egoistic or individualistic, and thus not strongly integrated into a primary group, may lead to suicide (Durkheim, 1951). We ponder such explanations, explore possibilities of others, and search for ways to test the explanations in research.

Theories close to observed data and empirical generalizations, such as that just described, are called *theories of the middle range* to distinguish them from *grand theories* that intend to explain universal relationships (such as Einstein's theory of relativity). Middle-range theories (Merton, 1968) are used by the newer sciences, such as sociology and nursing, and deal with *delimited* aspects of phenomena. Since nurses are close to observations of health and disease in daily practice, they may find the inductive method useful to explain carefully delimited aspects of nursing. It is less formidable a task to look for observed regularities between two or more variables, and to build a number of empirical generalizations from which nursing concepts and theory may be developed, than to hope for the creative leap that will produce a grand theory of nursing, explaining all of the facts observed in nursing.

Construction of Theory. Jacox (1974), discussing the construction of theory in nursing, summarizes the efforts to develop a theory in three steps: (1) specifying, defining, and classifying the concepts used to describe the phenomena of the field; (2) developing statements or propositions that propose how two or more concepts are related; and (3) specifying how all of the propositions are related to one another in a systematic way. In the first step, the emphasis is on concepts; in the second step, the emphasis is on the proposition (the empirical generalization); and in the third step, the propositions are related to one another in a theory. Thus, Jacox views theory construction as a process that begins with the description of observation, moves on to the invention of concepts and propositions, and culminates in the theory itself, a view that coincides with Figure 3–1.

In the same manner, Dickoff and James (1968) begin with description, but differ from approaches commonly used in science by calling this first step "theory." In addition, theory is given a broad definition—a mental invention for some purpose: to describe, explain, predict, or prescribe. This definition includes description as a basic level of theory, and prescription as the highest level of theory. In their view, theories may be constructed at four different levels: (1) factor-isolating theory; (2) factor-relating theory; (3) situation-relating theory; and (4) situation-producing theory. The lower levels are developed before, and provide a basis for, the higher levels of theory. Each of these levels will be examined in turn.

Levels of Theory. The first level of theory, *factor-isolating theory*, requires that the student first observe, next describe, and then look for ways to put similar descriptive data into categories. Finally, the student names the categories—i.e., creates concepts to stand for categories of information. Such data are produced by a qualitative research design (described in Part IV). Observations and descriptions lead the student to construct the factor-isolating or "naming theory."

Factor-relating theory, the second level of theory, relates the named concepts to one another. This level coincides both with Jacox's second step in theory construction—developing statements or propositions that propose how two or more concepts are related—and with the "empirical generalization" of Figure 3–1.

Situation-relating theory, the third level of theory, explains the interrelationships among concepts or propositions. This level coincides with both Jacox's third step and with the "theory" of Figure 3–1.

Situation-producing theory, the fourth of Dickoff and James' levels of theories, includes the prescription of the activities necessary to reach defined goals. This level goes beyond "theorizing," or thinking about theory, to proposed activity designed to reach a goal. However, the student who thinks about both ethics and malpractice insurance no doubt would include, as one of the first goals to be defined, the repeated testing of hypotheses derived from theory in ethical research.

Theories may be formulated from everyday observations in the clinical area. For example, the student may begin with a clinical problem or an unanswered question in nursing for which little information exists, and take the following steps: (1) attempt the difficult task of identifying patterns of related observations that as yet have no name—i.e., have not been conceptualized; (2) borrow a commonplace name or invent a new name that will stand for the related observations; (3) create a proposition that states the relationship between the newly named concept and another concept (for example, "degree of burnout varies with the workplace of the nurse" or, at a more abstract level, "degree of burnout varies with stress experienced by the nurse"); (4) test the proposition in research (by predicting that burnout associated with a particularly stressful workplace will be found over and over again); and (5) invent a middle-range theory (to explain stress in general in nursing practice).

This approach is similar to that of Glaser and Strauss (1966, 1967), who developed what they call *grounded theory* from their studies of dying in a hospital. Following Glaser and Strauss, the student begins by making lengthy and careful observation of patients dying in a hospital. Observations that are related to one another are then put in the same category. For example, two categories may include "awareness of the patient that she (or he) is dying" and "awareness of others that the patient is dying." Different types of awareness may be identified and named—an *open awareness*, when both patient and others know the patient is dying; *mutual pretense*, when the patient knows but others do not; *suspicious awareness*, when others know but the patient does not; and *closed awareness*, when no one knows. Once the researcher names the concepts and creates a statement (the empirical generalization) that states the relationship between concepts (such as "type of awareness" and "dying"), the student must then test the proposition over and over by first predicting (via hypotheses) what will be found in research concerning the awareness of dying: by various types of patients; in a variety of places; and of numerous maladies. Following the testing of each hypothesis, the student may then attempt to invent a theory that explains the general relationship between dying persons and the others involved with them in a number of situations. Van Gennep's *Rites of Passage* (1909, trans. 1960) includes the rites of separation, the ritual behavior at death among human groups everywhere.

In addition to beginning to construct theory with observation, the student may begin with a conceptual framework already invented. For example, nursing theorists such as Kim (1983), King (1981), Riehl and Roy (1980), Newman (1979), and others have devised conceptual frameworks essential to nursing and, at times, go beyond this to invent nursing theory.

The steps in the scientific inquiry may appear to be distinct but in actual fact may shade into one another, making it difficult to tell exactly when observations become empirical generalizations and when empirical generalizations become theories.

Deductive Reasoning: Creating Propositions to Test Explanations and Predictions. Deductive reasoning commonly begins with a theory, or general premise, and moves toward specific observations: it explains and predicts the data that we will observe. Deduction is the method used to convert theory into interrelated propositions and hypotheses that can be tested by observations. A simple example will illustrate the system.

First, a theoretical statement—called the *premise, proposition, postulate,* or *axiom*—is formulated or found in the literature. For example, a broad statement held to be true is, "All living things eventually die." This is a major premise. A second proposition, the minor premise, now states, "Man is a living thing." From proposition one and proposition two, a third proposition is deduced: "Therefore, all men must die." Put together in a system, the propositions are seen to be interrelated and to descend from the general proposition or premise to a specific proposition.

1. All living things eventually die.
2. Man is a living thing.
3. Therefore, all men must die.

Such a syllogism, or system of deductive reasoning, produces an hypothesis that we may test: if one is human, then one must die. We may test this hypothesis in several ways. For example, we can observe to see if humans do indeed die. Since we, too, are human, such direct observations are limited in time and space. To extend our observations, we can use other research methods to collect data. We can interview other persons directly or indirectly, by questionnaire, to determine if they have observed that humans die. Or, we can draw a random sample from a population of humans to see, retrospectively, which persons have died in the past, when, where, and of what. If the observations include even one person who has lived for centuries and appears to be immortal, then the theory must be revised to account for this fact. Thus, deductive reasoning begins with a theory and develops a system of interrelated propositions or hypotheses that predict what will be observed. These hypotheses may then be tested by using scientific research methods. However, formal systems of propositions are better-developed in the older sciences. New sciences, such as nursing, often develop hypotheses without recourse to a hierarchical system of logical propositions between theory and hypothesis.

Researchers also utilize assumptions and theories from allied disciplines to create hypotheses for use in nursing research. *Assumptions* are basic principles assumed to be true. They are statements whose correctness or validity is taken for granted. At times, a number of assumptions are used to deduce hypotheses, in the absence of formal deductive systems. Researchers are forced to make assumptions when the state of knowledge does not allow them to prove or disprove certain statements. Assumptions are found in a number of research studies, and these studies are helpful in identifying sound assumptions. For example, Rose (1980) proposed a number of assumptions on which to base studies of socialization. One assumption is as follows: "All persons are born into an ongoing society and are socialized into behavior that meets the expectations of the culture." Byrne and Edeani (1984) begin their article on the knowledge of medical terminology among hospital patients with an implicit assumption: "Effective communication between health-care provider and patient is essential for accurate and adequate information-gathering and dissemination." No proof is offered for the statement; instead, the authors note that few studies on communication patterns between health-care providers and patients are available.

A fruitful area for theories, and one that has been widely utilized by nurse researchers, is that developed by allied sciences: theories of learning, development, adaptation, and stress; systems theory; and social and cultural theories have been used and developed by nurse-researchers. (Each of these will be studied in the next two chapters.)

SUMMARY

The central element of scientific research is *observation*, watching and recording events in the selected research area. Observation must be related to *theory*, a general explanation of the relationship among observed facts, concepts, and propositions. *Facts* are empirically verifiable observations, which the mind orders into a *concept*—a word that stands for a complex idea or mental image formed from reality.

To relate theory and observation, the mind reasons either *deductively*, beginning with a theory, or *inductively*, beginning with observation. The relationship between logical thought and scientific observation may be depicted in a diagram that includes the elements of research—observation, proposition, and theory—and methods of reasoning—induction or deduction—that lead to constructing and testing theories. To test a theory, the mind utilizes *deduction* to reason from the theory to create a *proposition*, an *hypothesis* that predicts what will be found upon observation. To formulate a theory, the mind utilizes *induction* to reason from observation to theory by means of a proposition, an *empirical generalization*, that states an observed relationship between two concepts. Several related empirical generalizations or related concepts—called *constructs*—may be interrelated to one another in a general statement, or theory, that explains the relationship.

Basic terms of research include concepts and variables, the building blocks of empirical generalizations and hypotheses. Nursing concepts include nursing care and many other ideas at varying levels of complexity. Concepts, the mental images formed from reality, are transformed into observable and measurable *variables* by an *operational definition*, a step-by-step set of directions that specifies how to observe and measure the concept under study. Operational definitions enable scientists to test or replicate the work of one another and specify precisely what is to be observed and measured during the data-collection phase.

Variables are concepts that have been defined by operational definition in such a way that changes or variation can be observed and measured. Variables include the *independent variable*, the *dependent variable*, the *extraneous variable*, and the *attribute variable*. The independent variable is also known as the experimental, causal, stimulus, or treatment variable, while the dependent variable is known as the effect, the outcome, the response, or the criterion measure—that which is affected by, or responds to, the independent variable. The researcher manipulates the independent variable by introducing it into one group and withholding it from another group in order to study whether the independent variable made a difference. The change in behavior or outcome in the dependent variable that the researcher hopes to explain or predict is presumed to be caused by or associated with the independent variable. *Extraneous variables* are those present in large numbers that are not of interest to the researcher but that may interfere with the action of the independent variable or be mistaken for its action. *Attribute variables* are characteristics of the study subjects, such as age, race, or medical diagnosis, that pre-exist and that may act as extraneous variables.

Hypotheses are propositions formulated to predict a relationship between two or more variables that can be tested in research. Sources of hypotheses include theory, assumptions, observations, working experiences, and the literature. The formulation of hypotheses is a precise task that requires careful, critical work from the researcher. Testing hypotheses demands the careful collection and analysis of data, either for causality (a difficult task if human subjects are used) or for correlation, which indicates how factors vary together.

• *Views about the construction of theory* in nursing include that of Mathwig, who believes that theoretical knowledge of nursing must evolve from nursing alone; Johnson, and others, who view knowledge as useful across disciplines; and Diers, who suggests an evaluation and adaptation of all theory before use in nursing practice. Constructing nursing theory from observation by inductive reasoning involves observation, description, summarization, and creation of the empirical generalization in order to state a proposed relationship between two concepts. Theories are then created from a number of empirical generalizations. Jacox summarizes the construction of theory in three steps: the first emphasizes the specification, definition, and classification of concepts; the second emphasizes the proposition, the empirical generalization; and the third relates the propositions to one another in a theory.

Dickoff and James define theory as a mental invention designed to describe, explain, predict, or prescribe. Four levels of theory construction, each built upon the other, include: (1) observing, describing, and naming concepts; (2) relating named concepts to one another; (3) explaining the interrelationships among concepts or propositions; and (4) prescribing activities necessary to reach defined goals.

The clinical area is a fruitful one for formulating theory, beginning with clinical problems or unanswered questions, identifying and classifying patterns of observation related to the problems or questions, naming the classified categories, creating a proposition to state the relationship between the newly named concepts; testing the proposition in research over and over; and inventing a middle-range theory to explain observations and regularities.

Glaser and Strauss invented the term *grounded theory* to describe their approach to theory formulation. Beginning with lengthy and careful observation, the researchers proceeded in the manner similar to that described above for the clinical area: developing categories of observations, naming the categories, creating a proposition that states the relationship between concepts, testing and retesting the proposition, and inventing a theory to explain the general relationships that persisted. The researcher may also begin to formulate theory, utilizing conceptual frameworks already developed by various nursing scientists.

Deductive reasoning to test theory begins with that theory and creates a proposition—the hypothesis—that predicts what will be found upon observation. The formal system of propositions constructed between theory and hypothesis is more developed in the older sciences. Newer sciences, such as nursing, develop less often the hierarchical systems of logical propositions. At times, researchers may begin with assumptions, rather than theory, to create hypotheses. *Assumptions* are basic principles assumed to be true, statements whose correctness or validity is taken for granted. Assumptions are used when the state of knowledge does not allow well-developed theories to be utilized.

Theories from allied sciences, such as sociology, anthropology, social psychology, psychology, and physiology, are among those modified by nurses for use in research.

EXAMPLE FROM NURSING RESEARCH

Mary Shannahan and Barbara Cottrell (1985): Effect of the birth chair on duration of second-stage labor, fetal outcome, and maternal blood loss. Nursing Research, 34, 89–92.

The concepts utilized in the study included second-stage labor, duration of second-stage labor, birth chair, fetal outcome, and maternal blood loss. Definitions of the concepts were given with reference to what was found in the review of the literature.

1. The second stage of labor was defined as the duration of time between complete cervical dilation and delivery of the whole fetus.
2. Duration of second-stage labor was noted to vary, most investigators reporting a mean duration in primigravidas of 41 to 68 minutes, and multigravidas from 13 to 18 minutes. Nigerian women were reported to be in the second stage a much shorter time.
3. A modern birthing chair was defined as a molded plastic chair with footrests, motorized so that it can be elevated, lowered, and tilted. Birthing chairs were noted to have been used since 1450 B.C.
4. Fetal outcome was informally defined as the condition of infants as assessed by Apgar scores and umbilical artery pH, and included time of first cry of infants and umbilical-cord blood-gas analysis.
5. Maternal blood loss was informally defined as the postpartum hemoglobin and hematocrit values. The literature indicated that this may be higher for multigravidas in the birth chair.

The conceptual framework utilized the Roy Adaptation Model in which labor can be viewed as an environmental stimulus to which pregnant women must adapt during the process of childrearing. The focal stimulus is not manipulated first; therefore, the nurse manipulates contextual or residual stimuli. The upright position for delivery is a contextual stimulus. Since the birth chair is one way of achieving an upright position, hypotheses were developed to predict what would be observed in the use of the birth chair.

Propositions, stated as hypotheses, predicted the following: (1) Women who deliver in a birth chair will have shorter second-stage labor than women who deliver on a traditional delivery table. (2) Women who deliver in a birth chair will have a better fetal outcome than women who deliver on a traditional delivery table. (3) Women who deliver in a birth chair will have more blood loss than women who deliver on a traditional delivery table.

The method of study was a retrospective chart review of 60 primiparous women, 37–41 weeks' gestation, who gave birth in June or July 1983 in a medical center in north Florida. Thirty of the women delivered in a birth chair and 30 delivered on a traditional delivery table. Data collected from the charts included the type of delivery, episiotomy, laceration, anesthesia, analgesic within two hours before delivery, Apgar scores, hemoglobin and hematocrit upon admission and on first or second day postpartum, and duration of second-stage labor.

Findings included: no significant difference was found between the two groups for mean duration of second-stage labor; mean Apgar scores at one and five minutes were nearly identical. Statistically significant differences existed between the groups in mean maternal hemoglobin and hematocrit values. The birth chair group, while having higher mean hemoglobin and hematocrit upon admission, had significantly lower mean value after delivery. The birth chair is safe in terms of fetal outcome but presents no advantage to the mother in terms of shorter second-stage labor, and may be a disadvantage in terms of maternal blood loss. The researchers suggest further investigations, but no suggestions were given for theory.

STUDY QUESTIONS

1. Draw a diagram that shows the relationships among theory, propositions, and facts. What is the place of research in this model?
2. Find an article in *Nursing Research* or in another research journal. Does the author refer to a theory or a set of assumptions? Are concepts defined? Are operational definitions used? Does the researcher seek to establish and define correlation or causality? What nursing concepts can you identify? Does the researcher begin with observations or theory? Are hypotheses stated? Is inductive or deductive reasoning used?
3. Think of an observation that you have made in the course of nursing practice. Can you identify one or two concepts associated with the observation?
4. List all of the new terms that you have encountered in this chapter and define each.
5. Describe how observation and reasoning function to formulate or test theory.
6. Write an operational definition of some aspect of nursing care that you would like to study. What factors make it measurable and observable?
7. In nursing practice, you notice that seriously ill patients tend to respond to nurses touching them. Formulate an hypothesis that predicts the effect of touching on a seriously ill patient.
8. In 1897, Edward Jenner observed that dairy maids generally had good complexions, seldom showing the pockmarks of those who survived smallpox. Summarize Jenner's observations into an empirical generalization. Write an hypothesis deduced from the empirical generalization. How could the hypothesis be tested?

REFERENCES AND SUGGESTED READING

Abdellah, F. and Levine, E. (1965): Better Patient Care Through Nursing Research. New York: Macmillan, chap. 5.

Alderson, M. (1974): Effects of increased body temperature on the perception of time. Nursing Research, *23*, 44–49. *Clinical study of perception.*

Brill, E. and Kilts, D. (1980): Foundation for Nursing. New York: Appleton-Century-Crofts. *Textbook.*

Brown, J. et al. (1984): Nursing's search for scientific knowledge. Nursing Research, *33*, 26–32.

Byrne, T. and Edeani, D. (1984): Knowledge of medical terminology among hospital patients. Nursing Research, *33*, 178–181.

Charter, S. (1975): Understanding Research in Nursing. Geneva: W.H.O. Offset Pub. No. 14. *Relationship between concepts and principles is discussed.*

Code for Nurses (1977): American Journal of Nursing, *77*, 2581–2585. *Standards of practice.*

Coleman, L. (1980): Orem's self-care concept of nursing. In Riehl, J. and Roy, C. (eds.), Conceptual Models for Nursing Practice (2nd ed.). New York: Appleton-Century-Crofts, pp. 315–328. *Orem's self-care concept summarized and applied.*

Conant, J. (1947): On Understanding Science. New Haven: Yale University Press. *Definition of working hypothesis.*

Dailey, A. (1985): Burnout test. American Journal of Nursing, *85*, 270–271.

Dickoff, J. and James, P. (1968): Researching research's role in theory development. Nursing Research, *17*, 204–206.

Diers, D. (1979): Research in Nursing Practice. Philadelphia: J. B. Lippincott. *Clinical research emphasized.*

Downs, F. (1967): Ethical inquiry in nursing research. Nursing Forum, *6*, 12–20. *The problem of ethics in research is discussed.*

Downs, F. and Newman, M. (eds.) (1977): A Sourcebook of Nursing Research (2nd ed.). Philadelphia: F. A. Davis. *Eight nursing studies evaluate nursing intervention; seven explore indices of health.*

Downs, F. and Fleming, J. (eds.) (1979): Issues in Nursing Research. New York: Appleton-Century-Crofts. *Seven articles: trends, issues, and future of nursing research are discussed.*

Durkheim, E. (1951): Suicide. Spaulding and Simpson (Trans.). Glencoe, Ill.: The Free Press. *A classic study in research.*

Gebbie, K. (1976): Summary of the Second National Conference on Classification of Nursing Diagnoses. St. Louis: St. Louis University. *Currently accepted diagnostic nomenclature is discussed.*

Glaser, B. and Strauss, A. (1966): Awareness of Dying. Chicago: Aldine.

Glaser, B. and Strauss, A. (1967): Discovery of Grounded Theory. Chicago: Aldine.

Goode, W. and Hatt, P. (1952): Methods in Social Research. New York: McGraw-Hill. *Chapters 3–7 deal with science, values, concepts, and hypotheses.*

Gordon, M. (1979): The concept of nursing diagnosis. In The Nursing Clinics of North America. Philadelphia: W. B. Saunders, *Conceptualization of nursing diagnosis is discussed.*

Hardy, M. (ed.) (1973): Theoretical Foundations for Nursing. New York: MSS Information Corp. *Theories and concepts, including stress, crises, adaptation, and general systems theory.*

Henderson, V. and Nite, G. (1878): Principles and Practices of Nursing, (6th ed.). New York: Macmillan.

Jacobson, G., Thiele, J., McCune, J. and Farrell, L. (1985): Handwashing: Ring-wearing and number of microorganisms. Nursing Research, *34*, 186–187.

Jacox, A. (1974): Theory construction in nursing: An overview. Nursing Research, *23*, 4–13.

Johnson, D. (1968): Theory in nursing: Borrowed and unique. Nursing Research *17*. *Johnson discusses theory, noting that knowledge does not belong to any field of science exclusively.*

Kim, H. (1983): The Nature of Theoretical Thinking in Nursing. Norwalk, Conn.: Appleton-Century-Crofts.

King, I. (1971): Towards a Theory of Nursing. New York: Wiley.

Kuhn, T. (1962): The Structure of Scientific Revolutions. Chicago: University of Chicago Press. *Discusses how scientific knowledge accrues and changes.*

Lindeman, C. and Van Aernam, B. (1971): Nursing intervention with the presurgical patient—the effects of structured and unstructured preoperative teaching. In Downs, F. and Newman, M. (eds.), A Sourcebook of Nursing Research (2nd ed.). (1977): Philadelphia: F. A. Davis, pp. 45–63. *Clinical study reported.*

Mathwig, G. (1970): Nursing science—the theoretical core of nursing knowledge. Image, *4*, 20–23. *Presents the view that nursing theory should evolve from nursing rather than from other disciplines.*

McCorkle, R. (1981): Effects of touch on seriously ill patients. In Fox, D. (ed.), Readings on the Research Process in Nursing. New York: Appleton-Century-Crofts, pp. 114–125. *Clinical study; defines touch.*

Merton, R. (1968): Social Theory and Social Structure. New York: The Free Press. *Part I discusses theories of the middle-range.*

Newman, M. (1972): Nursing's theoretical evolution. Nursing Outlook, *20*, 449–453.

Olgas, M. (1974): Relationship between parents' health status and body image of their children. Nursing Research *23*, 319–324. *Olgas predicts a relationship between parents' health status and body image of child.*

Orem, D. (1971): Nursing: Concepts of Practice. New York: McGraw-Hill. *Framework for model of self-care.*

Riehl, J. and Roy, C. (eds.) (1980): Conceptual Models for Nursing Practice (2nd ed.). New York: Appleton-Century-Crofts. *Includes a number of theoretical models for nursing practice, such as Peplau, Neuman, Roy, Johnson, and Orem.*

Robischon, P. (1971): Pica practice and other hand-mouth behavior and children's developmental level. In Downs, F. and Newman, M. (eds.), A Sourcebook of Nursing Research (2nd ed.). Philadelphia: F. A. Davis. *States assumptions.*

Rose, A. (1980, orig. 1962): A systematic summary of symbolic interaction theory. In Riehl, J. and Roy, C. (eds.), Conceptual Models for Nursing Practice. New York: Appleton-Century-Crofts. *Assumptions.*

Rottkamp, B. (1981): A behavior modification approach to nursing therapeutics in body positioning of spinal-cord-injured patients. In Fox, D. (ed.), Readings on the Research Process in Nursing. New York: Appleton-Century-Crofts, pp. 107–113. *Develops hypothesis for her research study.*

Stevens, B. (1979): Nursing Theory: Analysis, Application, Evaluation. Boston: Little, Brown. *Specific theorists examined to familiarize reader with nursing theory.*

Van Gennep, A. (1909, trans. 1960): The Rites of Passage. Chicago: University of Chicago Press.

Van Ort, S. and Gerber, R. (1976): Topical application of insulin in the treatment of decubitus ulcers. Nursing Research *25*, 9–12. *Suggests causality.*

Wald, F. and Leonard, R. (1964): Toward development of nursing practice theory. Nursing Research *13*, 309–313. *Discusses the development of theory in practice.*

Wallace, W. (1971): The Logic of Science in Sociology. Chicago: Aldine. *Brief book examines theories, empirical generalizations, hypotheses, and observations; emphasizes their interrelations.*

PART II

Theory

4

Theories Utilized in Nursing Research

A theory summarizes what is known from past work and predicts what will be found on future observation. The student uses theory in research to provide a framework constructed from past ideas, understandings, and research findings, and as a foundation for the proposed research project. The student also uses theory to generate hypotheses that predict what will be found when data are collected and analyzed. The theoretical framework—the set of interrelated concepts and definitions—enables the student to contribute the findings of even a small project to the larger theoretical perspective that uses the same theoretical frame of reference.

The student identifies the theoretical framework to be used in the research project from an early review of the literature. However, the search for pertinent theories soon leads to the discovery that nursing lies at the theoretical crossroads of many disciplines. The challenge to the student is to determine which of these best explains the problem to be studied and which lends itself to research.

Upon completion of this chapter and the next, the student should be able to: (1) identify some of the major theories reported in the nursing research literature; (2) describe what the theory is explaining or predicting; and (3) report nursing research that has used various theories.

The primary objectives of this chapter and the next are to assist the student to identify theoretical frameworks used in published nursing research and to select a theoretical framework useful in a proposed research project.

According to Brown et al. (1984), theories can develop only when researchers are familiar with earlier research and with theoretical formulations relevant to their own findings. They found that researchers seldom discussed theoretical issues in the 1950s but have tended to include such discussion in recent years. However, as late as 1980, many of the authors of published articles failed to tie their findings into past work, thereby losing the opportunity to integrate their research into a larger whole. In addition, few research articles included suggestions for future study that would extend theory. Therefore, the student should keep in mind the need to become familiar with past research and theoretical formulations, to replicate good research, and to build upon a theoretical base, where possible.

MAJOR THEORIES REPORTED IN NURSING RESEARCH LITERATURE

Too many theories are reported in the nursing literature to examine in the space of two chapters. However, a number of the theories tend to fall into several categories: (1) learning theory; (2) development theory; (3) theories of adaptation, stress, and homeostasis; (4) systems theory; (5) social theories; and (6) cultural theories. The first four categories will be examined in this chapter, while social and cultural theories will be examined in the next.

　　Learning theory includes theories of conditioning, social learning, and Gestalt or cognitive theory. *Developmental theory* examines changes that occur through time in the physical, mental, psychological, and social structures. *Theories* of *adaptation*, *stress*, and *homeostasis* (often incorporated into many theories, including cultural theories) examine how individuals or groups survive and function in a particular environment. *Systems theory* is diverse, focusing at times on behavioral systems and at times on systems of interaction, communication, or adaptation. Each of these will be examined briefly to identify their major concepts and to note nursing theories and research that have utilized these perspectives.

LEARNING THEORY IN NURSING RESEARCH

A major concern of nursing is *learning*, a process in which past experience results in a lasting change in behavior, motivation, or perception. The predominant sources of learning theory are: (1) behaviorism, rooted in the conditioning theory developed by Pavlov and modified by Skinner and others; (2) social learning theory, closely associated with behaviorism but including social elements, such as imitation, modeling, and the locus of control; and (3) the cognitive theory of learning, proposed by Gestalt psychologists and modified by Piaget, Festinger, and others. Some theories include elements of all of these.

Conditioning

The theory of classical conditioning was developed by Pavlov (1928), who studied the effect of imposed learning upon innate reflexes. Pavlov used the instinctive behavior of hungry dogs (salivation when presented with food) to teach the dogs to salivate when they heard a buzzer. He accomplished this conditioning by introducing the sound of a buzzer simultaneously with the presentation of food. Salivation, the unconditioned response, came to be associated with the sound of a buzzer, the conditioned stimulus. Learning took place when the stimulus known to produce the response was presented, along with a new stimulus that the researcher wanted the subject to learn to associate with the response. The process was repeated over and over until the response was elicited from the new stimulus alone. Thus, the stimulus–response conditioning theory of learning was launched. *Stimulus* is broadly defined as an external or internal event that brings about an alteration in behavior; *response* is the alteration in the behavior. The theory proposes that behavior can be explained and predicted by examining the relationship between stimuli and response.

Operant Conditioning: Behaviorism

The classical theory of conditioning was modified by Skinner and others, who examined the relationship between learning and the action of the individual upon the environment. *Operant*, or instrumental, conditioning proposes that learning occurs as the individual acts upon the environment to obtain a reward or to reduce tension. The reward increases the likelihood that the desired response will occur. *Behaviorism*, as this approach is called, rejects the unobservable completely and is concerned only with human behavior in terms of observable and measurable responses to stimuli. In this view, all behavior is conditioned by habit and can be learned or unlearned. Behavior results from the association learned when the response to a stimulus is reinforced by rewards or extinguished by punishment or by failure to reward.

EXAMPLES FROM NURSING RESEARCH

Derived from operant conditioning and a body of experimental work, behavior modification has been used by O'Neil (1972) and Rottkamp (1976), among others, to study the effect of stimuli on various health problems. O'Neil examined the effect of three types of reinforcement in teaching a child with cerebral palsy to walk. The study consisted of 240 sessions of approximately 30 minutes each. Reinforcement included social reinforcement (saying, "Good, Nancy, good"); material reinforcement (giving Nancy marbles to play with); and food reinforcement (spoonfuls of ice cream). Results showed that the behavior modification techniques were effective in teaching Nancy to crutch-walk.

Rottkamp studied the effect of demonstration, shaping of body positions, and social reinforcement (attention from the nurse) on patients with spinal-cord injuries on improving their performance in body positioning. The experimental group of patients who received the behavior-modification techniques showed a greater difference in the frequency of patient-initiated changes of body position than did patients who did not receive the behavior-modification techniques. Rottkamp drew on stimulus-response theory to formulate her hypothesis that spinal-cord-injured patients with impairment in body-position behaviors would improve in their body-positioning performance to a measurable degree after receiving demonstration, shaping, and positive social reinforcement.

Operant conditioning principles have also been used to modify incontinence in neuropsychiatric geriatric patients (Grosicki, 1968) and to teach self-help activity to the profoundly retarded (Bensberg et al, 1965).

Social Learning

Theories of social learning that explain behaviors acquired through operant conditioning and through imitation are closely associated with the stimulus-response-reinforcement theory of learning but place emphasis on the social elements, such as the process of imitation and identification, or the "locus of control" concept developed by Rotter et al. (1972). *Locus of control* refers to the extent to which individuals believe that people in general have control over their own destiny and understand why they behave as they do.

EXAMPLES FROM NURSING RESEARCH

Cox (1985) utilized Rotter's theory to develop a Health Self-Determinism Index. She notes the assumptions underlying Rotter's theory as follows: An individual's motivation may be derived from either an internal or an external orientation toward self and the environment. Persons who are internally controlled are more likely to take the initiative in health care, be more knowledgeable about health, and adhere to prescribed health care regimens. In contrast, individuals who are externally controlled believe that health is a matter beyond their own control and that the state of health is due to outside controls, such as fate or luck.

Lamontagne (1984) examined the relationship between children's locus of control beliefs, as measured by the Nowicki-Strickland Locus of Control Scale, and their preoperative coping behavior. Results showed that children rated as active copers have a higher internal locus of control score than do children rated as avoidant or as a combination of avoidant–active.

Holaday (1974) used Rotter's theory to explain the perception and behavior of 24 chronically ill children. She found that the chronically ill children tended to view the success or failure of their achievement efforts as external; that is, as due to luck or to others. Windwer (1977) examined the relationships among locus of control, social desirability, and the psychoprophylaxis method of childbirth. Six hypotheses were formulated for study, none of which were supported. Lowery and DuCette (1976) examined the relationship between locus of control and patients' response to diabetes. Patients who viewed the locus of control as external were found to have less diabetic information but fewer diabetic problems over time, whereas patients who viewed the locus of control as internal had more information but showed no decrease in the number of diabetic problems.

Gestalt and Cognitive Theories of Learning

Gestalt is a German word that means form or pattern. A basic assumption of this approach is that the whole is greater than the sum of its parts. Learning occurs in the process of problem solving. The learner identifies similar patterns or categories, recognizes the relationship between the categories through insight, and draws conclusions. The brain gives a cognitive structure to sensations and perceptions. The thoughts, attitudes, beliefs, and behaviors of which a person is cognitively aware—that is, *knows*—are a result of active problem-solving and goal-seeking activity. Behavior is not molded by stimuli, responses, and reinforcement alone but includes the process of knowing, learning, and thinking.

EXAMPLES FROM NURSING RESEARCH

Lamontagne (1984) and Caty et al. (1984) utilized cognitive theory to examine coping behavior in a variety of situations. Lamontagne studied coping in preoperative children, while Caty et al. analyzed published case studies dealing with coping in hospitalized children.

Small (1980) used Piaget's theory of sensorimotor cognitive development in her research on visually impaired children to assess the spatial awareness and perceived body image of these children compared with normally sighted children. The relation of objects in space and the development of *object permanence*—searching for lost or hidden objects because the child knows that an unseen object is nonetheless permanent—are necessary states for the development of the child's body image and for awareness of the body and objects in the space surrounding the body. Small drew on the theory to develop hypotheses that predicted the relationship between being visually impaired and perceiving body images and spatial awareness. The findings revealed that there are overwhelming differences between the visually impaired child and the normally sighted child in spatial awareness and in perceived body images.

Festinger (1957) developed a theory of cognitive dissonance that explains how a person may simultaneously possess two cognitions, one the opposite of the other, called *dissonance*. This arises after an attempt to elicit overt behavior that is at variance with private beliefs. The individual tries to establish internal consistency or harmony among personal beliefs and knowledge. Stillman (1977) used the theory to examine the relationship between beliefs and preventive health behavior. Findings indicate that women who believe themselves to be susceptible to breast cancer practice breast self-examination more often than women who do not perceive themselves to be highly susceptible.

DEVELOPMENTAL THEORY IN NURSING RESEARCH

Developmental theory examines changes that occur through time, first on one level and then on another. Piaget's cognitive theory is a developmental theory that suggests that cognition proceeds through five phases, with a number of levels in each phase. The time span for the full development of formal operations is 15 years. In Freud's theory of personality, development begins at birth and includes a number of parallel processes that also continue over many years. Erikson's neo-Freudian theory of personality development incorporates the entire span of human life, as does Havighurst's task of development (Table 4–1). Therefore, studies of development must be either longitudinal studies (prospective or retrospective) or, if conducted at only one point in time, must deal with a cross-sectional segment of development, examined at that one period of time.

The concepts used in the developmental theories of Piaget, Freud, Erikson, and Havighurst have passed into nursing literature and research. However, the long time span required for observation discourages research, although particular phases are studied.

EXAMPLES FROM NURSING RESEARCH: NURSING RESEARCH AND THEORY DEVELOPMENT

Aamodt (1972) spent 13 months in the field observing the culture of the Papago in order to discover the development of cognitive patterns of meaning that could be related to health and healing. Among other things, she found the theme of "taking care of" in the Papago cultural system, a developmental model of the individual's life cycle. The patterns change as the child develops through adulthood and old age.

Robischon (1977) studied the relationship between the development of motor skills in children and *pica*, the habitual ingestion of nonedible substances. She found that motor development, reflected in the hand-to-mouth scores measured by the Denver Developmental Screening Test, was lower among children who practiced pica. Pica was viewed as a behavioral lag, a continuation of an earlier developmental phase in which oral environmental exploration was normal. This earlier phase had not been replaced by behavior more appropriate to the chronological age of the child.

Nolan (1985) conducted a retrospective time study of the development of work patterns of female nurses who had been graduated from one diploma nursing school in the 1950s and who were at midlife at the time of study. She identified four work patterns that developed over the years, including the stable pattern, the double-track pattern, the interrupted pattern, and the unstable pattern. Women appeared to simultaneously integrate numerous combinations of career, marriage, and childrearing, patterns that appeared to be unique for women when compared with men's careers.

Peplau (1952) elaborated a model of nursing roles to explain the development of interpersonal relations between the nurse and the patient. The model sought to describe and explain the changes that occurred in the role of the patient and nurse in simultaneous, but different, phases of interaction.

TABLE 4–1. THEORIES OF DEVELOPMENTAL PHASES

Age in Years	Piaget (Cognitive)	Erikson (Personality)	Freud (Personality)		Havighurst's Tasks
0	Sensori-motor	Phase I: Basic	Oral Stage	ID	Learning:
1	Phase	Trust			to walk
					to talk
2			Anal Stage	Ego	to control body
3	Precon-ceptual	Phase II: Sense of			sex differences
			Phallic	Super-	simple concepts
4	Phase	Autonomy	Stage	Ego	to relate emotionally
					right from wrong
5	Intuitive-Thought	Phase III: Sense of			to play
			Latency		games
6	Phase	Initiative	Stage		gender roles
					to read, write, calculate
7					Developing:
					concepts for living
8	Concrete Operations				morality, values
					attitudes
9	Phase	Phase IV: Sense of			Achieving:
10		Industry			personal independence
					peer-relationships with
11					both sexes
			Genital		sex roles
12	Phase of Formal	Stage			emotional independence
13	Operations	Phase V: Sense of			Accepting:
14		Identity			the physical body
					Preparing:
15					for a career
					for economic independ-
16					ence
					for marriage and family
					for civic competence
17					socially responsible
					behavior
18					norms and values
					Selecting a mate
					Marriage and adjustment
		Phase VI:			Expanding a family
		Sense of Intimacy			Rearing a family
Adulthood		Sense of Generativity			Adjusting to middle and old age
Late adult-hood		Sense of Integrity			

In the first phase, the patient entered the *orientation* phase, assessing the new environment and assuming a dependent role like that of an infant. At this time, the nurse was in the assessment phase, listening as the patient expressed needs and feelings and assuming a reciprocal role as a surrogate mother. In the second phase, *identification*, the patient developed a sense of belonging, but, like a child, identified with the nurse. In this phase, the nurse interacted with the patient as a sibling surrogate, identifying with the patient but, at the same time, making a nursing diagnosis and formulating nursing-care plans. In the third phase, *exploitation*, the patient developed an identification with the nurse and, like an adolescent, made use of the services offered. In this phase, the nurse acted the role of a resource person and took steps to intervene so as to help both patient and nurse reach mutual goals and intended consequences. In the fourth phase, *resolution*, the patient developed an adult independence from the nurse. At this point, the nurse evaluated the growth that had occurred in both people and assumed the reciprocal adult role in interaction with the patient.

Nordal and Sato (1980) utilized the Peplau model to examine three cases of developmental growth and maturity of both the patient and the nurse. However, Roy (1980), using the Peplau model to study the interaction of patient and nurse, found that both were anxious and felt threatened, with little development of therapeutic interpersonal relations.

THEORIES OF ADAPTATION, STRESS, AND HOMEOSTASIS IN NURSING RESEARCH

People adapting to the environment is a central theme in the work of nursing theorists such as Roy (1980) and is a factor in the work of Neuman (1980) and others.

Adaptation is a process in which persons adjust in a particular environment in order to function and survive. Successful adaptors are those who survive and leave offspring to carry on the genetic and social characteristics that enabled survival. However, individuals who would have died in the past now survive and function. Phenylketonuria, an inborn error of metabolism, was formerly severely handicapping. If recognized early, it can now be successfully treated with a special diet. The individual adapts to various stressors in the external and internal environment using compensatory mechanisms in the physiological and psychosocial structures.

Stress, the tension resulting when changes occur in the physical and social environment, is a factor in all states of illness. The relationship between adaptation and stress has been explored by Selye (1956), who developed a theory to describe and explain the relationship. Selye defines *stress* as a state manifested by the "General Adaptation Syndrome." The syndrome evolves in three stages, as the body attempts to adapt to stressors. The first stage is *alarm*, arising when agents such as disease or injury call forth an increase in the vital activity of the body to resist. The second stage is *resistance*, marked by the full adaptation of the body to the stressor. The final stage is *exhaustion*, arising during the course of lengthy resistance to severe stressors. The body's energy is finite; therefore, if not reversed, this stage leads to death.

Adaptation and homeostasis are related in theories of equilibrium–disequilibrium. *Homeostasis*, a term coined by physiologist Walter Cannon (1939), means "staying the same." The process of homeostatic regulation involves the theory of a system maintained by negative feedback—every deviation from the normal triggers a response to correct it (Fig. 4–1). The simple system in the figure is maintained at a normal state through the process of negative feedback, which stimulates processes to correct excesses or deficiencies when these arise. Negative feedback systems are at work both inside and outside the individual.

EXAMPLES FROM NURSING RESEARCH

Roy (1980) develops her model of an adaptive system with reference to theories developed in psychology, sociology, and physiology. The person, as a patient, is viewed as being comprised of parts linked together. Strains may arise both within the linked system or from the external environment. The linked elements of the system include four subsystems: *physiologic needs*, *self-concept*, *role function*, and *interdependence*. The four subsystems function by adapting: the person adapts according to physiological need; the person adapts self-concept in interaction with others; the role is adapted in response to outside stimulation; and finally, the person adapts according to the subsystem of interdependence. The nurse's role is to act as an external regulator so as to modify adverse stimuli affecting adaptation.

Cowan and Murphy (1985) investigated the relationship between bereavement following the volcanic eruption of Mount St. Helens in 1980 and subsequent life stress, social support, and illness. The theoretical basis of the study included bereavement constructs and the association among life stress, social support, and illness. There were six variables, including gender, age, concurrent life stress, perception of the prior relationship between the bereaved and deceased as central or peripheral, perception of catastrophic

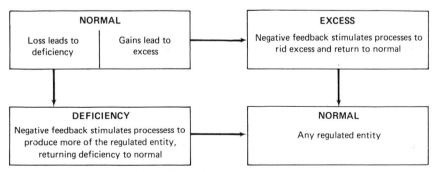

Figure 4–1. Model of homeostasis.

death as preventable or unpreventable, and perception of social support. The researchers looked for an association between the variables and health outcomes, including depression, somatization, and physical health status.

Two complex research questions included the following: (1) Is there a significant association between life stress (and other factors) and state of physical health, depression, and somatization 11 months postdisaster? and (2) To what extent can life stress and other factors predict health outcomes 11 months postdisaster? The researcher found concurrent negative life stress to be the most important single predictor in all three health outcomes: depression, somatization, and physical health status.

Farr et al. (1984) used a physiological conceptual model to study stress. The researchers sought to determine if a relationship existed between the degree of circadian alteration and the subject's reentrainment to typical circadian profiles. They measured alteration in level, timing, and coupling of circadian excretion of catecholamine metabolites, adrenal cortical hormones, sodium, potassium, creatinine, and vital signs in acute-care surgical patients. Data indicated that certain circadian rhythms of hospitalized subjects were altered and uncoupled from external stimuli.

DeWalt and Haines (1977) were interested in the effect of stressors on the human body and in the function of nursing intervention to render the stressors less harmful. They examined the effects of specified local stressors, such as oral breathing, oxygen flow, and intermittent mechanical suction, on healthy oral mucosa. During the first stage, the alarm reaction, there was evidence of increased salivation and paling and drying of the mucosa. During the second stage, the adaptive reaction, decreased salivation and increased dryness of the mucosa were noticed, together with other signs. During the third stage, the exhaustive reaction, a numbness and loss of taste and a breaking in the continuity of the lip mucosa were noted. Oral hygiene given twice during the fifth and final hours of the experiment seemed to minimize the effects of the stressors.

Downs (1977) studied the effects of stressful conditions on the newborn. Study subjects were women of low socioeconomic status. The data supported the contention that environmental stress was related to neonatal pathology.

SYSTEMS THEORY IN NURSING

A *system* is an organization of parts that are interrelated in such a manner that a change in one part brings about a change in all parts. A system constantly changes as it interacts with the external environment—adaptations and adjustments continuously occur, although these may be subtle and difficult to observe. A system differs from each of its parts and is greater than the sum of its parts. In addition, a number of subsystems form a larger and more complex system. The concept *system* stands for a number of differing ideas. For example, a social system is not the same as a general system. A social system may be a small constellation of roles, such as those in the family (husband–wife–child, or mother–father–

brother–sister), or it may be the interrelated systems of an entire society. On the other hand, a general system is a complex adaptive system characterized by an elaboration or evolution of organization that depends on disturbances and variety in the environment to keep it informed.

General systems theory is the end result of a culmination of shifts in the scientific perspective over the past few centuries. First, a system was viewed as one of equilibrium–disequilibrium. The *equilibrium model* depicts a system of simple organization that functions to reach stability and remain steady within a narrow condition of disturbance. Next, a system was viewed as homeostatic. The *homeostatic model* applies to more complex systems, such as those of the body, that tend to be highly organized in spite of infections or injuries that threaten to reduce the level of organization. The *general system model* is characterized by a complex adaptive system that changes organization in response to changes in the environment. General systems theory is quite complex but centers upon cybernetic processes as crucial in self-correction and change.

The types of system used by nursing scholars vary from one theorist to another. Johnson (1980) uses a behavioral-system approach, while Neuman (1980) proposes a system comprised of an individual interacting holistically with stress and with reaction to stress.

Johnson's Behavioral System

Johnson (1980) developed her model of behavioral systems for nursing from an interdisciplinary body of theoretical literature and empirical data drawn from psychology, ethology, anthropology, and general systems theory.

The model depicts the patient as a behavioral system, in a manner similar to that of the physician who views the patient as a biologic system (Fig. 4–2). Johnson defines *system* as a "whole which functions as a whole by virtue of the independence of its parts." The parts of Johnson's system are seven subsystems of behavior: (1) the attachment or affiliative subsystem; (2) the subsystem of dependence; (3) the ingestive; (4) the eliminative; (5) the sexual; (6) the aggressive; and (7) the achievement. An eighth subsystem, restoration, is added later by other theorists using the Johnson behavioral system, but Johnson (1980) rejects this addition.

Each of these subsystems functions to carry out a specialized task for the system as a whole, and each subsystem is structured by a set of behavioral responses organized around a motivational structure. The elements of the motivational structure include observed behavior, drive, set, and choice. *Drive* is associated with goal-directed behavior, while the individual's *set* refers to the predisposition to act in a particular way with reference to the goal. The *choice*, or *behavioral repertoire*, is the set of behaviors available to the individual to achieve a particular goal. Johnson suggests that the cross-cultural prevalence of the subsystems indicates that the behavioral response, or the releasers for such behavior, are ge-

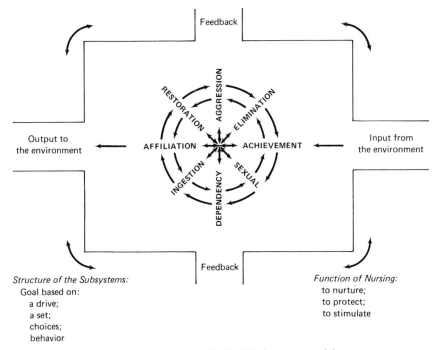

Figure 4–2. Johnson's behavioral system model.

netically programmed. At the same time, she notes that the variability found in human responses indicates the significance of social and cultural factors.

Johnson notes that each of the subsystems must be protected from noxious influences and malfunctions and that each must be stimulated to grow. The function of nursing is to help restore the balance of each subsystem when it is disturbed and to act to prevent future imbalances.

Johnson summarizes the functions of each of the behavioral subsystems:

1. The attachment, or affiliative, subsystem functions in both survival and security, and is critical. Likewise, it has empirical consequences for other functions, such as social inclusion, intimacy, and bonding. This subsystem is one of the first to develop and is rooted in the mother-child dyad.

2. The dependency subsystem functions to obtain nurturant responses by manifesting succoring behavior—that which solicits aid, assistance, attention, recognition, and approval. Dependency behavior undergoes a developmental process, progressing from total dependence, seen in infants and ill persons, to dependence on self and interdependence on the social group.

3. and 4. The ingestive and eliminative subsystems, intimately associated with the biological system, are controlled by social norms that prescribe the rules for proper eating and elimination.
5. The sexual subsystem functions to procreate and gratify, and is rooted both in biology and in social norms that influence when, where, and with whom sex is allowed. It also influences gender-role identity.
6. The aggressive subsystem functions to protect and preserve, although collective life limits self-protection to include the protection of the group.
7. The achievement subsystem functions to master or control intellectual, physical, creative, mechanical, and social skills.

Research is needed to study the system and subsystems and to identify, clarify, and explain problems encountered in nursing that are associated with disturbances in the systems.

EXAMPLES FROM NURSING RESEARCH

A number of scholars, such as Auger (1976) and Small (1980), use the Johnson model to describe and assess the activity within each subsystem.

Auger uses the case study method to examine and describe the systems of a hospitalized patient. First, she describes the activity in each of the subsystems; then, she discusses the impact of hospitalization upon each subsystem. Finally, she predicts what behavior patterns the patient must learn by the time of discharge.

Small (1980) first completes research on the perceived body image and spatial awareness of visually impaired children, then uses the Johnson model to identify problems in the behavioral subsystems of both the visually impaired and their parents. Small notes that the eye contact deemed to be important in maternal-infant bonding may be missing in cases of visual impairment. The task of the nurse is to encourage the mother to substitute other behaviors, such as touch and vocalization, for the impaired subsystem.

Criticizing Johnson's theory, Stevens (1979, p. 72) notes that attention is upon the subsystems, while the nursing processes to be applied are less well-formulated. Nor are the relationships among the subsystems of behavior fully explored and described. For example, the relationship between achievement behavior and affiliative behavior has yet to be adequately explained. In Stevens' view, Johnson's theory is one of equilibrium–disequilibrium. The equilibrium sought is that of behavior.

Neuman's Health-Care System

Neuman's health-care system draws on systems theory, Gestalt theory, and adaptation theory to present a *total-person approach* to the patient problem. The individual is seen as an open system in interaction with the total interface of the environment. The person adjusts to stress and defends against tension-producing stimuli that may cause disequilibrium,

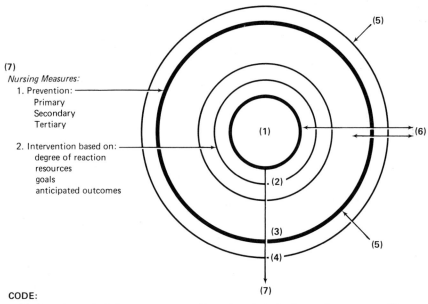

(7)
Nursing Measures:
  1. Prevention:
     Primary
     Secondary
     Tertiary

  2. Intervention based on:
     degree of reaction
     resources
     goals
     anticipated outcomes

CODE:
  (1) *Central core* — basic factors common to all organisms, including temperature range, genetic structures, response patterns, organ strength, weaknessess, ego structure, and knowns or commonalities.
  (2) *Lines of resistance* — interval factors that help defend against a stressor.
  (3) *Normal lines of defense* — variables such as coping patterns, life-style, stage of development.
  (4) *Flexible lines of defense* — a dynamic protective buffer against stressors.
  (5) *Stressors identified and classified* — includes loss, pain, change, sensory deprivation.
  (6) *Reaction* — individual intervening variables, such as time, resistance.
  (7) *Nursing prevention and intervention measures* — primary, secondary, tertiary prevention; intervention based on resources, goals, anticipated outcomes, and degree of reaction.

Figure 4–3. Neuman's health-care system.

crises, or stress. Variables that influence the adjustment process include basic physiological condition, sociocultural background, state of development, cognitive skills, age, and sex. The interacting variables determine the amount of resistance that an individual can demonstrate to any stressor. The stressors may be intrapersonal (conditioned responses), interpersonal (role expectations), or extrapersonal (financial circumstances).

The model is depicted as a series of concentric rings surrounding a central structure—the basic survival factors common to all human beings (Fig. 4–3). Surrounding the core structure, a series of rings depict the *flexible line of resistance*—internal factors that help defend against a stressor. The next ring, *lines of defense*, includes variables such as the individual's coping patterns, lifestyle, developmental stage, and other factors of resistance. *Flexible lines of defense*, surrounding the lines of defense, are dynamic factors that alter rapidly and act as protectors.

Multiple stressors, or negative factors (such as loss of sleep), can reduce defenses and can evoke a reaction to stress.

Nursing intervention includes primary prevention to strengthen flexible lines of defense; secondary prevention to treat symptoms, strengthen resistance, and rank need-priorities; and tertiary prevention to maintain adaptation.

EXAMPLES FROM NURSING RESEARCH

Craddock and Stanhope (1980) conducted a study to test the usefulness of the Neuman model in nursing practice. The study sample included registered nurses and clients in a private, nonprofit home-health-care agency. Each nurse chose clients from his (or her) caseloads, which one of the researchers assessed using the Neuman approach. The researcher then interviewed each of the nurses to compare perceptual differences between the nurse providing care and the client receiving care. The results of the study suggested that the Neuman model has the ability to categorize data for assessment and planning.

Dunbar (1982) utilized the Neuman model to study the stress that occurs when a patient is transferred from the critical-care environment. Patients/clients who were nearing transfer were interviewed to determine nursing diagnoses for those clients.

SUMMARY

The theoretical framework summarizes what is known from past work and predicts what will be found in the future.

A number of theories are used in nursing research, including learning, development, adaptation, systems, social, and cultural theories.

Learning theory includes theories of conditioning, behavior, and social learning. Conditioning, or stimulus–response theory, suggests that learning takes place when a stimulus known to produce a response is presented along with a new stimulus that the researcher wants the subject to learn to associate with the response. Operant conditioning, or behaviorism, proposes that learning occurs as an individual acts upon the environment to obtain a reward or reduce tension. Social learning theories are closely associated with the stimulus–response–reinforcement theory but place considerable emphasis on social elements, such as imitation, associated with learning.

The Gestalt, or cognitive, theories of learning propose that learning occurs in association with knowing and thinking on the part of the individual. In this view, the whole picture is more than the sum of its parts.

Developmental theory seeks to explain changes that take place through time, first on one level and then on another. Piaget's cognitive theory suggests that knowing proceeds through five phases of development, reaching from birth to the 15th year of life. Freud's theory is that personality development begins at birth and continues throughout life. Erikson's theory incorporates the entire span of human life, as does Havighurst's theory of the tasks of development. Peplau explains that the development of interpersonal relationships between patient and nurse occurs in four phases, during which the nurse assumes reciprocal roles in relation to the patient's roles.

Theories of adaptation, stress, and homeostasis explain the process by which persons adjust internally and externally in order to function and survive, often in the face of disease and stress. Selye defines *stress* as a state manifested by the General Adaptation Syndrome. The syndrome evolves in three stages: alarm, resistance, and exhaustion. The third stage must be reversed or the individual will die. Adaptation and homeostasis are related, in that the organism reacts to gains and to excesses or deficiencies by negative feedback that triggers the homeostatic process to correct the imbalance.

Systems theory explains the organization of parts and their interrelationships. A system differs from each of its parts and is greater than the sum of its parts, but a change in one part brings about a change in the whole system. Systems may consist of a simple level of organization, such as the equilibrium model, or it may be as complex as the general systems model. The general systems model is a complex adaptive system that changes organization in response to changes in the environment and in the subsequent cybernetic process in the system. Widely used in nursing, Johnson's behavioral system depicts the patient as a system of seven interacting behavioral subsystems. Each subsystem carries out a specialized task for the system as a whole. The nurse nurtures, protects, or stimulates needed systems. Neuman's health-care system also incorporates elements of Gestalt and adaptation theories.

TWO EXAMPLES FROM NURSING RESEARCH: EXAMPLES UTILIZING STRESS-COPING THEORY

Diane W. Scott, Marilyn Oberst, Marilyn Bookbinder (1984): Stress-coping response to genitourinary carcinoma in men. Nursing Research, 33, 325–329.

The authors present a descriptive study of 30 men with chronic genitourinary cancer. They utilize theory, former research reports, and a model invented by Scott, Oberst, and Dropkin (1980) to study stress-coping responses in men with cancer. The research is a partial replication of an earlier study of women by Scott (1983) that examined the anxiety, critical thinking, and information processing of women during and after breast biopsy.

The researchers designed the study to examine stress response in men to periodic monitoring of the genitourinary carcinoma. Specifically, the researchers sought to evaluate anxiety level and problem-solving ability of the men prior to cystoscopy and six to eight weeks following, and to determine the relations among these measures and concurrent stressors, coping methods, and degree of problem resolution following hospitalization.

The authors rely on the stress-coping model of Scott et al., based (in part) on the paradigm developed by Lazarus and others (1972), to examine the relationship among cognition, stress, coping, and anxiety. *Cognition* is viewed as the understanding of experience—the combining of external circumstances with the traits, beliefs, and styles characteristic of the individual. *Coping* is defined as a combination of intrapsychic processes and direct psychomotor behavior, the outward display of coping. Successful coping may include the capacity to deploy attention, appraise a situation, and control the autonomic outcomes of anxiety.

In addition to the theoretical framework, the authors include previous findings from studies of cancer patients by Weisman and Worden (1976) and by Mages and Mendelsohn (1979), who reported gender differences in coping behavior. Men tend to smoke and drink more, to use blame, to be neglectful of medical regimen, to be irritable and fearful, and to alienate or withdraw from social networks of support. These investigators concluded that personal assessment of cancer is partially a function of gender: men respond more intensely to threats to self-reliance and are less in touch with their bodies than are women.

The conclusions of Scott et al. included the following: men with higher education, higher problem-solving ability, lower anxiety, and less concurrent stress in their lives seemed to cope most effectively with in situ carcinoma of the urinary bladder. These men tended to describe their hospitalization as a respite from the "real" strains in their lives—they could be dependent in the hospital, since they trusted their physicians to keep the disease under control. Most of these men focused on current nonhealth-related problems as predominant concerns. However, the researchers raised questions about the extent to which these men may have minimized the cancer experience due to denial and stoic submission. Implications for nursing practice included helping patients to cope, patient education, family participation, and preparation for follow-up of each case.

Suzanne Caty, Mary Ellerton, Judith Ritchie (1984): Coping in hospitalized children: An analysis of published case studies. Nursing Research, 33, 277–282.

These authors used a different method (content analysis), a different sample (published articles), and a different objective (to develop a category system), but the same theoretical framework as Scott et al. They examined the range of coping behavior identified by authors of 39 case studies of hospitalized children, aged 20 months to 10 years, published in *Maternal–Child Nursing Journal* between 1972 and 1982. The explicit theoretical framework utilized to analyze the patterns of coping was that of Lazarus's (1980) stress-and-coping paradigm. *Coping*, as defined by Lazarus and Launier (1978, p. 311), is the effort, both action-oriented and intrapsychic, to manage environmental and internal demands (and conflicts among them) that tax or exceed a person's resources. This definition also includes all attempts to manage the problem, deal with emotions, and arrive at adaptations. Four modes of coping include information seeking, direct action, indirect action, and intrapsychic processes. The conclusion of the authors was that a category system based on Lazarus's stress and coping paradigm can provide a framework to allow logical analysis of a child's coping-behavior pattern. Recommendations for further research included answering the question "Coping with what?" In addition, the authors suggested that research include a search for a mechanism to determine whether the category system is sensitive to variations in coping behavior across various stressful situations.

STUDY QUESTIONS

1. Why is theory useful in nursing research?
2. Describe what nurse-researchers need to do in terms of theory in research.
3. Which category of theory would be useful to test the use of behavior modification?
4. Identify a nursing problem that you would like to study and the theory that would assist you.
5. Using either Johnson's or Neuman's systems theory, formulate a nursing problem that would use one or both of these theories.
6. Suggest a longitudinal research project based on developmental theory.
7. Select one of the studies above to analyze in terms of the use of theory and former research findings in nursing research.

REFERENCES AND SUGGESTED READINGS

Aamodt, A. (1972): The child's view of health and healing. In Batey, M. (ed.), Communicating Nursing Research. Boulder, Colo.: Western Interstate Commission for Higher Education. *The Papago child's view of health and healing.*

Abbey, J. (1980): FANCAP: What is it? In Riehl, J. and Roy, C. (eds.), Conceptual Models for Nursing Practice (2nd ed.). New York: Appleton-Century-Crofts. *A mnemonic device for teaching, using general system theory and Selye's general adaptation syndrome.*

Auger, J. (1976): Behavioral Systems and Nursing. Englewood Cliffs, N.J.: Prentice-Hall. *Chapters two and three include systems theory.*

Bell, J. (1977): Stressful life events and coping methods in mental-illness and -wellness behavior. Nursing Research, *26*, 136–141. *Selye's stress theory used.*

Bensberg, G. et al. (1965): Teaching the profoundly retarded self-help activities by behavior shaping techniques. American Journal of Mental Deficiency, *69*, 674–679. *Uses language theory to change behavior.*

Blake, M. (1980): The Peplau developmental model for nursing practice. In Riehl, J. and Roy, C. (eds.), Conceptual Models for Nursing Practice (2nd ed.). New York: Appleton-Century-Crofts. *Developmental theory.*

Brown, J. et al. (1984): Nursing's search for scientific knowledge. Nursing Research, *33*, 26–32.

Buckley, W. (1967): Sociology and Modern Systems Theory. Englewood Cliffs, N.J.: Prentice-Hall. *Modern systems theory explained.*

Cannon, W. (1939): Wisdom of the Body (rev. ed.). New York: Norton. *Cannon identifies and names the concept homeostasis.*

Caty, S., Ellerton, M. and Ritchie, J. (1984): Coping in hospitalized children: An analysis of published case studies. Nursing Research, *33*, 277–282.

Cowan, M. and Murphy, S. (1985): Identification of postdisaster bereavement risk predictors. Nursing Research, *34*, 71–75.

Cox, C. (1985): The health self-determinism index. Nursing Research, *34*, 177–183.

Craddock, R. and Stanhope, M. (1980): The Neuman health-care systems model: Recommended adaptation. In Riehl, J. and Roy, C. (eds.), Conceptual Models for Nursing Practice (2nd ed.). New York: Appleton-Century-Crofts. *Summarizes the theory behind the Neuman model.*

DeWalt, E. and Haines, A. (1977): The effects of specified stressors on healthy oral mucosa. In Downs, F. and Newman, M. (eds.), A Sourcebook of Nursing Research (2nd ed.). Philadelphia: F. A. Davis. *Stress theory used.*

Diers, D. (1979): Research in Nursing Practice. New York: J. B. Lippincott. *Chapters two and three include theory for nursing research.*

Downs, F. (1977): Maternal stress in primigravidas as a factor in the production of neonatal pathology. In Downs, F. and Newman, M. (eds.), A Sourcebook of Nursing Research (2nd ed.). Philadelphia: F.A. Davis, pp. 129–139. *Uses stress theory.*

Downs, F. and Newman, M. (eds.) (1977): A Sourcebook of Nursing Research (2nd ed.). Philadelphia: F. A. Davis. *Fifteen research reports, many of which state theoretical orientation.*

Dunbar, S. (1982): Critical care and the Neuman model. In Neuman, G. (ed.), The Neuman Systems Model. Norwalk, Conn.: Appleton-Century-Crofts, pp. 297–301.

Erikson, E. (1950): Childhood and Society. New York: Norton. *Neo-Freudian developmental theory.*

Farr, L., Keene, A., Samson, D., and Michel, A. (1984): Alterations in circadian excretion at urinary variables and physiological indicators of stress following surgery. Nursing Research, *33*, 140–146.

Festinger, L. (1957): A Theory of Cognitive Dissonance. Stanford, Calif.: Stanford University Press. *Presents Festinger's cognitive dissonance theory.*

Fielo, S. (1975): A Summary of Integrated Nursing Theory (2nd ed.). New York: McGraw-Hill. *Summarizes various theories.*

Freud, S. (1938): The Basic Writings of Sigmund Freud. New York: Random House. *Psychoanalytic theory.*

Glaser, B. and Strauss, A. (1967): The Discovery of Grounded Theory. Chicago: Aldine. *Used in nursing theory.*

Goslin, D. (1969): Handbook of Socialization Theory and Research. Chicago: Rand McNally. *Sources for developmental theory.*

Grosicki, J. (1968): Effects of operant conditioning on modification of incontinence in neuropsychiatric geriatric patients. Nursing Research, *17*, 304. *Operant conditioning theory in research and practice.*

Hardy, M. (ed.) (1973): Theoretical Foundations for Nursing. New York: MSS Information Corp. *Eight articles including general systems theory, stress, adaptation.*

Havighurst, R. (1952): Developmental Tasks and Education. New York: Longmans, Green. *Developmental theory.*

Holaday, B. (1974): Achievement behavior in chronically ill children. In Nursing Research, *23*, 25–30. (1980): Implementing the Johnson model for nursing practice. In Riehl, J. and Roy, C. (eds.). Conceptual Models for Nursing Practice (2nd ed.). New York: Appleton-Century-Crofts, pp. 255–263. *Uses Johnson's system model and Piaget's developmental model to assess a case study.*

Johnson, D. (1980): The behavioral system model for nursing. In Riehl, J. and Roy, C. (eds.), Conceptual Models for Nursing Practice. New York: Appleton-Century-Crofts, pp. 207–216. *Johnson presents the theory behind her systems model.*

King, I. M. (1981): A Theory for Nursing Systems, Concepts, Process. New York: Wiley.

Lamontagne, L. (1984): Children's locus of control beliefs as predictors of pre-operative coping behavior. Nursing Research, *33*, 76–79.

Levine, M. (1967): The four conservation principles of nursing. Nursing Forum, *47*, 45. *Principles of nursing proposed.*

Lowery, B. and DuCette, J. (1976): Disease-related learning and disease control in diabetes as a function of the locus-of-control. Nursing Research, *25*. *Locus-of-control theory.*

Neuman, G. (1980): The Betty Neuman health-care system model. In Riehl, J. and Roy, C. (eds.), Conceptual Models for Nursing Practice (2nd ed.) New York: Appleton-Century-Crofts, pp. 119–134. *Systems theory.*

Nolan, J. (1985): Work patterns of mid-life female nurses. Nursing Research, 150–154.

Nordal, D. and Sato, A. (1980): Peplau's model applied to primary nursing in clinical practice. In Riehl, J. and Roy, C. (eds.), Conceptual Models for Nursing Practice (2nd ed.). New York: Appleton-Century-Crofts.

O'Neil, S. (1972): The application and methodological implication of behavior modification in nursing research. In Batey, M. (ed.), Communicating Nursing Research. Boulder Colo.: WICHE. *Stimulus-response-reinforcement theory.*

Pavlov, I. (1928): Lectures on Conditioned Reflex (trans. W. H. Gantt). New York: International Publishers. *Classical conditioning theory.*

Peplau, H. (1952): Interpersonal Relations in Nursing. New York: G. P. Putnam's Sons. *Utilizes developmental theory.*

Piaget, J. (1926): The Language and Thought of the Child. New York: Harcourt, Brace, and World. *Theory of development and perception.*

Riehl, L. and Roy, C. (eds.)(1980): Conceptual Models for Nursing Practice. (2nd ed.). New York: Appleton-Century-Crofts. *Three theoretical models presented.*

Robischon, P. (1977): Pica practices and other hand-mouth behavior and children's development level. In Downs, F. and Newman, M. (eds.). A Sourcebook of Nursing Research. Philadelphia: F. A. Davis, pp. 152–170. *Developmental theory.*

Rottkamp, B. (1976): A behavior modification approach to nursing therapeutics in body positioning of spinal-cord-injured patients. Nursing Research, *25*, 181–185. *Behavior modification theory.*

Rotter, J. et al. (1962): Internal versus external control of reinforcement: A major variable in behavior theory. In Washburn, N. (ed.), Decisions, Values and Groups. New York: Pergamon Press, pp. 473–516. *Locus of control theory.*

Scott, D., Oberst, M. and Bookbinder, M. (1984): Stress-coping response to genitourinary carcinoma in men. Nursing Research, *33*, 325–329.

Selye, H. (1956): The Stress of Life. New York: McGraw-Hill. *Widely used stress syndrome and theory.*

Skinner, B. (1953): Science and Human Behavior. *Basis for behavior modification procedures, based on operant conditioning theory.*

Small, V. (1980): Nursing visually impaired children with Johnson's model as a conceptual framework. In Riehl, J. and Roy, C. (eds.), Conceptual Models for Nursing Practice (2nd ed.). New York: Appleton-Century-Crofts, pp. 264–275. *Use of system theory.*

Stevens, B. (1979): Nursing Theory. Boston: Little, Brown. *A critique of nursing theory.*

Stillman, M. (1977): Women's health beliefs about breast cancer and breast self-examination. Nursing Research, *26*, 121–127. *Cognitive dissonance theory.*

Wallace, W. (1971): The Logic of Science in Sociology. Chicago: Aldine. *Brief book includes examination of theory.*

Windwer, C. (1977): Relationship among prospective parents' locus of control, social desirability and choice of psychoprophylaxis. Nursing Research, *26*, 96–99. *Locus of control theory.*

5

Social and Cultural Theories Used and Developed by Nurse-Researchers

Social theories, such as theories of social stratification, demography or population, social networks, social support, and symbolic interaction, are frequently used in nursing research to explain the relationships between poverty and disease, morbidity rates in various social contexts, and social roles and social structures in modern Western society. Cultural theories, which overlap with social theories, differ in emphasizing traditional ways of life of both Western and non-Western societies. Theories include studies of cross-cultural institutions, transcultural nursing, cultural diversity and relativity, value orientations of Western and non-Western societies, and cultural ecology. Each of these will be examined briefly.

SOCIAL THEORIES UTILIZED IN NURSING RESEARCH

Social Stratification Theory

Theories of social stratification explain the ranking of individuals and groups in terms of property, power, and prestige. The rich have property, power, and access to the best systems of health care, while the poor have none of these. The best single indicator of social class is occupation. Occupational prestige suggests levels of social class (Table 5–1). Anthropologists (such as Warner) and sociologists (such as Myrdal) have developed a number of models that identify the basis of stratification in terms of occupation, education, property, lineage, affiliation, reputation, and race. Warner (1963) proposed a six-class system based on his study of Appalachia (Table 5–2).

TABLE 5-1. OCCUPATIONAL PRESTIGE RANKS

Occupation	Rank	Occupation	Rank
U.S. Supreme Court Justice	1.0	Undertaker	44.0
Physician	2.0	Welfare worker for city	44.0
Scientist	3.5	Policeman	47.0
State governor	5.5	Bookkeeper	49.5
College professor	8.0	Insurance agent	51.5
Chemist	11.0	Carpenter	53.0
Lawyer	11.0	Mail carrier	57.0
Dentist	14.0	Plumber	59.0
Architect	14.0	Automobile mechanic	60.0
County judge	14.0	Barber	62.5
Psychologist	17.5	Corporal in regular army	65.5
Minister	17.5	Truck driver	67.0
Mayor of large city	17.5	Clerk in store	70.0
Priest	21.5	Lumberjack	72.5
Banker	24.5	Filling station attendant	75.0
Biologist	24.5	Coal miner	77.5
Instructor in public schools	27.5	Night guard	77.5
Captain in regular army	27.5	Restaurant waiter	80.5
Accountant for a large business	29.5	Taxi driver	80.5
Building contractor	31.5	Janitor	83.0
Railroad engineer	39.0	Garbage collector	88.0
Electrician	39.0	Shoeshiner	90.0
Trained machinist	41.5		

Based on Hodge et al.: Occupational prestige in the United States 1925-1964. American Journal of Sociology, 70, 286-302, 1964.

TABLE 5-2. WARNER'S SIX-CLASS MODEL

	Social Class	Characteristics of People
I	Upper-upper class	Old families; old aristocracy; people with money
II	Lower-upper class	Aristocracy but not old families; people with money
III	Upper-middle class	Nice, respectable people with little money
IV	Lower-middle class	Good people but "nobody"; don't have money
V	Upper-lower class	Poor whites, poor but honest people
VI	Lower-lower class	Poor whites; no-account lot; shiftless people

Myrdal (1944) noted that, in comparison with white people, few black people ever make the money or have the property and prestige characteristic of the middle class. And the number of blacks in the upper class is so low as to be without consequence.

Whether blacks or whites, the poor of the United States tend to be migrant farm laborers, elderly living on a fixed and inadequate income, ghetto and slum dwellers, and skid-row people. Families occupying the bottom of the class system include those handicapped by unemployment, mental illness, alcoholism, illegitimacy, desertion, chronic illness, crime, and ignorance. Harrington (1962) estimated that such poor people comprised between 30 and 40 million during the 1960s.

EXAMPLES FROM NURSING RESEARCH

Kitagawa and Hauser (1973) reported a recent, massive, nationwide study of mortality, noting that persons in lower classes have higher morbidity and mortality rates for almost every disease or illness. And the gap between the social classes may be increasing. Persons from the lower class usually have a limited education, which interferes with their understanding of the health-care system. For example, the language of doctors and nurses may be difficult for them to interpret, and they may hesitate to ask for explanations.

Byrne and Edeani (1984), studying the knowledge of medical terminology among hospital patients, reviewed studies from 1961 to 1980. Earlier studies (from 1961) indicated that the level of comprehension of medical vocabulary among hospital patients was less than was expected by medical personnel. Poor understanding was increased if the patient was a member of an ethnic group, from a low-social-class environment, or poorly educated. Studies in 1980 indicated that race, education, and age predicated the level of understanding of hypertensive terminology. Byrne and Edeani found in their study that, while knowledge of most medical terms has increased since 1961, there were some terms for which no significant increase was noted, and that knowledge of some terms, such as abdomen, showed a significant decrease.

Examining the characteristics and perceptions of low-income women, Triplett (1970) noted that the poor not only have more health problems but also receive less care. She drew on theories of social class to design an exploratory study to determine whether or not lower-class women perceive health workers as threatening. Forty white women who lived in an urban area and who had at least one preschool child were interviewed. Among the findings, Triplett noted that poor users of preventive health services tended to be heads of their households, to receive welfare assistance, and to have more children than good users of such services. On the other hand, good users tended to have lower self-esteem, to be more socially isolated, and to admit feelings of loneliness.

Ailinger's study (1982) of hypertension knowledge in a Hispanic community in Virginia used the Hollingshead Index (1957) to compute the socioeconomic class of the sample. She found that 17 percent of the Hispanic respondents were in the upper class for this sample, 64 percent were in the middle, and 19 percent were in the lower class.

Demographic Theory

Demography is the study of population variables, such as age, sex, and race. Population changes, reflected in birth rates, death rates, and disease rates, are also of primary interest. Many research projects include demographic variables as part of their data collection; at times, the entire research focuses on demographic characteristics or epidemiological studies.

EXAMPLE FROM NURSING RESEARCH

Nakagawa (1972) conducted an epidemiological study of changes in psychiatric symptoms over a 26-year span. She examined trends in the complaints of patients in the context of changing sociocultural environment and psychiatric treatment. Findings indicate that recent complaints tended to center around drug overuse, somatic problems, and sociocultural problems. On the other hand, the number of persons exhibiting thought-process disorders declined over the years. Nakagawa suggests that such approaches may be useful in searching for ways to improve nursing.

Theories of Social Networks and Social Support

Social network refers to the web of social relations that each person builds, including family, friends, and others who share similar interests at work and in clubs or other voluntary associations. The social network forms the social environment of primary and secondary groups and, likewise, provides the means by which the individual or group is integrated into society as a whole. The network of an individual or family varies over time as children are born, grow up, and disperse to form their own family networks, as well as their own networks of friends and associates, which may not coincide with those of other family members. Social networks of an individual are minimum when the person is a very young child; networks expand as a working adult interacts with many friends, colleagues, and family members. The networks shrink again when the person becomes sick, aged, or isolated. According to Bott (1957), family and social networks may be loose-knit, in which few of a person's friends and colleagues know and interact with one another. Or, the networks may be close-knit, in which case, most of the persons with whom an individual interacts also know and interact with one another. Loose-knit networks are typical of the mobile middle class, while close-knit networks are more typical of the sedentary lower class, who are often born, reared, marry, work, and die within the same community or city.

Social support is the extent to which an individual or family can depend on primary and secondary groups, such as members of family, neighborhood, and church groups. In crises or disasters, persons usually turn first for help to those who have a legal relationship with them, such as parents or spouse. Next, the social network of the family or individual is called upon for aid. Finally, social agencies are the only resort. However, remote bureaucracies, such as those that administer Social Security and Medicare, are becoming more and more important in the lives of families with elderly members. The concepts of social network and social support assume significance in cases of dependent, isolated persons who are in need or disabled by sickness or handicap. The social support provided by primary groups is then in inverse proportion to that provided by social agencies, such as the hospital or other health associations charged with such functions.

EXAMPLES FROM NURSING RESEARCH

Nursing research that has utilized the theories of social network and social support include Cronenwett (1985) and Hubbard et al. (1984). Cronenwett reports a study of 50 primigravid fathers and mothers who were respondents to a questionnaire designed to measure social network characteristics and perceived social support during the third trimester of pregnancy and again at 6 weeks postpartum. Relationships among network factors, perceived support, and postpartum outcomes were documented. Findings included the fact that emotional and instrumental support were important variables in explaining six-week postpartum outcomes.

Hubbard et al. (1984) conducted two studies to investigate the relationship between individuals' perceived level of social support and their performance of specific and positive health practices. The findings indicated that a strong positive association was found between the social-support and health-practices variables. It was also found that married participants among senior-center participants scored significantly higher on both the social support and health practices instruments than did their nonmarried counterparts and that senior-center participants who had a confidant had higher scores on both the social support and health practices instruments than those without.

Symbolic Interaction: Role Theory

Symbolic interaction focuses on the meanings that roles, symbols, and interaction have for the actors. Symbolic interaction is a dynamic process in which roles change and adjust over time. The theory is often used to study childhood socialization and to examine roles learned in adult life.

The theoretical foundations of symbolic interaction appear in the work of Cooley (1902) and Mead (1934). Cooley formulated the concept of the *looking-glass self* to designate the process by which the child develops a self-image by imagining what other people are thinking of the child. Each to each, Cooley notes, is a looking-glass: we see ourselves reflected in the eyes of the others around us. The looking-glass self emerges in three steps: first, we imagine how we appear to the other person; then, we imagine the judgment that the person makes of our appearance; finally, we get a feeling, such as pride or mortification, as we imagine the person's judgment of us. Our self-image is a social image, created symbolically as each puts him- or herself in the place of others and views him- or herself objectively through their eyes. The nurse acts as a looking glass to the children, patients, and clients, who see themselves reflected in the nurse's role behavior. And the nurse sees her or his own image reflected in their eyes.

Mead views the "self" as a social phenomenon, but he stresses the process of communication in language, play, and games. In the use of language, the child comes to see her- or himself as an object: the *I* and the *me* and the *other*. To put him- or herself in the place of the other is to play that role and look back at oneself as the other must. Thus, the child or the adult sees her- or himself objectively.

The self emerges first in the child's egocentric play and then in games with others. In team games, the person must not only take the role of significant others but must have expectations of roles in general. The roles can be rehearsed in imagination before they are played in fact.

A number of nursing perspectives and studies are based on the role of the nurse and patient and on self-image. For example, Riehl's model (1980) uses the perspective of symbolic interaction to examine the role of the patient vis-a-vis the nurse: to understand the role assumed by the patient, the nurse attempts to put himself or herself in the patient's role; that is, role taking. Then the nurse attempts to understand how the patient acts in response to attitudes of others and the person's self-image.

Rose (reprinted in Riehl and Roy, 1980, pp. 38–50) views symbolic-interaction (role) theory as a supplement to the behaviorist and Gestalt theories. He discusses five assumptions of symbolic-interaction theory: (1) Humankind lives in a symbolic environment and can be stimulated to act by symbols as well as by physical stimuli; (2) through symbols, the individual has the capacity to stimulate others in ways other than those in which the individual is stimulated; (3) through communication of symbols, individuals can learn large numbers of meanings, values, and ways of acting from others; (4) symbols, and the meanings and values to which they refer, do not occur only in isolated bits, but in clusters, sometimes large and complex; and (5) thinking is the process by which possible symbolic solutions and other future courses of action are examined and assessed for advantages and disadvantages.

In terms of the socialization of the individual child, Rose proposes four assumptions:

- *Assumption 1.* Society (a network of interacting individuals), with its culture (the related meanings and values by means of which individuals interact), precedes any existing individual. All persons are born into an ongoing society and are socialized into behavior that meets the expectations of the culture.
- *Assumption 2.* The process by which socialization takes place can be thought of as occurring in three stages: In the infant, the first

stage includes learning roles through conditioning, trial and error, or habit. The second stage arises when a blockage occurs in the habit; for example, the infant is hungry but the mother does not appear, and the image of the incompleted act arises in the mind of the infant. The third stage appears when the infant integrates the image with a word or words.

- *Assumption 3.* One is socialized into both the general culture and into various subcultures; e.g., a person may be both American and Italian.
- *Assumption 4.* The cultural expectations, meanings, and values of "old" groups may be temporarily dropped but are not forgotten.

EXAMPLES FROM NURSING RESEARCH

Woods' study (1985) examined the relationship of socialization and stress to perimenstrual symptoms, disability, and menstrual attitudes. The sample included 179 women from five city neighborhoods with a variety of races and socioeconomic statuses. Participants were interviewed in their homes using several instruments, including the Index of Sex-Role Orientation. The researchers found that traditional socialization, intense negative affect symptoms, and related disability all influenced menstrual attitudes.

O'Shea (1982) explored the relationship between role orientation and role strain, and the relationship of both to selected professional and experiential characteristics. *Role strain* was defined, following Goode (1960), as "a felt difficulty in meeting role obligations." Since an individual engages in several role relationships with different individuals, role strain is considered normal. The problem is how to allocate personal resources to make the whole role system manageable. A survey of teachers collected the data, which were analyzed by computer, using the Statistical Package for the Social Sciences. Results indicated that role orientation is a steady state unrelated to the variables tested. However, role strain was influenced by age, amount of teaching experience, and formal preparation for teaching. The data suggest that younger, less-experienced faculty report greater role strain. Recommendations for further research included making studies of the clinical teaching faculty and a comparative study to investigate the relationships between teacher preparation and role orientation in several health-care professions.

Hayden et al. (1982) published a study of the factors that facilitate or inhibit implementation of the emergency-nurse-practitioner role without any reference to theory. However, a literature review gave the history of the emerging role; the intent of the role; and the structural controls that may affect the role, role development, and the function of the role.

THEORIES OF CULTURE UTILIZED IN NURSING RESEARCH

Broadly defined, *culture* is a traditional way of life that has been learned and passed on from one generation to another. Theories of culture used in nursing research include: (1) Leininger's theoretical perspectives of transcultural nursing; (2) theories utilizing cultural relativity; (3) Kluck-hohn's theory of value orientation; and (4) the theory of cultural ecology. Many studies that utilize theories of culture developed in anthropology are qualitative studies, although a number include quantitative aspects, such as the calculation of frequency and other techniques that allow a statistical analysis of data.

Leininger's Theory of Transcultural Nursing

Leininger (1978, p. 8) defines *transcultural nursing* as the subfield of nursing that focuses upon a comparative study and analysis of different cultures and subcultures in the world with respect to their caring behavior; nursing care; and health–illness values, beliefs, and patterns of behavior. The goal of transcultural nursing is to develop a scientific and humanistic body of knowledge in order to provide culture-specific and culture-universal nursing care practice. Transcultural nursing has as its major focus the humanistic and scientific study of all people from different cultures in the world, with thought to the ways in which the nurse can assist people with their daily health and living needs.

Transcultural nursing theory refers to a set of interrelated cross-cultural nursing concepts and hypotheses that take into account individual and group caring behaviors, values, and beliefs based upon their cultural needs (Fig. 5–1). Leininger defines the essence of nursing as caring and proposes a number of hypotheses useful to the nurse to collect and analyze data. These include the following (abridged):

1. Differences in caring values and behaviors lead to differences in the nursing-care expectations of care-seekers.
2. Differences in caring values and norms exist between societies of high and low technology.
3. Nurses with different values who work in other cultures can create conflict and problems.
4. Nurses' dependence on technology can increase interpersonal distance and client dissatisfaction.
5. Differences between folk values and Western nurses' values are reflected in conflict and stress.
6. Culture-specific nursing will elicit more satisfaction from clients than will nonculturally oriented services.

EXAMPLES FROM NURSING RESEARCH

Leininger (ed., 1978) includes a number of research studies that utilize theories of transcultural nursing. For example, Horn (1978, pp. 223–238) reports her studies of transcultural nursing and child-rearing patterns of the Muckleshoot people of the Muckleshoot Indian Reservation located at Auburn, Washington. Aamodt (1972, pp. 239–249) writes about her observations of the Papago children and adolescents living in Tohono in the center of the Papago

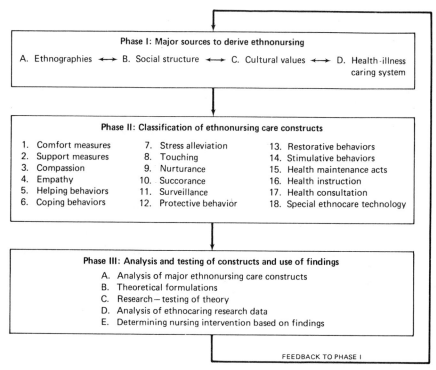

Phase I: Major sources to derive ethnonursing

A. Ethnographies ⟷ B. Social structure ⟷ C. Cultural values ⟷ D. Health-illness caring system

Phase II: Classification of ethnonursing care constructs

1. Comfort measures
2. Support measures
3. Compassion
4. Empathy
5. Helping behaviors
6. Coping behaviors
7. Stress alleviation
8. Touching
9. Nurturance
10. Succorance
11. Surveillance
12. Protective behavior
13. Restorative behaviors
14. Stimulative behaviors
15. Health maintenance acts
16. Health instruction
17. Health consultation
18. Special ethnocare technology

Phase III: Analysis and testing of constructs and use of findings
   A. Analysis of major ethnonursing care constructs
   B. Theoretical formulations
   C. Research—testing of theory
   D. Analysis of ethnocaring research data
   E. Determining nursing intervention based on findings

FEEDBACK TO PHASE I

Figure 5–1. Leininger's conceptual and theory-generating model (1978).

Indian reservation in southern Arizona, while Steffen and Francis (1978, pp. 283–297) report their efforts to apply transcultural principles to nursing practice with Chicano, Kickapoo, and Navajo migrant workers of Utah. Leininger (pp. 299–316) studied witchcraft practices in the course of providing psychocultural therapy to four Spanish-speaking families and two Anglo-American families. At the same time, she studied other families that were not receiving psychocultural therapy. She found that ingroup tensions, problems of acculturation, and other stresses were attributed to the witches in a known outgroup. These witches were believed to act upon the bewitched victim (the scapegoat) in the ingroup. Thus, witchcraft practices were considered important mechanisms for coping with ingroup problems.

EXAMPLES FROM NURSING RESEARCH

Research Utilizing the Theory of Cultural Diversity and Relativity

Cultural relativity is an approach to the understanding or explanation of a society by emphasizing its particular system of values as a part of its own internal cultural systems without making a judgment of the culture in terms of better or worse. For example, Olade (1984) evaluated the Denver Developmental Screening Test, one of the most widely used screening tools in "advanced" countries, to assess its usefulness as a tool to assess Nigerian children of various ethnic groups. She concluded that the test was culturally biased and was not sensitive in areas where sociocultural environments differed. Among specific items were those dealing with naming colors and playing games.

Johnston (1977, pp. 77–86) studied 200 mothers representing four ethnic groups: Anglo, English-speaking Mexican-Americans, Spanish-speaking Mexican-Americans, and black Americans. A questionnaire was designed to elicit their "folk beliefs" about the efficacy of taking vitamins, whether vitamins were viewed as "medicine or magic." It was found that expectations for supplemental vitamins were higher for Spanish-speaking and black mothers, while Anglos had less belief in vitamin efficacy. The author noted surprise upon finding that there were no ethnic group differences expressed by parents of male children, although differences were expressed by mothers of female children, who held magical expectations for vitamins (such as making the baby happier, prettier, and more graceful).

Chung (1977, pp. 67–75), who studied the cultural implications of being an Oriental maternity patient in an American cultural milieu, reported that it was a shocking experience for the Oriental patient to undergo the process of pregnancy and childbearing in this country. Cultural barriers included language problems, beliefs associated with various foods, and differing concepts of delivery and postpartum care.

Primeaux (1977, pp. 55–65) used a case study to illustrate the health care practices of Native American Indians from a cross-cultural perspective. The contrasts between the cultures of the Indian and the Anglo were brought into focus when an Indian child was admitted to the hospital. Hospital staff members were ignorant of cultural taboos, such as the cutting of an infant's hair, and denied all attempts by the Indians to use their traditions in coping with the child's illness.

EXAMPLES FROM NURSING RESEARCH

Research Utilizing Kluckhohn's Theory of Value Orientation

Value-orientation is a theoretical construct developed by anthropologist Florence Kluckhohn (1971) to identify the distinctive profile of a particular culture. It centers upon what Kluckhohn calls universal problems faced by human beings and the solutions to these problems by individual cultures, which (together) create the distinctive profile of a particular culture. Brink (1984) used this construct as an assessment tool in studying cultural diversity in Nigeria, finding that Nigerians stressed "being over doing," "group over individual," and "the present over the future" (see the research example at the end of the chapter).

In the United States, the Southern Appalachian subculture, with its accompanying values, beliefs, behavior, and health needs, was studied by Tripp-Reimer and Friedl (1977, pp. 41–54), who modified the value-orientation tools developed by Kluckhohn. The researchers found that the culture of middle-class America contrasted sharply with that of the Appalachians. For example, middle-class Americans thought that humankind had a variable human nature that was nonetheless perfectable, while Appalachians believed that human beings are inherently evil and that this fact was immutable. In addition, the Appalachians believed that humankind is subjugated to nature, while the middle class believed that humankind has, or should have, control over nature. The time orientation of Appalachians is the present, while the middle class values the future. The Appalachians value "being"; middle-class Americans value "doing." The relational aspect of life for the Appalachians is that of the group of kin and friends, while middle-class Americans stress the individual over the group.

The Theory of Cultural Ecology

Cultural ecology is a theoretical approach developed by anthropologists to study the relationship of a culture (simply defined as the traditional way of life of a people) to the environment. It includes the features of the environment itself and the cultural arrangements by which human beings exploit the environment. Cultural arrangements include: (1) technology (the tools and the know-how to use the tools) and economic organization (the way goods and services are produced, distributed, and consumed); (2) social structures (the ways in which parts of a society are put together, such as the family, the class structure, and the political and economic systems); and (3) belief system or ideology.

Jerome, Pelto, and Kandel (1980, p. 14), interested in the relationships among nutrition, culture, and the environment, developed a model based upon an ecological approach that integrates biological, psychological, social, cultural, and economic factors (Fig. 5–2).

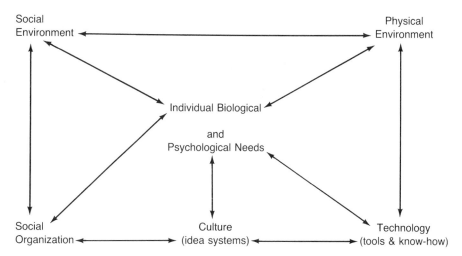

Figure 5–2. An ecological model. *(Modified from Jerome, Kandel, Pelto, 1980, p. 14.)*

EXAMPLES FROM NURSING RESEARCH

Flaskerud (1984, p. 190) used the theory of cultural ecology in a study that compared the perceptions of problematic behavior by six minority groups and by mental-health professionals. She was interested in the belief systems that arose in response to the social environment; in particular, the social structures of a culture. It was her view that an *emic* view of behavior (i.e., from the native's point of view) provides mental-health nurses with explanations of behavior that are culture-compatible, thereby enabling the nurse to intervene and manage the behavior in a culture-compatible way. Her research questions included the following: (1) Is there a difference between groups in the application of the label "mental illness" to the same sets of behaviors? (2) Is there a difference between groups in suggested management of such behaviors? Her hypotheses stated the following: (1) There will be a significant difference between groups in the application of the label "mental illness" to the behaviors described in ten vignettes; and (2) there will be a significant difference between groups in suggested management of the behaviors described in the ten vignettes.

The research design was a comparative survey. Working with Flaskerud were 12 nurse-investigators in different parts of the country who sampled and interviewed each of the minority groups and professional groups. The sample of 227 persons was selected by convenience sampling (use of readily available persons as subjects) and consisted of two parts. The first part included 68 mental-health professionals—psychiatrists, psychologists, psychiatric social workers, and psychiatric nurses. The second part included 159 minority-group members from six minority groups—persons from Appalachia, blacks, fundamentalists, Native Americans (Indians), Chinese-Americans, Filipinos, and Mexican-Americans.

Each researcher interviewed the subjects in English or, if English was not the native language, the interviewers used a questionnaire that had been translated into the subject's native language. The instrument used was a structured interview schedule consisting of two parts: the first part asked for biographic and demographic data, while the second part consisted of ten vignettes, each a short story that told of a person who experienced problems. The respondents were read the stories or read the stories themselves from the questionnaire. The interviewers or the questionnaire asked three questions: (1) What do you think of this person's behavior? (2) Do you think anything should be done about it? (3) If so, what?

The data were analyzed by putting responses into the following categories: (1) mental illness/no mental illness and (2) psychiatric treatment/no psychiatric treatment. Findings were not reported, as the research is still in progress.

SUMMARY

Social theories, such as theories of social stratification (class, caste, and power), explain the observations of the researcher on the basis of social forces that are external to, and that coerce, the individual. The forces of stratification place the individual and his or her family in a social class or caste, which determines the individual's chances of becoming sick, dying, or getting well. Stratification also influences the individual's style of living, including the ability to obtain health care, information, and nutrition.

Demographic theories examine human populations and the rates at which their members are born, get sick, die, and migrate.

Social-network and social-support theories examine the relationships between an individual (or family) and all of those persons with whom the individual or family have interacted over the years. The emphasis is on those upon whom persons/families can depend in times of sickness or other need.

Symbolic interaction theories focus on the meanings that roles, symbols, and interactions have for the actors. Taking the roles of the other and looking back upon oneself as an object is a central focus of symbolic interaction.

Culture is the traditional way of life that has been learned and shared by groups of people. Theories of culture utilized in nursing research include Leininger's theoretical perspectives of transcultural nursing, theories of cultural relativity, theories of value orientations and, more recently, the theory of cultural ecology. *Transcultural nursing theory* refers to a set of interrelated cross-cultural nursing concepts and hypotheses that take into account the behaviors, values, and beliefs of selected groups. *Cultural relativity* is an approach that emphasizes the particular system of values that makes up the internal cultural system of a people, without judging the people or their institutions as better or worse than that of the observer's. The theory of *value orientation* identifies the distinctive profile of a particular culture in terms of human nature, the relation of humankind with nature, the time orientation of a culture, and its values of being or doing. *Cultural ecology* is a theoretical approach developed by anthropologists to study the relationship between a people/culture and the environment. It involves a complex of environmental factors, including the physical and social environments, social organization, technology, culture, and the individual needs of the persons studied.

EXAMPLE FROM NURSING RESEARCH

Evelyn Shaw (1985): Female circumcision. American Journal of Nursing, 85, 685–687.

Female circumcision is defined as an operation on the female genitalia, classified according to degree of severity. *Sunna circumcision* is the removal of the prepuce and/or excision of the tip of the clitoris. *Excision* or *clitoridectomy* may include excision of the clitoris, the labia minora, and the labia majora. *Infibulation* includes removal of part or all of the clitoris, labia minora, and medial aspect of the labia majora. The raw areas on both sides are pulled together over the vagina and held with suture, thorns, or paste. A small opening is left for urinary and menstrual flow. The operation is performed at a young age, usually when the child is seven, but may be performed earlier or later. After the operation, the child's legs are tied together to immobilize the wound, usually for three weeks. Upon marriage, women who have been infibulated must be forcibly penetrated with the penis of the husband, his knife, or some other sharp instrument. During childbirth, the scar tissue must be cut and the opening enlarged, or the mother and infant may die. Many other serious physical complications have been reported, and prolonged pain and coital problems are not uncommon. Emotional symptoms include severe anxiety and frigidity.

Female circumcision is still a widespread practice in some parts of the world, such as the Sudan, Somalia, and Egypt. Women from these areas who visit the United States with their husbands for months or years often need health care from local practitioners who are neither familiar with such practices nor skilled in the care of circumcised women.

To collect data on female circumcision, Shaw used a variety of research methods. She used unstructured interviews to collect data from 11 circumcised women who lived in Shaw's college community; she communicated with health professionals in Africa, and reviewed the literature.

According to reports, about 74 million girls and women in Africa have been circumcised to date. Belief in female circumcision is held by several religions, including Christians, Muslims, and Jews. The rationale for female circumcision includes economic factors, sexual control, cultural beliefs concerning childbirth and infant care, religious beliefs and traditions, and cosmetic or curative beliefs.

Of the 11 women interviewed, all were from the upper or upper-middle socioeconomic classes and ranged in age from 18 to 34. One woman had had a clitoridectomy, and 10 had been infibulated. Four of the women had had urinary-tract infections during pregnancy, and four had had the scars torn during childbirth. Several themes emerged during the interviews, including the need for health-care providers to be familiar with the practice of female circumcision and the need for women to provide the health care. Many of the women were Muslims and were forbidden by their religion to have any bodily contact with a man other than their husband, except in a dire emergency. Concerns expressed by the women included: (1) a fear that health-care providers would not have knowledge about either the cultural beliefs or results associated with female circumcision; (2) whether women would be available as health providers; (3) whether their physician would know how to open the scar for birth and how to avoid postpartum complications; (4) fear of painful pelvic examinations; (5) fears that modesty would not be protected; and (6) concerns over the high cost of health care in the United States.

Recommendations included that the health-care practitioner establish trust and a positive working relationship with the husband, since the male family member makes the ultimate decisions, and that the nurse be sensitive to the woman's preferences—a woman who has been circumcised may not share all of her culture's customs and values; many espouse the latest Western birthing customs.

STUDY QUESTIONS

1. What is the difference in the ways that a social class (such as middle-class Americans) and a subculture within America view time, nature, and social relationships? What implications for nursing does this theory have?
2. You have been asked to help with a new research project to study the health care problems of Cubans and Vietnamese who have just arrived in the United States. What theories would be useful?
3. You have obtained a job in the inner city working at a prenatal clinic. What theory would be helpful to understand the relationships between the poor and their way of life?
4. The post-World War II baby boom that began in the late 1940s brought about a change in the population structure of the United States. What implications does this have for nursing in the decade of the 1990s? The next century?
5. Discuss the various ethnic groups in the United States. What does the theory of cultural relativism explain in terms of health beliefs?
6. What theory is most appealing to you for use in research? Why?

REFERENCES AND SUGGESTED READINGS

Aamodt, A. (1972): The child's view of health and healing. In Baley, M. (ed.), Communicating Nursing Research. Boulder Colo.: Western Interstate Commission for Higher Education pp. 239–249. *The Papago child's cognitive view of health and healing.*

Ailinger, R. (1982): Hypertension knowledge in a Hispanic community. Nursing Research, *31*, 207–213. *Research using social class index.*

Bott, E. (1957): Family and Social Network. London: Tavistock Publications.

Brink, P. (1984): Value orientation as an assessment tool in cultural diversity. Nursing Research, *33*, 198–203.

Brown et al. (1984): Nursing's search for scientific knowledge. Nursing Research, *33*, 26–32.

Byrne, T. and Edeani, D. (1984): Knowledge of medical terminology among hospital patients. Nursing Research, *33*, 180–181.

Chung, H. (1977): Understanding the Oriental maternity patient. Nursing Clinics of North America, *12* (1), 67–75. *Oriental culture.*

Cooley, C. (1902): Human Nature and the Social Order (rev. ed., 1922). New York: Scribner's. *Describes the looking-glass self, a concept of symbolic interaction theory.*

Cox, C. (1985): The health self-determinism index. Nursing Research, *34*, 177–183. *Index to measure self-determinism and health.*

Cronenwett, L. (1985): Network structure, social support, and psychological outcomes of pregnancy. Nursing Research, *34*, 93–99.

Downs, F. and Newman, M. (eds.) (1977): A Sourcebook of Nursing Research

(2nd ed.). Philadelphia: F. A. Davis. *Fifteen research reports, many of which state theoretical orientations.*

Field, S. (1975): A Summary of Integrated Nursing Theory (2nd ed.). New York: McGraw-Hill. *Summarizes various theories.*

Flaskerud, J. (1984): A comparison of perceptions of problematic behavior by six minority groups and mental health professionals. Nursing Research, *33*, 190–194. *Use of theory of cultural ecology.*

Glaser, B. and Strauss, A. (1966): Awareness of Dying. Chicago: Aldine.

Glaser, B. and Strauss, A. (1967): The Discovery of Grounded Theory. Chicago: Aldine. *Used in nursing theory.*

Goode, W. (1960): A theory of role strain. American Sociological Review, *25*, 483–493. *Stress in roles explained.*

Goslin, D. (1969): Handbook of Socialization Theory and Research. Chicago: Rand McNally. *Sources for socialization and developmental theory.*

Hardy, M. and Conway, M. (eds.) (1978): Role Theory: Perspectives for the Health Professions. New York: Appleton-Century-Crofts. *Role theory used as a unifying theoretical approach in nursing.*

Harrington, M. (1962): The Other America. New York: Macmillan. *Poverty in the United States.*

Hayden, M., Davies, L. and Clore, E. (1982): Facilitators and inhibitors of the emergency nurse practitioner role. Nursing Research, *31*, 294–299.

Hodge et al. (1964): Occupational prestige in the United States. American Journal of Sociology, *70*, 286–302. *Ranking of occupations by prestige.*

Horn, B. (1978): Transcultural nursing and child-rearing of the Muckleshoot people. In Leininger, M. (ed.), Transcultural Nursing. New York: Wiley, pp. 223–238. *Uses transcultural theory.*

Hubbard, P., Muhlenkamp, A. and Brown, N. (1984): The relationship between social support and self-care practice. Nursing Research, *33*, 266–270.

Jacox, A. (1974): Theory construction in nursing: An overview. Nursing Research, *23*, 4–13.

Jerome, N., Pelto, G. and Kandel, R. (1980): An ecological approach to nutritional anthropology. In Jerome, N., Dandel, R. and Pelto, G. (eds.), Nutritional Anthropology. Pleasantville, N.Y.: Redgrave, pp. 13–45.

Johnston, M. (1977): Folk beliefs and ethnocultural behavior in pediatrics, medicine or magic. Nursing Clinics of North America, *12* (1), 77–84.

Kim, H. (1983): The Nature of Theoretical Thinking in Nursing. Norwalk, Conn.: Appleton-Century-Crofts. *Develops a typology of three domains: client, environment, and nursing action.*

King, I. M. (1981): A Theory for Nursing: Systems, Concepts, Process. New York: Wiley. *King's theory updated.*

Kluckhohn, F. (1971): Dominant and variant value orientations. In Kluckhohn, C. and Murray, H. (eds.), Personality in Nature, Society, and Culture (2nd ed. revised). New York: Knopf, 342–357.

Lamontagne, L. (1984): Children's locus of control beliefs as predictors of preoperative coping behavior. Nursing Research, *33*, 76–79.

Leininger, M. (ed.) (1978): Transcultural Nursing. New York: Wiley. *A series of articles using transcultural theory.*

Levine, M. (1967): The four conservation principles of nursing. Nursing Forum, *47*, 45. *Principles of nursing proposed.*

Mead, G. (1934): Mind, Self and Society. Chicago: University of Chicago Press. *The classic dynamic approach to role theory.*

Merton, R. (1957): The role-set. British Journal of Sociology, *8*, 106–120.

Myrdal, Gunnar et al. (1944): An American Dilemma. New York: Harper & Row. *Social stratification theory with reference to race.*

Nakagawa, H. et al. (1972): An epidemiological study of psychiatric symptom pattern change: Pilot study findings. In Batey, M. (ed.), Communicating Nursing Research. Boulder, Colo.: WICHE. *An epidemiological approach to nursing research.*

Newman, M. (1979): Theory Development in Nursing. Philadelphia: F. A. Davis.

Nolan, J. (1985): Work patterns of midlife female nurses. Nursing Research, *34*, 150–154.

Nursing Theories Conference Group. Nursing Theories: The Base for Professional Nursing Practice. Englewood Cliffs, N.J.: Prentice-Hall.

Olade, R. (1984): Evaluation of the Denver development screening test as applied to African children. Nursing Research, *33*, 204–207.

O'Shea, H. (1982): Role orientation and role strain of clinical nurse faculty in baccalaureate programs. Nursing Research, *31*, 306–310.

Peplau, H. (1952): Interpersonal Relations in Nursing. New York: G. P. Putnam's Sons.

Primeaux, M. (1977): American Indian health care practices. Nursing Clinics of North America, *12* (1), 55–65.

Quint, J. (1967): The Nurse and the Dying Patient. New York: Macmillan.

Riehl, J. and Roy, C. (1980): Conceptual Models for Nursing Practice (2nd ed.). New York: Appleton-Century-Crofts.

Rogers, M. (1970): An Introduction to the Theoretical Basis of Nursing. Philadelphia: F. A. Davis.

Rose, A. (1980, orig. 1962): A Systematic Summary of Symbolic Interaction Theory. In Riehl, J. and Roy, C. (eds.), Conceptual Models for Nursing Practice. New York: Appleton-Century-Crofts, pp. 38–50. *Assumptions underlying symbolic interaction theory.*

Roy, C. (1980): A case study viewed according to different models. In Riehl, J. and Roy, C., Conceptual Models for Nursing Practice (2nd ed.). New York: Appleton-Century-Crofts, pp. 381–392.

Roy, S. and Roberts, S. (1981): Theory Construction in Nursing: An Adaptation Model. Englewood Cliffs, N.J.: Prentice-Hall.

Shaw, E. (1958): Female circumcision. American Journal of Nursing, *85*, 685–687. *Describes female circumcision, and problems associated with circumcised females.*

Steffen, M. and Francis, J. (1978): Transcultural nursing experience and care with migrating children. In Leininger, M. (ed.), 1978 Transcultural Nursing. New York: Wiley, pp. 283–297.

Stevens, B. (1979): Nursing Theory. Boston: Little, Brown. *Includes a critique of nursing theory.*

Triplett, J. (1977): Characteristics and perception of low-income women and use of preventive health services: An exploratory study. In Downs, F. and Newman, M., A Sourcebook of Nursing Research. New York: Appleton-Century-Crofts, 94–106. *Uses social class theory.*

Tripp-Reimer, T. (1982): Barriers to health care: Variation in interpretation of

Appalachia client behavior by Appalachian and non-Appalachian health professionals. Western Journal of Nursing Research, *4*, 179–191. *Subculture of Appalachia.*

Tripp-Reimer, T. and Friedl, M. (1977): Appalachians: A neglected minority. Nursing Clinics of North America, *12* (1), 41–54.

Van Gennep, A. (1909; trans. 1960): The Rites of Passage. London: Routledge and Kegan Paul Ltd. *Rituals associated with changes in status, including death, on cross-cultural perspective.*

Warner, W. (ed.) (1963): Yankee City. New Haven, Conn.: Yale University Press. *Subculture of Appalachia. Social class.*

Woods, N. (1985): Relationship of socialization and stress to perimenstrual symptoms, disability and menstrual attitudes. Nursing Research, *34*, 145–149. *Urban women of various classes and races studied.*

PART III

The Research Proposal and Report

6

Phases and Steps in the Research Process

The student who seeks to initiate a research project for the first time often wonders where to begin. This chapter provides a simple model to help answer that question (Fig. 6–1). The model is a calendar wheel, a diagram of the phases and steps of research placed in a temporal framework. However, the particular time framework of each project must be individually determined. The circular design of the model suggests the unending process of research: the communication of research findings that concludes one project provides the springboard for further research.

Upon completion of this chapter, the student should be able to: (1) depict and explain a model of the phases and steps of the research process; (2) state briefly what occurs in each phase and step; (3) identify chapters in this book that deal with each step; and (4) construct a model that includes the time framework of his or her own research.

THE MODEL

The model provides at a glance the phases of the research project. The student should understand the model for several reasons: (1) to gain an overview of the project from beginning to end; (2) to learn to prepare a timetable that allocates the time reasonably spent at each phase; (3) to anticipate what must be done in early steps in order to be prepared for later ones; (4) to examine the research literature more effectively by comparing the research reports of others; and (5) to write a rough draft of the research paper step-by-step by documenting the work in each phase of the model. In addition, the model provides a guide to the organization of this book—reference to pertinent chapters is made at each step.

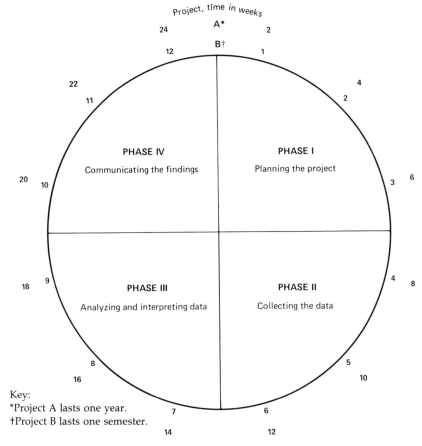

Figure 6–1. Calendar wheel: four phases of the research process in a temporal framework.

ꞏ As each phase is discussed, the steps within individual phases of the model are added. However, every research project is unique. The sequence and number of steps within each phase, and the time spent at each step, may vary according to the individual research project. But the four phases of research remain stable. The student always begins with Phase I, planning. Then, in Phase II, the student collects the data and, in Phase III, describes, analyzes, and interprets them. Finally, in Phase IV, the student presents findings in written or oral form, communicating the results of the research.

The student must carefully calculate the time to be spent in each of the phases. A project to be completed in one year or semester requires a rigorous division of the time available. Phases of approximately six weeks each (three weeks for semester projects) may be realistic, but this depends upon whether the study is descriptive or explanatory. Descriptive studies may require more time for collecting data, while explanatory projects may require more time for planning. However, both of these phases must come to an end in time to analyze and interpret the data and to write (and rewrite) the research report. Projects that take place in the summer or that allow longer periods for the research require their own timetable. Using the model as a guide, each researcher should construct a calendar wheel and should check off each step as it is completed and documented. Each of the four phases, and the steps that usually occur in each phase, will now be examined briefly. (Later chapters will explore each of the steps in greater detail.)

PHASE I: PLANNING THE RESEARCH PROJECT

During Phase I, the student completes most, if not all, of the following steps: (1) identify a researchable problem; (2) formulate the research proposal; (3) define concepts and variables; (4) state objectives or hypotheses; (5) examine possible ethical implications of the research proposal; (6) review pertinent literature; (7) identify the theory, assumptions, and limitations of the proposal; (8) describe the research design; (9) describe the methods of research, including sampling, data collection, instruments to be used, and method of data analysis; (10) obtain informed consent from subjects to be studied in the pilot study; (11) conduct the pilot study and revise the proposal in light of the findings; and (12) plan how to communicate the findings (Fig. 6–2). Each of these steps will now be examined.

Step 1. Identify a Researchable Problem in Nursing

The first step is to select an area that is of interest to the student and of importance to nursing, and then to delimit this to a specific, circumscribed problem that is researchable and that identifies exactly what the student plans to study (see Chap. 7). The student who is uncertain about what to do or who would like to replicate a good study (if possible) may begin immediately with an initial review of the literature. Good research reports state the general importance of the study early in the report and follow this immediately with a statement of the specific problem that was studied. For example, in her report of maternal stress and neonatal pathology, Downs (1977) states in the opening paragraph why the study is important for nursing: the former steep decline in perinatal mortality has decreased, and nursing needs to study factors (such as stress) that may contribute to this undesirable state. Johnson (1975) identifies a potential nursing problem: pulmonary complications following general anesthesia. She then specifies what she plans to study: the outcome criteria that evaluate respiratory function during the postoperative period. Such studies for-

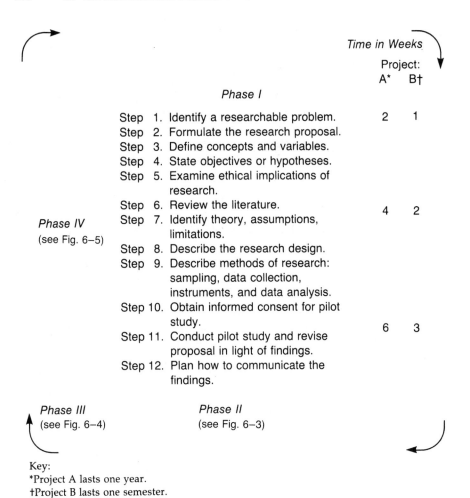

Key:
*Project A lasts one year.
†Project B lasts one semester.

Figure 6–2. Phase I: Steps in planning the research project.

mulate and delimit a significant research problem, narrowing the general question down to a manageable form.

Step 2. Formulate the Research Proposal

Proposition.

The research proposal is a written summary of steps one through nine, stating what the student intends to do, how he or she plans to do it, who or what comprises the study sample, when and where the study is to be done, and the timetable for the study. The proposal is often written for the approval of a professor or committee, but it assists the student as well. The proposal begins with the identification of the problem and moves step-by-step through all elements of the planning stage, which are pre-tested in the pilot project. As the student moves through the steps, the research proposal is often written and rewritten many times in order to refine the proposal (see Chap. 7). The final writing is usually done after the pilot study is completed, when changes may be incorporated in light of any weaknesses and strengths identified at that time.

Step 3. Define the Concepts and Variables

The student must define each concept or variable early in the study, not only to understand what is to be examined, but to be able to communicate this information to others. This is not always an easy task. Bloch (1974) expresses her frustration in the search for definitions, coming face-to-face with a "semantic jungle." Where definitions are confused, the student must spend time defining and communicating, with clarity, the meaning of each concept. In particular, operational definitions require careful work, as these describe how the variable under study is to be observed and measured. Definitions found in the literature that have already been developed and tested in research should be used whenever possible.

Step 4. State Objectives or Hypotheses

Objectives are what the student proposes to accomplish in the research —the specific, short-term, measurable goals to be met. For example, a specific objective may be to describe a phenomenon such as child abuse. The student may plan to develop (or may find in the literature) an operational definition that defines how to observe and measure child abuse. At the conclusion of the study, both the reader and the researcher can determine whether the objectives of the study were met.

Hypotheses are statements formulated to predict a relationship between two or more variables. The student who has defined a researchable problem and formulated the research proposal has identified a relationship between nursing concepts or variables to be tested in research. For example, Schmitt and Wooldridge (1981) tested the hypothesis that extra preparation for surgery would decrease the stress and anxiety experienced by patients and would lead to a more rapid postoperative recovery. McCorkle (1981) predicted that "touching and verbally stimulating a seriously ill patient [would] produce an increase in the number of positive acceptance responses." The student who wishes to use an hypothesis may examine the literature to find a similar study whose hypothesis is stated and whose variables are defined.

Step 5. Examine the Ethical Implications of the Research

At this point, the student is wise to examine the ethical implications of the study. Should the research proposal deal with problems too complex to solve in the time available, it is possible to modify it without losing too much time and effort. An ethical study is one that does not harm the study subjects. All subjects are carefully informed concerning the following: the purpose of the study; their part in it; any possible discomfort; how privacy will be guarded; their right to refuse to participate or to stop participating without penalty; and the manner in which data will be used. The student must also gain the approval of committees that investigate studies using human subjects and must receive the written, informed consent of each study subject (see Chap. 2).

Step 6. Review the Literature

An initial review of research publications often takes place early in the project, as soon as the general area of interest is defined. Such an early review helps to identify a researchable problem and to formulate the research proposal. However, the initial review must be followed by a more critical review that concentrates on the strengths and weaknesses of each study (see Chaps. 8 and 9). The review should be as complete as time allows. The student should examine definitions of concepts, objectives, and hypotheses; identify competing theoretical frameworks and research studies that support or refute these; and compare research designs. The student should also examine how the study sample was selected, how the data were collected, and what instruments and methods of data analysis were used. The student may find a study to replicate or a well-written study to use as a guide.

Step 7. Identify Theory, Assumptions, and Limitations

All research benefits from a clear statement of the theory or assumptions to which the research proposal is related. The goal of all research is to provide scientific explanations for what is observed and to predict what will be observed under given circumstances. Nursing has drawn on a broad range of theories from the natural, behavioral, and social sciences. Currently, nurses are seeking to produce theory peculiar to nursing practice (see Chaps. 4 and 5). Theories of stress, behavior, transcultural nursing, learning, development, and systems are often found in basic nursing textbooks. Research articles usually specify the theory or assumptions upon which the study is based. *Limitations* are aspects of the research that were not studied. For example, a study of the behavior of hospitalized children may be limited to a particular age group or to those children having a common diagnosis. The student may summarize the use of theory, assumptions, and limitations as he or she examines the research literature.

Step 8. Describe the Selected Research Design

Research designs include the qualitative and quantitative; descriptive and historical; the experiment; the survey; and the ex post facto and correlational (see Chaps. 10–13). An experiment often examines how a treatment or stimulus (the independent variable) affects subjects exposed to the treatment (the dependent variable). The experimental design describes, step-by-step, how the research will be conducted. Crucial elements of the experiment include how the research subjects are selected and how controls are used (see Chap. 12). A survey is a research design that uses questionnaires and interviews. Important elements of the survey include, not only how the subjects are selected, but also their willingness to answer the questionnaire or interview. The number of returns from a questionnaire, and the ability of the respondent to answer the questions, determine the extent to which the design is successful. The proper development of the questionnaire form and interview schedule are also crucial.

The historical and documentary designs use material already in existence, such as public and private records. Gaining access to the material, finding records that are complete and legible, and discovering whether or not the writer recorded material accurately are important.

Other research designs include *field studies*, in which the researcher investigates the phenomenon in its natural setting. The researcher may live and work on the site, collecting data in a community, mental hospital, or health clinic. The descriptive case-study design centers upon an in-depth investigation of one unit—a patient, a disease, a group, or an institution.

The student selects the research design that is ethically appropriate and describes the design carefully, using a step-by-step plan as a guide.

Step 9. Describe the Research Methods

The methods of sampling, data collection, and analysis and interpretation are the heart of every research project. *Sampling* is the selection of study subjects from the target population under study (see Chap. 14). Precise methods must be used so as to be able to apply research findings from a small sample to the population from which it was drawn.

Methods of data collection include observing, questioning, and measuring, or a combination of these (see Chaps. 15–17). Observation is a basic method of collecting data. When the phenomenon under study cannot be observed, the researcher asks questions, either face-to-face (in an interview) or by using questionnaires. *Measuring* is the set of rules that assigns numbers or values to objects to represent the variation of some attribute. For example, to measure weight, the rules designate that the object be placed on a scale that records pounds, ounces, or grams. To measure height, other rules are used. To measure attitudes, quality of patient care, degree of pain, or condition of a patient is more difficult. Qualitative scales have been developed to approximate quantitative measures.

To collect data using a specific method requires careful description of the instrument being used. At times, several methods may be used simultaneously. For example, to measure the effect of touch on seriously ill patients, McCorkle (1975) used observation, questioning, tape recorders, and electrocardiographs. In addition, she developed a special work sheet to record nonverbal responses.

To analyze data, frequencies are counted and descriptive statistics are used to summarize findings (see Chap. 19). If specific sampling techniques are used, inferential statistics are used to infer from the sample to the population from which the sample was drawn (see Chap. 20). To test data, computers are the fastest and most accurate means. The microcomputer is the newest tool for researchers (see Chap. 21).

Step 10. Obtain Informed Consent from Study Subjects to Be Used in the Pilot Study

As we saw in Step 5, *informed consent* is the voluntary consent given by the study subjects after they are fully informed of every detail of the proposed research, including the rights to participate or not and to withdraw from the study at any time without penalty. Thorough comprehension of the proposed participation is a crucial factor of informed consent (see Chap. 2). Informed consent must be obtained from subjects in both the pilot study and the actual research study. Permission for both may be sought at the same time by using identical forms.

Step 11. Conduct the Pilot Study

The pilot study is a small-scale dress rehearsal that proceeds as if it were the actual study, except for the fact that subjects who will participate in the actual study are not used. However, they may be selected at this point. The primary objective of the pilot study is to test as many elements of the research proposal as possible, in order to correct any part that does not work well. For example, the pilot study tests whether the variables defined by operational definition are actually observable and measurable. Instruments and scales are likewise tested to determine if each actually measures what the researcher intends it to measure. If a questionnaire is used, the pilot study reveals any problems that the respondents have with either the instructions or the wording. If an interview schedule is used, the pilot study answers many questions, including the following: Is a proper place available for the interview? How much time is needed to ask all of the questions? Is more than one interviewer needed? Are they properly trained? Do the subjects understand the wording of the questions?

The time and effort spent to conduct a pilot study are well worth it. Pitfalls and errors that may prove costly in the actual study may be identified and avoided.

Step 12. Plan How to Communicate the Research Findings

Although the communication of research findings may seem far away at this point, it is helpful to spend a few hours to consider how the research findings will be communicated. Research reports are often required as a part of course work. The written report and oral presentation may be the first steps in reaching a broader audience. The student may wish to investigate the possibility of presenting the paper at a professional meeting or locating a journal that publishes student papers. Whether it is published or not, the well-prepared research paper may enable the student to communicate the experience as a researcher to graduate schools or to prospective employers. Careful work in research makes a contribution to the profession, and experience in certain areas of research is reflected in the scientific practice of nursing. Chapter 22 discusses more fully the communication of research.

PHASE II: THE COLLECTION OF DATA

Phase II implements all of the plans made in Phase I to collect the data. If the study subjects have not been selected from the target population, this is the first step, as Figure 6–3 indicates. The second step is to contact the subjects, as well as any agencies involved, in order to explain the study and obtain their informed consent. The sampling process is a crucial element of the research design. It determines from whom or from what the data are to be collected, which (in turn) influences the method of data analysis that can be used. If sampling uses a process that affords each unit in the target population an equal chance of being chosen for study, then many methods of data analysis may be used. Any other kind of sampling limits the type of analysis but may be useful in descriptive or exploratory studies. The method by which data are collected varies by research design. An experiment observes and measures two groups (experimental and control); the survey involves questioning and measurement; and the record review requires asking questions of data. The student may observe, question, or measure—the most frequently used methods —and may use instruments to help perform these methods. In addition, classification is a means of data collection that may be useful. This method requires that the student develop categories into which observations will fall. For example, if the student is studying high blood pressure, she or he may construct categories such as age, race, sex, place of residence, and socioeconomic status. A tally sheet containing these categories enables the student to fill in the information quickly and efficiently.

Once the data-collection phase is finished, or is stopped for practical reasons, the phase of data analysis and interpretation begins.

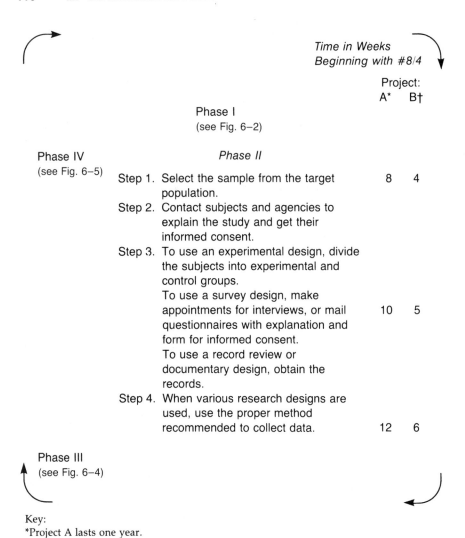

Time in Weeks
Beginning with #8/4

Project:
A*   B†

Phase I
(see Fig. 6–2)

Phase IV
(see Fig. 6–5)

Phase II

		A*	B†
Step 1.	Select the sample from the target population.	8	4
Step 2.	Contact subjects and agencies to explain the study and get their informed consent.		
Step 3.	To use an experimental design, divide the subjects into experimental and control groups.		
	To use a survey design, make appointments for interviews, or mail questionnaires with explanation and form for informed consent.	10	5
	To use a record review or documentary design, obtain the records.		
Step 4.	When various research designs are used, use the proper method recommended to collect data.	12	6

Phase III
(see Fig. 6–4)

Key:
*Project A lasts one year.
†Project B lasts one semester.

Figure 6–3. Phase II: Steps in collecting the research data.

PHASE III: ANALYZING AND INTERPRETING THE DATA

The task in Phase III is to summarize, analyze, and interpret facts and observations (Fig. 6–4). The first step is to examine raw data for completeness and accuracy. An incomplete or inaccurately completed questionnaire must be discarded. Next, the raw data must be transferred to a general tally table or worksheet, in order to bring categories of data together. The categories may be male/female; categories of ages; or public

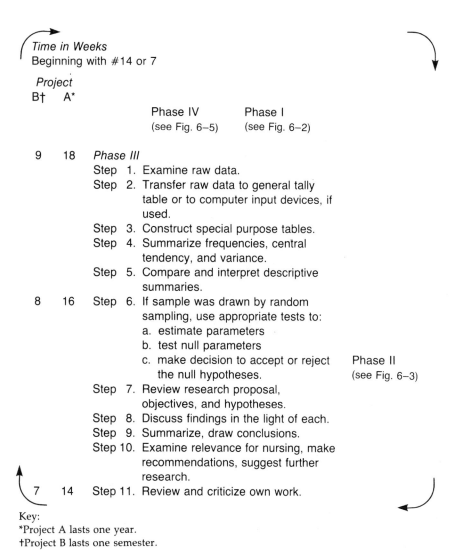

Figure 6–4. Phase III: Steps in analyzing and interpreting data.

patients/private patients, depending entirely on what information was collected. The tally marks are then counted, and the counts are summarized. In addition, special-purpose tables help summarize data (see Chap. 19).

Rates, ratios, and percentages are used to summarize data such as occupation, marital status, or type of illness. For quantitative data, summary measures such as mean, median, and mode are used. These are descriptive summaries and may be used to compare and interpret data from descriptive or exploratory studies.

Time in Weeks

Project		Phase IV
B†	A*	Communicating Findings‡

12	24	Step 1. Select method and means of communications.
		Step 2. Complete tables and graphs in finished form.
		Step 3. Write introduction, including problem statement, definitions, objectives, hypotheses, assumptions, and limitations.
		Step 4. Write review of literature, summarizing polar theories and research findings.
		Step 5. Designate the theoretical framework or findings of previous research to which study is addressed.
		Step 6. Relate theory or former research to problem statement or hypotheses.
		Step 7. Discuss research methods, with particular attention to sampling methods, how instruments were judged to be reliable and valid, and problems.
11	22	Step 8. Present findings.
		Step 9. Relate findings to problem statement and hypotheses.
		Step 10. Summarize research project.
		Step 11. Criticize research project.
		Step 12. Draw conclusions: relation to theory or prior research; relevance for nursing.
		Step 13. Complete bibliography, abstract, and give title to paper.
		Step 14. Submit final draft to colleague for criticism.
		Step 15. Present paper or submit for publication.
10	20	Step 16. Revise and resubmit, if necessary.

Key:
*Project A lasts one year.
†Project B lasts one semester.
‡Please note that Step 1 begins with either Week 20 (year project) or Week 10 (semester). The steps are listed from top to bottom for sake of convenience in reading.

Figure 6–5. Phase IV: Steps in communicating findings of the research project.

If the sample has been drawn randomly, a process that affords each unit in the population an equal chance of being chosen, inferential statistics may be used to analyze data, estimate parameters, and test null hypotheses (see Chap. 20).

The student examines the research findings and applies these to the research proposal, interpreting the findings in light of the stated objectives or hypotheses. Then the student summarizes the research findings and draws conclusions from the summaries. Next, the student discusses the importance of the research findings for nursing, states recommendations, and makes suggestions for further research. The student should now carefully review and criticize the work, noting any weaknesses that may be corrected by future research.

PHASE IV: COMMUNICATING THE RESEARCH FINDINGS

The final phase of the research process is the communication of findings. The research report, either written or oral, must communicate each step (see Fig. 6–5). It is usually wise to complete tables and graphs, since these aid in the process of communication. The structure of the report may follow Figure 6–5. Chapter 22 is also devoted to writing the research report. The report should be well-organized and in enough detail to inform but, at the same time, it should be succinct. Whether professors, other scientists, or laypersons, the audience to be reached determines how the report is presented. The student should also become familiar with the publication policies of various journals, since each has its own guidelines. The goal of the report should be kept in mind, together with appropriate writing style. The confidentiality of subjects and agencies should also be protected.

SUMMARY

A model may be devised that depicts the phases and steps of the research process. The calendar wheel (Fig. 6–1) is a model that divides the process into phases and steps and that assists the student in preparing a timetable that allocates the time to be spent in each phase. The model also suggests the unending process of scientific research: the conclusion of one project provides the data upon which another may be based.

The four phases of research include planning, collecting data, analyzing and interpreting data, and communicating the findings of the research. Each phase may be divided into various steps, which may differ in some ways from project to project. Common steps in Phase I require the researcher to: (1) identify a researchable problem; (2) formulate the research proposal; (3) define concepts and variables; (4) state objectives and hypotheses; (5) examine ethical implications of research; (6) review the literature; (7) identify theory, assumptions, and limitations; (8) describe the research design; (9) describe the methods of sampling, data collection, instrumentation, and data analysis; (10) obtain informed consent for a pilot study from agencies and study subjects; (11) conduct a pilot study and revise the research proposal in light of the findings; and (12) plan how to communicate the findings.

Phase II, the collection of data, relies heavily on two central processes: (1) selecting the sample from which the data are to be collected and obtaining informed consent from study subjects and involved agencies; and (2) selecting the method best-suited to collect data in light of the research design being used. Both the sampling process and the methods are complex issues intimately related to research designs, as well as to the ability to generalize from the small sample under study to the larger population from which the sample was drawn. The student needs to think carefully about these matters in terms of all of the factors involved, including time. Specific chapters in this book deal with each of these elements of the research process.

Phase III, the summarization, analysis, and interpretation of data, begins with an examination of raw data and transforms it into summaries, including frequencies, measures of central tendency and variance, and tables or graphs. Studies that have used random sampling can use inferential statistics to estimate parameters and to test null hypotheses. Once data summaries and estimates are concluded, the student can analyze these in the light of the research proposal, including objectives. The student draws conclusions from the analysis and discusses what these mean to nursing in general. Next, the student may make recommendations that are relevant for practice, administration, or teaching, or may suggest further research. Finally, the student carefully reviews and criticizes the research project, in preparation for communicating the findings.

Phase IV is concerned with communicating the research by oral presentation or written report. The organization and substantive approach depend, in part, upon the audience. The student reexamines the goals of the research and organizes the content in the proper format, using a writing style that is appropriate for the prospective readers, whether scientists or laypersons.

The temporal model presented is an idealized paradigm of the research process, which the student modifies with assistance from pertinent chapters of the book.

EXAMPLE FROM NURSING RESEARCH

Patricia Hubbard, Ann Muhlenkamp, Nancy Brown (1984): The relationship between social support and self-care practices. Nursing Research, 33, 266–270.

The researchable problem was to investigate the relationship between individuals' perceived level of social support and their performance of specific, positive health practices. The research proposed to explore the relationship between what people do to promote healthy lifestyles and how they perceive their level of social support.

Concepts were defined as follows: Social support is a multidimensional construct consisting of people as interpersonal resources who provide gratification of basic human needs in relationships. *Positive health practices* were defined as specific activities performed that may affect one's health, including nutrition, exercise, relaxation, safety, substance use, and prevention practices.

The primary hypothesis stated that a positive association will be found between the social-support and health-practice variables. (The researchers did not report possible ethical implications of the research proposal.)

The review of the literature included 16 studies, dating from 1974 through 1983, that reported converging and conflicting views, and research reports of social support and health characteristics.

Theory was not explicitly stated. However, it was implicit in the selection of authors and concepts to review in the literature, and in the hypotheses that were stated. In the review of the bibliography, nine of the 31 citations dealt with concepts of social support, five with the related theory of social networks, and three with related theories of social status.

The authors identified the research design as being a descriptive survey with two distinct samples. The sample in Study 1 consisted of 97 volunteers from an urban senior-citizen's center and, in Study 2, consisted of 133 individuals attending an urban health fair held at two shopping malls. Data were collected by survey utilizing two questionnaires. Instruments used included a Personal Resources Questionnaire, which was used to measure social support and which had reliability and validity reported from other studies.

Methods of data analysis included counting, calculating percentages, and using measures of central tendency including the mean, standard deviation, and range. A pilot study was not reported by the authors. The findings were communicated to a large audience by submitting the article for publication.

STUDY QUESTIONS

1. If you were to study any nursing problem you could, what would it be?
2. Identify the central concepts of your problem (above).
3. Examine the following problem: Radical mastectomy in women is an instance of the general phenomenon of changes in body image. This problem offers an opportunity to investigate the process of adjustment that takes place when a woman is faced with a loss of the breast, a symbol of femininity and motherhood. What are the concepts in the problem that need definition? Is this a researchable problem?
4. Do you foresee any ethical implications of the proposed research problem?

5. If you were to undertake the study of such a problem, what objective would you plan to meet?
6. Given the information in question three (above), where would you begin a review of the literature?
7. Have you encountered any theory that would be helpful in such a study?
8. Beginning with the assumption that surgical disfigurement alters a person's self-concept, what could you predict you would find if you observed or questioned a woman who had had a mastectomy 2 weeks previously?
9. If you were to develop a research design or plan to study patients with mastectomies, what would be the four phases of the research design?
10. What is a pilot project?

REFERENCES AND SUGGESTED READINGS

Abdellah, F. and Levine, E. (1965): Better Patient Care Through Nursing Research. New York: Macmillan, chap. 5. *The steps in the research process.*

Bloch, D. (1974): Some crucial terms in nursing: What do they really mean? Nursing Outlook, *22*, 689–694. *Cites the difficulty of finding consensus on the definition of concepts.*

Brink, P. and Wood, M. (1978): Basic Steps in Planning Nursing Research: From Question to Proposal. North Scituate, Mass.: Duxbury Press. *Each chapter explains a step in research.*

Downs, F. (1977): Maternal stress in primigravidas as a factor in the production of neonatal pathology. In Downs, F. and Newman, M. (eds.), A Sourcebook of Nursing Research. Philadelphia: F. A. Davis.

Fox, D. (1976): Fundamentals of Research in Nursing (3rd ed.). New York: Appleton-Century-Crofts. *Chapter 3 includes nineteen stages in a three-part plan of research.*

Hubbard, P., Muhlenkamp, A., and Brown, N. (1984): The relationship between social support and self-care practices. Nursing Research, *33*, 266–270.

Johnson, M. (1975): Outcome criteria to evaluate postoperative respiratory status. American Journal of Nursing, *75*, 1474–1475. *Formulation of a significant problem for nursing.*

Lin, N. (1976): Foundations of Social Research, New York: McGraw-Hill. *Chapter 1 includes eight phases of research.*

McCorkle, R. (1981): Effects of touch on seriously ill patients. In Fox, D. (ed.), Readings on the Research Process in Nursing. New York: Appleton-Century-Crofts. *Instruments used include observation, questionnaire, tape recorder, etc.*

Polit, D. and Hungler, B. (1978): Nursing Research: Principles and Methods. Philadelphia: J. B. Lippincott. *Chapter 3 includes 15 steps in the research process.*

Schmitt, F. and Wooldridge, P. (1981): Psychological preparation of surgical patients. In Fox, D. and Lesser, I. (eds.), Readings in the Research Process in Nursing. New York: Appleton-Century-Crofts.

Selltiz, C. et al. (1976): Methods in Social Relations (3rd ed.). New York: Holt, Rinehart & Winston, pp. 12–14. *Brief treatment of the major steps in research.*

Simon, J. (1978): Basic Research Methods in Social Science. New York: Random House, chap. 7. *Includes the steps in an empirical research study.*

7

The Research Proposal

A research proposal is a written summary of what the researcher intends to do, how, and why. The research proposal is forward-looking. It describes the anticipated plan of research for the approval of the supervising professor, committee, or funding agency. A well-written proposal is a valuable tool for the student, well worth the time and effort put into its development. The proposal anticipates as many of the elements of the research process as possible and provides a model that helps the student write the research report. The research proposal is written during the planning phase of research, implemented during the phases of data collection and analysis, and described in the communication phase.

This chapter is designed to help the student to identify a researchable problem and to write a research proposal. Upon completion of the chapter, the student should be able to: (1) identify a significant problem in nursing; (2) state the characteristics of a researchable problem; and (3) write a research proposal that includes what the researcher intends to study and why, objectives and hypotheses, ethical considerations, theoretical viewpoints, design, and methods.

SOURCES OF SIGNIFICANT RESEARCHABLE PROBLEMS IN NURSING

Nursing problems become research problems when the researcher can identify what to observe, what questions to ask, or what to measure. Sources of significant problems in nursing are the clinical area, the literature, experienced professionals, and the student's own interest. The researcher may observe a problem in the clinical area and then examine pertinent research reports for further information. Or, the researcher may begin with the literature. Advice from professors and practitioners of nursing may point the way to a stimulating research project already underway that the student can join. However, the interest of the student is the most fruitful source of nursing problems. The student's curiosity and energy light the fire necessary for sustained commitment throughout the project.

The Clinical Area

The clinical area of nursing is one in which patients or clients are observed, treated, cared for, advised, and/or taught. It is a fertile area for identifying problems in practice, teaching, or administration. To identify problems in the clinical area, Diers (1979) suggests that we begin by asking a series of questions: (1) "I wonder why . . ."; (2) "What is this?"; (3) "What is happening here?"; and (4) "What happens if . . .?"

1. *The nurse who wonders why he or she observes certain events in nursing may be noting a discrepancy: things are not the way the nurse thinks they should be.* Or else, what the nurse knows varies from what she or he needs to know. For example, Dee et al. (1965) noticed that certain patients were receiving excellent nursing care, while others seemed uncomfortable and unattended. She wondered why this was so. Upon investigation, she found that patient care seemed related to the way that nurses felt about the patients: those regarded favorably received good care, while those regarded unfavorably did not, a discrepancy in the way things were and the way they should be. Noting discrepancies is a major step in the identification of a clinical nursing problem, which then may be described or explored.

2. *The nurse who wonders what it is that he or she is observing is searching for the name of the problem.* For example, what is the name of the needs of a grieving spouse in the hospital setting (Hampe, 1974)? What is the name of the feeling that families have when a psychiatric patient is returning home? What are the names of the various processes associated with dying in the hospital (Glaser and Strauss, 1966–1968)? Searching for a name leads the nurse to describe, classify, and name nursing phenomena. Nursing diagnoses are the names given to the descriptions and classification of nursing observations. The nurse who isolates specific factors from observations in order to describe and name these factors is using *naming theory,* an explanation for the classification of nursing data.

3. *The nurse who wonders what is happening here is searching for relationships between named variables.* In this case, the names of the concepts or variables are known, but the relationship between

them is not. For example, Brown et al. (1977) wondered about the relationship between drug interactions and the consequences of these interactions for elderly patients in nursing homes who were prescribed these drugs. Williams (1972) wondered what factors were related to the incidence of decubitus ulcers among hospitalized patients; and Ambron (1976) was interested in which of 22 clinical signs were most related to the need for tracheo-bronchial suctioning. Beginning with observation, all such problems lead inductively to the formulation of factor-relating theory.

4. *The nurse who wonders what would happen if . . . seeks to predict a relationship between variables.* He or she may wonder how factors vary in terms of one another (correlation), or if one factor causes the other (causation). For example, what happens if a person smokes? Is the person at risk to get cancer? Is smoking correlated with cancer? What happens if there is a rise in fever, and is it associated with changes in the perception of time passage (Alderson, 1974)? What is the effect of nursing on the incidence of postoperative vomiting (Dumas and Leonard, 1963)? What happens when the nurse prepares a patient for surgery by precise teaching methods? Will the patient be able to deep-breathe and cough more effectively? Will the patient stay in the hospital less time and need analgesics less frequently (Lindeman and Van Aerman, 1977)?

The nurse can find significant problems in the clinical area by asking the right questions or by reviewing the literature.

The Nursing Literature

Nursing literature is a readily available source of important research problems in nursing (see Chap. 8). Abdellah et al. (1960), over two decades ago, identified 21 areas of patient needs from which problems may be identified. More recently, Abbey (1980) developed the acronym FANCAP (*F*luids, *A*eration, *N*utrition, *C*ommunication, *A*ctivity, *P*ain) to provide a mnemonic device for reminding nurses of possible problem areas. Roy (1980) identifies problems of adaptation, including physiologic needs of patients, self-concept, and role and relations of interdependence. Roy's model reveals the kind of problems found when deviations from the desired state occur. Lindeman (1975) published a list of areas that nurses themselves identified as problem areas needing research: patient care and education; alleviation of stress and pain; indicators to measure quality nursing care; and the nursing process. Each of these defines sources of problems in the clinical area, in teaching, or in administration.

Fox (1976, p. 214) suggests a significant problem for both nursing service and education: to delineate *what* needs to be measured and to devise instruments to measure the phenomenon. For example, what characteristics should nurses measure to define good nursing care? What can be measured to predict the reaction of patient X when nurse Y enters the room? What identifies the freshman student who will be a functioning nurse of the future? These are challenging questions.

Stress is a problem area that received considerable attention following Selye's (1965) publication, *The Stress of Life*. Kjervik and Martinson (1979) examined a number of areas stressful to women that should be the concern of nursing: childbearing, poverty, pain, and the loss associated with divorce, desertion, or widowhood. Many books contain articles specifically related to nursing problems: Downs and Newman (1977); Downs and Fleming (1979); and Verhonick (1975, 1977). The journal *Nursing Research* is a fertile source of problems. For example, a series of articles published during 1977 is concerned with research in nursing specialties, such as maternal-child nursing, community health, and psychiatric nursing. Each article suggests significant areas for research.

Suggestions of Experienced Professionals

Professors, clinical specialists, and experienced nurses are important resources to aid the student in identifying significant nursing problems. It is a rare professional that does not welcome the interest of a student in his or her area of research or clinical specialty. At times, it is possible for the professional to invite the student to participate in ongoing research. Such participation provides the student with an exceptional opportunity to examine the research proposal, instruments, recording processes, and ethical implications of a sophisticated research project.

Student Interest

Student interest is often the best source of a problem for study. A burning interest in a particular area of nursing practice, education, or administration is vital to make the research come alive. It transforms what could be a routine and demanding chore into a stimulating and rewarding experience. The student's fresh approach to nursing enables her or him to identify nursing procedures that often are ritualistic and useless, at best, and that may be costly and traumatic. The student views the profession from a new and vital perspective—a resource of considerable importance to nursing.

CHARACTERISTICS OF A RESEARCHABLE PROBLEM

Several characteristics define a researchable problem for study: (1) availability of data, (2) feasibility, (3) importance, and (4) general applicability. A research proposal is no better than the problem that it proposes. Therefore, the problem must be, not only sound, but researchable.

Availability of Data

Not all data are equally accessible to all researchers. For example, an undergraduate student may have difficulty gaining access to certain subjects, such as rape victims, patients undergoing a sex change, or patients involved in child abuse. The subjects may object, or the hospital or supervising personnel may protest the study of sensitive areas such as these. If reliable and valid instruments are not available, data may also be difficult to collect. In addition, the collection of cultural data may require more hours of observation than the researcher can afford. If the researcher plans to obtain data by asking questions in interviews or by questionnaire, the willingness and ability of the respondent to answer the questions must be assessed. To obtain data from records, the records must be available and complete, and the data must have been accurately and legibly recorded. To obtain data from an experiment involving human subjects, ethical questions must be answered and permission obtained from various committees concerned with the protection of human rights.

Therefore, a good research question that does not have a dependable and available source of data may begin and end with the question itself.

Feasibility of the Research

The second characteristic of a good research proposal is its suitability or practicality. What is practical for one researcher may not be so for another. Nevertheless, certain criteria apply to nearly all projects. Those of special concern include time, money, space, equipment, cooperation of agencies and personnel, and the personality of the researcher. Each of these will be examined briefly.

Time. Every study needs a timetable, although this may vary in terms of the researcher's status and the project's funding. Undergraduate nurses must integrate research with other courses and course work with the number of weeks in the academic semester or year. Graduate students have a similar problem, which may be complicated if a supporting grant has deadlines of its own. The nurse in practice must consider time for research, in addition to the regular schedule for work. Therefore, it is expedient to examine the research problem and proposal in terms of the length of time necessary to complete each step of the study. It may be necessary to reduce the scope of the problem or to reduce the number of variables under study. A second dilemma arises from the times that data must be collected. For example, a study of pain during childbirth must consider, not only when the patient may go into labor (day or night), but likewise, the changing rhythms of labor. Another problem is observing several women simultaneously in labor. A good research proposal allows for a practical timetable in terms of both the researcher's program of study or work and the time necessary for proper data collection.

Money. The simplest research project costs money. Costs of small items such as index cards, paper, pencils and pens, typewriter ribbons, paper clips, rubber bands, and file folders soon add up. It is a rare study that does not also include the purchase of books and journals or the reproduction of articles. If a questionnaire is to be used, postage both to send and to return the questionnaire must be calculated, as well as the cost of envelopes and paper. Interviews may call for transportation and, at times, long-distance phone calls. If the use of a computer is necessary to analyze data, service charges must be calculated. A good research question is one that falls within the financial ability of the researcher to pay and produces results that reimburse the researcher or the granting agency.

Space and Equipment. Certain research projects, such as a survey or questionnaire, need little space or equipment beyond a desk, paper, and pencil. Others may require instruments to measure physiological functioning and special rooms for conducting experiments. A simple interview needs privacy and quiet in order for the interviewer and respondent to be able to communicate freely. Audiovisual aids of various types, such as recorders, cameras, and projectors, offer considerable assistance but may be beyond the resources of the neophyte researcher. A sound research question involves no more need for space and equipment than can be met within the limits of time and money available to the investigator.

Cooperation of Agencies and Personnel. Cooperation of others may often depend upon legal and ethical considerations, as well as availability of unrestricted data. For the undergraduate nurse, the length of time required to obtain permission to collect data in schools, industries, nursing homes, or hospitals may exceed the time available. And permission may be denied. A letter or phone call by a high official or influential person in the field may help, but these persons must be available to the researcher. The nurse in practice is in an enviable position—the collection of data may occur in the course of practice. However, consent of supervisors and subjects is necessary and ethical. In order to test whether a research question is feasible in terms of cooperation of crucial agencies or persons, permission should be obtained as early in the research process as possible.

Personality of the Researcher. Certain nurses seem better-suited for certain kinds of research than others, although difficulties in this area are not always easily foreseen. An experienced investigator in the same field may be able to predict the success of a particular nurse. Often, a pilot project may point up difficulties that otherwise would be unpredictable. An aggressive personality may do better with a questionnaire survey than with an interview, although a timid nurse may find it difficult to knock on doors and interact with strange persons. A good research proposal must take into account both the personality of the researcher and the variables we have examined.

Importance of the Research Proposal

The most important nursing questions deal with the nursing care of the sick, maintenance of the health of the well, and evaluation of health care. Moreover, the frequency with which problems in health care are occurring is important. For example, how often do hospitalized patients get bedsores? How frequently are illegitimate children born prematurely? How often are clinic appointments broken? How frequently do patients know the side effects of the drugs that they take? The frequency of a problem not only affects the health of the population but also increases the cost of health services. For example, frequent infection of surgical wounds means a longer and more costly stay in the hospital for the patient.

General Applicability of the Findings

Research proposals are generally applicable when they can be related to theory and when the subjects to be studied are selected from the target population by a method of random sampling (see Chap. 14). Some theories used in nursing research are the systems theory, theories of human development, the stress theory, and theories of adaptation (see Chaps. 4 and 5). The theoretical framework helps the researcher explain the relationships among the facts observed during the data-collection phase.

FORMULATING THE RESEARCH PROPOSAL

The research proposal is intimately related to the research problem. Research problems become research proposals when the student can precisely state the following: (1) what is to be studied and why; (2) the objectives and/or hypotheses of the study; (3) the ethical implications, if any; (4) the theoretical viewpoints, assumptions, and limitations; and (5) the research design, sampling, and methods. As the student reviews the literature related to the problem and attempts to obtain a proper sample of study subjects from a target population, a research proposal may go through many revisions. A well-formulated research proposal repays the researcher for the time and effort that it takes, and it informs the reviewers. The anticipated plan of research is summarized, the extent to which the findings may be generalized to other times and places is made apparent, and the potential for application in the clinical area becomes evident.

What the Researcher Intends to Study

The researcher states the problem to be studied in the opening paragraph of the research proposal. The general area of study is first introduced, its importance to nursing is indicated, and then the exact problem is specified. The following example illustrates these points:

> The general effect of hospitalization upon the emotional and mental health of children is a question of importance to nurses who must daily assess the condition of their patients. The relationship between hospitalization and the emotional and mental status of children has been well-studied by Bowlby (1965) and others. Nurses such as McGillicuddy (1977) have investigated the effect of hospitalization on the child if the mother stays in the room with him. Does the mother's rooming-in with her child make a difference in the child's subsequent behavior? This research proposes to study that question, to examine the effect of the mother's rooming-in with her child on his subsequent behavior after he has left the hospital.

This brief introductory paragraph has identified the general problem area, suggested its importance to nursing, referred the reader to examples in the general literature and the nursing literature, and specified exactly what the researcher is proposing to study.

What the researcher intends to study must now be explained further by defining each major concept by operational definition, which clarifies what is to be observed and measured. Definitions should be drawn from the literature to strive for a consensus in the meaning of nursing concepts and variables. Drawing on a similar but more extensive study by McGillicuddy, the student defines the concepts as follows:

1. *Rooming-in*. The mother remains with the child 24 hours a day during the first 2 days and at least 10 hours daily thereafter until discharge.
2. *Child*. Those children who are 14 months or older but not yet 49 months old; who are hospitalized for minor surgery, including eye surgery and tonsillectomy.
3. *Behavior*. Selected ways of behaving by the child, including eating, sleeping, and toilet behaviors.
4. *Effect*. The effect of the mother's rooming-in with her child on the child's subsequent behavior, as measured by the mother's response to the questionnaire answered after the child has been home for a month and compared with the mother's response to a questionnaire answered on the day of her child's admission to the hospital.

The researcher who uses hypotheses not only specifies what is to be studied, but also predicts a relationship between the variables:

If the mother rooms-in with her child during hospitalization for minor surgery, then the child will manifest increased maturity in selected areas of behavior compared with the child whose mother does not room-in.

Objectives

An *objective* is an intent, a statement of what the student proposes to accomplish in the research. It denotes observable, measurable attributes that make it possible to determine whether the objective has been met. To be meaningful, the stated objective must communicate to the reader the exact intent of the researcher. The most important characteristic of an objective is to identify the tasks the researcher plans to perform during the study. As the following examples drawn from different research reports demonstrate, each objective expresses only one intended outcome:

- An objective of this research is to compare the communication patterns of elderly male and female patients.
- An objective of this study is to record the words that various patients use to describe the functions of their bodily organs.
- An objective of this study is to state factors that increase the opportunities for mothers of hospitalized children to participate in their care.

When several objectives are developed, these should be stated in their order of importance. Each objective should be related to the research design and methods. Descriptive or exploratory studies rely on objectives more often than explanatory studies, which tend to rely on hypotheses.

Ethical Implications

At some point in the research proposal, the researcher must inform the reviewer of the ethical implications of the study and how these will be handled. Forms of informed consent may be attached to the proposal, and forms indicating the protocol for research on human subjects may be included, together with any other information required by the human investigations committee that a particular school may have. Both agencies and subjects must be considered in the plan to obtain informed consent.

Review of the Literature

The review of the literature may either be interwoven into the identification of the problem, the definition of concepts, the theoretical section, the research design and methods; or it may be presented in a section of its own. The review should identify pertinent studies about what is known and what remains to be learned. It should provide a background of the problem to be studied and convince the reviewer that the researcher has explored significant studies and has a grasp of the theory and research findings relevant to the proposed research. The preliminary proposal that the student submits for the first tentative approval may not include all citations, but the finished proposal should demonstrate a thorough grasp of the studies documented in the literature.

Theory, Assumptions, and Limitations

A theory provides the explanation for observed facts and relationships, predicts what the researcher will observe, and summarizes what is known about the topic under study. The researcher states the theory used to deduce the hypotheses and refers the reader to any previous research relevant to his or her proposal. In the absence of well-developed theory, the researcher states the assumptions that underlie the proposal. Assumptions are statements whose validity can be found in the literature or are considered to be self-evident. Some examples of assumptions are:

- Child development proceeds as an integrated system in interaction with the environment (Robischon, 1977, p. 155).
- The development of mothering ability is determined by the mother's previous experience, her current life situation, and the inborn behavior of the infant (Durand, 1975).

Limitations establish the parameters, i.e., the boundaries, of the research. Ability to include limitations in the proposal enhances the quality of the proposal. Some examples of limitations are:

1. The sample of this study will be limited to one child with Down's syndrome.
2. This investigation will be limited to children between 19 and 24 months.
3. The sample will be limited to children living in intact family units.

Limitations should not stop with the statement of the population sampled but should include the researcher's opinion about the ability to generalize or apply the study's results beyond the study sample. In addition, the researcher should assess the ability of any instruments to be used to measure what the researcher intends to measure. If an instrument is not valid, the researcher should delay the proposal until an instrument of demonstrated validity is found (Fox, 1976, p. 292).

Research Design

The research design is often described in a single paragraph that indicates whether the design is qualitative or quantitative, descriptive, historical, experimental, partially experimental, a survey, or of another type.

- This experimental study will determine whether a causal relationship exists between the amount of touching a seriously ill patient receives and the number of positive responses that the patient makes.

- A three-group experimental design will be used to test the hypothesis.
- Two of the groups will be control groups and one will be experimental.
- The researcher intends to use a record review to collect data on the birth weights of babies born to primiparas who smoke and those who do not smoke.
- The design of research is a descriptive survey that uses a questionnaire to measure the tendency of operating-room nurses to desire friendly interaction with others.
- The research design is an exploratory survey (interview) to determine whether poor women perceive health workers as threatening.

Research Methods

The researcher reports the method to be used to collect data, whether by observation, questioning, measuring, or a combination of the three. The following examples suggest a few of the various combinations.

1. Data will be collected by direct observation of two observers.
2. A questionnaire will be administered by an observer. A tape recorder will record any verbal interactions.
3. Data will be collected using measures of blood pressure, pulse rates, and temperature readings.
4. Data will be collected by interviewing patients to determine how much they know about the side effects of medications they are taking.

Instruments. The instruments used to collect data may be described in a manner similar to the following:

1. The instrument to be used to measure psychological stress response is the Zuckerman's Affect Adjective Check List, consisting of 61 adjectives that have emotional overtones. The subjects will check every word that describes their present feelings.
2. Heart-rate measurement instruments include a two-channel direct writer that will record ECG.
3. A questionnaire of 27 items will be used to assess behavioral changes.

Sampling

An important part of the research proposal is how the sample is to be selected. The following examples illustrate some of the sampling methods used in research:

1. A sample of 100 seriously ill patients will be selected from a 1000-bed general hospital in Central City. An alphabetical list of seriously ill patients in intensive care and coronary care will be obtained weekly. Those patients who are oriented to their surroundings, who can hear well and do not have speech problems, and who are between 20 and 60 years of age will be included in the sample. These patients will be alternately assigned to an experimental or control group, beginning with a flip of a coin to designate the initial assignment.
2. A random sample of 800 nurses will be chosen from a list of nurses registered with the West Virginia State Board of Nurse Examiners at the time of the survey.
3. Data will be collected during the intensive study of one case of Down's syndrome.
4. The sample will be comprised of patients admitted for surgery in which general anesthesia will be used. Patients admitted during one month will serve as the control group, while patients admitted during the next month will serve as the experimental group.

Methods of Data Analysis

Numerous methods of data analysis may be selected, including the plan to develop various categories for descriptive data; to use descriptive statistics appropriate to the scale used to summarize and compare data; or to use inferential statistics to test hypotheses. If the use of a computer is planned, this should be noted in the proposal.

SUMMARY

A research proposal summarizes what the researcher intends to do, how it will be done, and why it is important for nursing. The proposal anticipates as many elements of the research process as possible. It is written during the planning phase, implemented during the data collection phase, and described during the communication phase.

To write a sound research proposal, the student must be able to identify a significant problem in nursing, state the characteristics that are researchable, and use this information to write that portion of the research proposal that specifies the general area of study and the specific problem to be studied.

Sources of significant researchable problems in nursing include the clinical area, the literature, experienced professionals, and the student's own interest. Problems in the clinical area can be identified by asking questions such as, "I wonder why?"; "What is this?"; "What is happening here?"; and "What happens if . . .?" A number of books and journals in the nursing literature, such as *Nursing Research*, include helpful information about nursing problems. Experienced professional nurses may be engaged in ongoing research that the student may be invited to join. However, the best source of a research problem is often the student herself (or himself).

Characteristics of researchable problems include available data and feasible or practical research, in terms of time, money, space, equipment, cooperation of others, and the personality of the researcher. All of these should be carefully weighed before selecting a problem for study. The importance of the proposed research to nursing must be examined, such as nursing care of the sick, maintenance of good health in the well, evaluation of health care, and the frequency with which the problem occurs.

Once the problem is selected, the student is launched. The formulation of the research proposal begins with a brief paragraph that describes what the researcher intends to study and its importance to nursing. This is followed by a definition of the major concepts used in the study. Operational definitions then clarify what is to be observed and measured.

The objective of the study defines what the student intends to accomplish in the research project. The most important characteristic of the objective is to identify the tasks the student will perform during the research. Hypotheses are used in explanatory research to predict what will be found in research.

A section of the proposal must be devoted to a thorough description of the research design, whether it will be an experiment, a survey, or an historical documentary review of records. The research methods and instruments that will be used to select a sample and collect data receive particular scrutiny from the reader and require a careful exposition by the student.

The assumptions of the study—statements documented in the literature, or ideas considered to be correct—should be clearly stated to demonstrate the student's grasp of theory and research. The limitations of the study, or those aspects of research that will not be studied, should be noted to enhance the quality of the research proposal.

A brief but significant review of the literature provides a background for the study and helps convince the reader that the student understands what has been discovered and what remains to be learned.

Ethical implications must be anticipated and dealt with in a professional manner. Proper forms should be processed, and the student should be ready to proceed, once permission is obtained from all necessary agencies and subjects.

EXAMPLES FROM NURSING RESEARCH

Examples of Applied Research

Suzanne Caty, Mary Ellerton, Judith Ritchie (1984): Coping in hospitalized children: An analysis of published case studies. Nursing Research, 33, 277–282.

The authors in the second paragraph of their article note that the project underway was designed in three parts with the objective of developing and testing a category system of coping behavior used by hospitalized children. The first study was to develop a category system; to test the system in a series of three studies; and then to use it as the basis of an observation instrument. The study reported in this paper used this category system to analyze published case studies of hospitalized children.

A second study was planned to analyze previously collected process recordings of totally unstructured observations as described by a participant observer; and a third study was planned to observe hospitalized children in specific hospital situations.

The questions under investigation in this paper were: What range of coping behaviors do authors identify in 39 published case studies of hospitalized children aged 20 months to 10 years? What pattern of coping is revealed when the behaviors are analyzed according to a category system based on the Lazarus (1980) paradigm?

Thomas Knapp (1985): Validity, reliability, and neither. Nursing Research, 34, 189–192.

The author in the second paragraph of his article cites the purpose of the paper: to call attention to a number of misuses of the terms "validity" and "reliability" that have appeared in the pages of *Nursing Research*, other nursing journals and books, and psychometric reports in other disciplines. He found that certain studies categorized as validity or reliability studies should not be subsumed under either term.

Deborah McGuire (1984): The measurement of clinical pain. Nursing Research, 33, 152–156.

The author begins by defining clinical pain as "the perception of unpleasant stimuli arising from sensory alterations associated with a disease process and/or therapeutic and diagnostic procedures." She then notes the paper will review the following: (1) problems encountered in measuring clinical pain; (2) existing instruments with recommendations of studies in which they may be used; (3) advantages and disadvantages of the existing instruments; and (4) factors to consider when selecting a measuring instrument.

STUDY QUESTIONS

1. You have just received a large grant to study a nursing problem of your own choosing. What will you study?
2. If you are uncertain about what to study, name three sources of significant nursing problems.
3. In your own case, what identifies a problem that is researchable and one that is not?
4. What ethical consideration must be given to nursing research in general?

5. What are the ethical implications of the nursing problem you selected in Question 1?
6. Name and discuss four characteristics of a good nursing problem and research proposal.
7. Identify the what, who, how, when, and where of your proposal.
8. Define the central concepts of your problem.
9. Establish four or five clear objectives for your proposed study.
10. Select one of the examples from nursing research literature cited previously. Can you formulate a research proposal from the statement given by the author? What did the researcher intend to study? Were there ethical implications? What were the objectives? Can you determine the research design used? The research methods? Sampling?
11. How would you rewrite Knapp's purpose as a research proposal (see above)?

REFERENCES AND SUGGESTED READINGS

Abbey, J. (1980): FANCAP: What is it? In Riehl, J. and Roy, C. (eds.), Conceptual Models for Nursing Practice (2nd ed.). New York: Appleton-Century-Crofts, pp. 107–118. *Mnemonic device to identify possible patient problems.*

Abdellah, F. et al. (1960): Patient-Centered Approaches to Nursing. New York: Macmillan. *The identification of patient needs suggests problem areas for research.*

Alderson, M. (1974): Effect of increased body temperature on the perception of time. Nursing Research, *23*, 43–49. *An example of a clinical problem.*

Ambron, S. (1976): Clinical signs associated with amount of tracheo-bronchial secretions. Nursing Research, *25*, 121–126. *A problem in the clinical area.*

Bowlby, J. (1956): Maternal-child separation. In Soddy, K. (ed.), Mental Health and Infant Development. New York: Basic Books. *Maternal bonding is discussed.*

Brown, M. et al. (1977): Drug–drug interactions among residents in homes for the elderly. Nursing Research, *26*, 47–52. *A problem in health care of the elderly.*

Caty, S., Ellerton, M., and Ritchie, J. (1984): Coping in hospitalized children. Nursing Research, *33*, 277–282.

Dee, F. et al. (1965): Self-acceptance of nurses and acceptance of patients: An exploratory investigation. Nursing Research, *14*, 345–350. *Observation detects a problem in the clinical area.*

Diers, D. (1979): Research in Nursing Practice. Philadelphia: J. B. Lippincott. *Nursing problems in the clinical area identified.*

Downs, F. and Fleming, J. (eds.) (1979): Issues in Nursing Research. New York: Appleton-Century-Crofts. *Seven articles examine research issues.*

Downs, F. and Newman, M. (eds.) (1977): A Sourcebook of Nursing Research (2nd ed.). Philadelphia: F. A. Davis. *Fifteen articles evaluate nursing intervention and explore indices of health.*

Dumas, R. and Leonard, R. (1963): The effect of nursing on the incidence of postoperative vomiting. Nursing Research, *12*, 12–15. *Seeks to predict a relation between variables; the problem: patient anxiety.*

Durand, B. (1975): Failure to thrive in a child with Down's syndrome. Nursing Research, *24*, 272–286. *Assumptions stated.*

Fox, D. (1976): Fundamentals of Research in Nursing (3rd ed.). New York: Appleton-Century-Crofts, pp. 25–26, 292. *Problem areas discussed.*

Glaser, B. and Strauss, A. (1966): Awareness of Dying. Chicago: Aldine. (1967): The Discovery of Grounded Theory. Chicago: Aldine. (1968): A Time for Dying. Chicago: Aldine. *A variety of problems associated with dying.*

Hampe, S. (1974): Needs of grieving spouse in a hospital setting. Nursing Research, *24*, 113–120. *Problems identified from needs.*

Kjervik, D. and Martinson, I. (eds.) (1979): Women in Stress: A Nursing Perspective. New York: Appleton-Century-Crofts. *Twenty articles examine stress in various situations.*

Knapp, T. (1985): Validity, reliability and neither. Nursing Research, *34*, 189–192.

Lindeman, C. (1975): Delphi survey of priorities in clinical nursing research. Nursing Research, *24*, 434–441. *Problems given priorities in nursing.*

Lindeman, C. and Van Aernam, B. (1977): Nursing intervention with the presurgical patient—the effects of structured and unstructured preoperative teaching. In Downs, F. and Newman, M. (eds.), A Sourcebook of Nursing Research. Philadelphia: F. A. Davis, pp. 45–63. *Identifies problems in the clinical area.*

McGillicuddy, M. (1977): A study of the relationship between mothers' rooming-in during their children's hospitalization and changes in selected areas of children's behavior. In Downs, F. and Newman, M. (eds.), A Sourcebook of Nursing Research. Philadelphia: F. A. Davis, pp. 64–77. *Includes definition of concepts.*

McGuire, D. (1984): The measurement of clinical pain. Nursing Research, *33*, 152–156.

Robischon, P. (1977): Pica practice and other hand-mouth behavior and children's development level. In Downs, F. and Newman, M. (eds.), A Sourcebook of Nursing Research. Philadelphia: F. A. Davis, pp. 152–170. *States assumptions.*

Roy, C. (1980): The Roy adaptation model. In Riehl, J. and Roy, C. (eds.), Conceptual Models for Nursing Practice. New York: Appleton-Century-Crofts, pp. 179–188. *Problems of adaptation.*

Selye, H. (1965): The Stress of Life. New York: McGraw-Hill. *Problems of stress.*

Verhonick, P. (ed.) (1975): Nursing Research I Boston: Little, Brown. *Articles on the problems that nurses study.*

Verhonick, P. (ed.) (1977): Nursing Research II. Boston: Little, Brown. *Articles on problems in the clinical setting.*

Williams, A. (1972): Study of factors contributing to skin breakdown. Nursing Research, *21*, pp. 238–243. *Problem factors in the clinical area.*

8

A Critical Review
of the Literature

Review of the literature refers to an extensive, thorough, and systematic examination of publications relevant to the research project. *Critical review* refers to the examination of the strengths and weaknesses of appropriate publications. The review of the literature is usually divided into two parts: first, the student locates as many of the important publications as is feasible; then the student reviews critically those publications of particular significance to the project.

Upon completion of this chapter, the student should be able to: (1) state reasons why a review of the literature is an essential part of every research project; (2) describe how to conduct a literature review; (3) state how to identify and summarize pertinent publications; and (4) describe how to conduct a critical review of the research literature.

THE LITERATURE REVIEW: AN ESSENTIAL PART OF EVERY RESEARCH PROJECT

The review of the literature is an essential part of every research project for many reasons: First, the student is able to determine the extent to which theory and research are developed in the field under study, the opposing theoretical perspectives, and the research that supports or does not support opposing perspectives. Second, the student can identify the definition of concepts and variables already established in the literature and can examine elements of research used by others, such as designs, methods, scales, instruments, measures, and techniques of data analysis that may prove useful in the proposed project. Third, the student can discover what is known and what remains to be learned in the field, and may identify a study that can be replicated or whose findings may be compared and contrasted with the proposed study. Fourth, the student may become aware of difficulties experienced by others, which may save time, money, and error and which may identify ethical problems. Finally, the student may find a research report that is so well-structured and easy to read that it will be useful as a guide in writing the research report.

The Preliminary Review of the Literature

The first stage of the review of the literature is a general, preliminary search that attempts to locate all pertinent publications for a quick perusal. The second stage, a more critical review of the major works, is designed to identify the merits, strengths, weaknesses, and shortcomings of each. As the researcher gains experience, he or she may conduct a critical review as a part of the preliminary review and may immediately discard publications that do not meet the researcher's standards. A review of the literature may precede, accompany, or follow the initial formulation of the research proposal. The student may go to the literature first, write a tentative proposal, and then examine the literature; or the student may have a research report in hand, formulate an initial research proposal, and then conduct a more intensive search of the literature. The two processes work intimately together, each influencing the other.

The preliminary review generally includes three steps: (1) to identify and locate important publications; (2) to summarize and record the content of publications; and (3) to compare related elements, such as the theoretical perspective, definitions, research designs, methods, instruments, and findings. Each of these will be examined.

Identification of Important Publications

The first step in the preliminary review of the literature is to identify what has been published in the field, when, and by whom. The best place to begin is with the most recent publications. These often summarize and criticize earlier work, report contemporary research, and provide bibliographies for further perusal. The most recent publications are found in journals, since articles can be written and published well in advance of books. Such publications may be located in two ways: by a computer search of the literature (provided by most health science libraries), and by manual search of the local library.

The most rapid access to citations for current journals is obtained by a computer search of the literature. *MEDLARS*—medical literature analysis and retrieval system—is designed to achieve rapid access via the computer-based bibliographic processing system to hundreds of thousands of journals in the National Library of Medicine in Bethesda, Maryland. *MEDLINE*—an "on-line" computer search—provides immediate (if limited) references, while the more extensive "off-line" searches are more expensive and slower, being sent by mail. Other acronyms designed to refer to specific subject areas include *CATLINE*, which provides a list of books on a proposed topic; *CANCERLINE*, which provides literature on cancer; *SOCIAL SCISEARCH*, corresponding to the publication *Social Science Citations Index*; *SOCABS*, corresponding to *Sociological Abstracts*; *SCISEARCH*, corresponding to *Science Citations Index*; *ERIC*, corresponding to *Current Index to Journals in Education*; and many others that the medical librarian can explain.

The researcher should begin a computer search by conferring with the librarian designated to work in these areas, who will explain how the request for a literature review is matched against the citations in a particular data base; he or she will also explain the mechanics involved in making a request for information. The steps are simple but important: First, the researcher states the information completely and accurately, using the terms from *MeSH*, the medical subject headings. Next, the researcher manually searches the *Index Medicus* to identify publications whose bibliographies may be helpful. Third, the researcher carefully completes any further information required by the library.

MEDLARS and *MEDLINE* provide access to journals but not to books. A search of journals over the past 2 to 3 years is sufficient in most cases, although these data bases date back to 1963. The system is programmed to subjects, not authors. Authors, like books, theses, Ph.D. dissertations, and technical reports, require a manual search. *MEDLARS* is especially useful when coordinating several related subjects or finding citations on a single subject. It is important to note that precise information is required. Due to vague or improperly stated requests, many researchers have obtained long lists of citations not pertinent to their work. Consultation with the librarian beforehand saves later frustration, especially when the researcher is pressed for time. "Off-line" requests may take more than a week to process and mail.

Manual searches to identify relevant publications include an examination of the card catalog, indexes, abstracts, and various reference sources. It is helpful to begin a manual search by first consulting with the librarian, who will help familiarize the researcher with both the physical plan of the library and the resources available. The librarian will expedite the manual search within the local library and will arrange for an interlibrary loan of materials that the local library does not have.

The *card catalog* is an alphabetical arrangement of all of the publications held by a particular library. The catalog includes authors, subject headings, and publication titles. Authors are filed by surname, in alphabetical order, and by given name, where a number of surnames (such as *Smith*) are the same. When searching the card catalog, it is wise to have the author's complete name. Titles are filed by the first word, unless the first word is an article (such as *the* or *an*), in which case, the second word of the title is used. To locate publications by subject, the researcher begins with the broad heading such as *Nursing* and then looks for subcategories under the general term. Information on the card that helps identify pertinent work includes dates and places of publication, publisher, cross-references, number of pages, and call number. The call number is used to locate the book physically in the library. Two systems of call numbers are used: the *Dewey Decimal System* (numbers only), and the *Library of Congress System* (letters and numbers). To find materials not listed in the card catalog, the researcher turns to indexes, abstracts, directories, and bibliographies.

An *index* is a list of books and articles about topics; likewise, it is the list of authors and subjects commonly found in the back of a book. Nursing indexes include the *Nursing Studies Index*, by Virginia Henderson et al., a four-volume annotated index that lists all studies reported from 1900 to 1959. The *Cumulative Index to Nursing Literature* reports work from 1956 forward, while the *International Nursing Index* includes worldwide nursing literature from 1966 forward. Other indexes are published by various journals, such as *Nursing Research, Nursing Outlook,* and the *American Journal of Nursing.* The journal indexes are both annual and cumulative, combining subject and author listings. Other useful indexes are the monthly *Index Medicus,* whose January issue lists Medical Subjects Headings by name of article, author, and date; the *Abridged Index Medicus*; the *Science Citation Index,* which lists an author followed by those citing the author; and the *Hospital Literature Index.*

Abstracts are short statements giving the main ideas of an article or book. These have appeared in *Nursing Research* since 1959, the articles being classified by both author and subject headings. "Abstracts of Studies in Public Health Nursing, 1924–1965" appears in *Nursing Research* (Spring 1959, p. 45–115), listing monographs and articles from 21 periodicals. Other abstracts may be found in *Excerpta Medica, Psychological Abstracts,* and *Sociological Abstracts.*

Reference sources for nurses are found in *Nursing Outlook* (May 1972, "Reference Sources for Nurses," pp. 338–343) and in *Canadian Nursing* (March 1972, "Information Resources for Nursing Research," pp. 40–43). Other useful reference works include Blake and Roos' (eds.) *Medical Reference Works* (1967) and Gates' *Guide to the Use of Books and Libraries* (1969).

Once a list of useful books and articles is in hand, a search is made to locate and scrutinize these. It is always desirable to use primary sources whenever possible. *Primary sources* are first-hand accounts of events, such as diaries, patient charts, letters, eyewitness accounts, journals, autobiographies, research reports, and information collected by interview and questionnaire. *Secondary sources* are second-hand accounts, such as histories, biographies, textbooks, and other materials that give secondary analysis of the data found in primary records. The careful researcher never relies solely on secondary sources, although these often furnish valuable leads to primary works. If possible, the researcher reviews the primary work in order to judge and analyze the data. The use of primary sources acts as a check against errors that may have crept into a secondary source and that may have been perpetuated by dependence upon these sources alone.

Books and articles not available in local libraries may often be obtained by interlibrary loan. However, requests should be made early, since the process tends to be slow and since the time available to scrutinize these sources is limited.

The amount of time spent in a preliminary search of the literature varies according to the nature of the research study, the amount of material available, and the length of time that may reasonably be allocated to the search. For a circumscribed study of one year, four weeks may be all of the time available for both the preliminary search and the critical review of the literature. Such limitations should be kept clearly in mind, since it is easy to be led into interesting by-paths not strictly related to the research question.

Summarizing and Recording

Once the researcher identifies and locates the pertinent literature, then he or she makes a record of the sources studied and summarizes the pertinent information found in each. A systematic procedure for recording the information pays dividends in the long run, although it is a rare researcher that does not resort to scribbling on scraps of paper from time to time, only to regret it later when the scraps have disappeared.

The most common and useful method for recording bibliographical information is to write the complete information for each publication on a separate 3×5-inch card. Information should include: (1) the surname of the author or authors, followed by the complete given name; (2) the complete title and subtitle of the book or article; (3) the date, publisher, place of publication, and edition; (4) the journal in which the article appears, date in detail, and pages of the article; (5) the bibliography or index, whether or not it is present and extensive; and (6) the call number of the local library (a time-saver when the book must be checked in and out). The bibliography cards should be kept in alphabetical order in a permanent file specifically for that purpose. This file will then be available as a ready source to cite relevant work in the body of the research report, as well as in the final bibliography. It is also a resource that will grow over the years, as the researcher records new publications.

An orderly system must be devised for recording the substance of an article or book. A number of ways are useful, and individuals often devise their own unique system. The long-term benefits of establishing a concise, yet flexible, system are considerable. An author of many books and publications suggests the following system.* Obtain a number of 3×5 slips of pastel-colored paper or mark a number of 3×5-inch cards with a color code in the upper-right-hand corner, such as orange, blue, and green. Use the pale orange slips or cards marked with an orange marker only for direct quotes from the literature. When definitions of concepts are used or specific hypotheses are noted, direct quotes are especially necessary. Use blue slips to summarize information directly from an article or book, without criticism or comment. Use green slips to record insights, ideas, or criticisms of the publications (such original thoughts are often lost unless immediately documented). Use white slips for other researchers' criticisms of an article or book. This system is a foolproof one for avoiding the dangers of plagiarism, for separating the content of the book or article from the reader's opinion, and for preserving the insight and ideas of the reader.

Prepared index cards for literature reviews are also available from commercial sources. These cards have rows of holes around the edges, which may be coded and notched. Together with more complex coding schemes, these may be developed if the project is an extensive one and if the publications are numerous and broad. The most important approach is an orderly and systematic one that summarizes an article or book with the same format each time. This enables the researcher to make quick comparisons. The following system may be helpful:

1. To select a pertinent book or article from a general review of the literature, examine the book or article quickly. For a book, examine the title page, which gives the author's credentials; then scan the table of contents, the index, the bibliography, and the charts and tables. Read the preface rapidly to determine the author's purpose; then thumb through the chapters quickly to assess their substance. If the book is promising, keep it for a critical review. For an article, examine the author's credentials, quickly scan the problem statement and the hypotheses, and then focus on the methods of research used, especially how the sample was selected and the data analyzed. Read conclusions and summaries, and note the use of theory and of other research studies. Retain sound and pertinent literature for summary and critique.

2. To summarize and record information, first note the author, title of article, and year of publication. If further information is needed, this immediately refers the reader to the bibliography card.

3. Record information from a research report in the following order: (1) problem statement; (2) definition of concepts (direct quotes on orange-coded slips or cards); (3) hypotheses, if any; (4) theories or

---

*Personal advice from Professor Edgar Thompson of Duke University.

assumptions used; (5) method of research, including how the sample was drawn; (6) instruments and scales used; (7) type of research (descriptive or explanatory); (8) methods and findings of data analysis; (9) interpretation of data, especially whether hypotheses were supported or rejected; and (10) recommendations and suggestions for further research, if any. Make special note of implications for nursing practice or theory.

4. Note data that were *not* included, such as limitations that were not noted; means of establishing the validity and reliability of instruments that were not given; theory that was not used; or former studies that were not examined.

Comparison of Content

Upon completion of the summaries, the student can compare the different approaches of the individual scientist to the same problem. The definition of concepts, for example, not only reveals the degree of concensus among nursing scholars, but at the same time, enables the student to document the source of his or her own definitions. A comparison of the theory utilized helps uncover competing theories used to explain the same phenomenon —information that the student can include in his or her own review of the literature. Research reports, in addition, cite previous studies that support (or do not support) the selected theory and derived hypotheses.

A comparison of research designs allows the student to consider whether a qualitative or quantitative design, a survey (questionnaire or interview), a record review (historical or documentary approach), or an experiment is most suitable for the proposed project. Comparing the different designs also allows the student to compare the research method used to collect data—observation, questioning, measuring, or a combination of these. In addition, the student may find valid instruments and techniques of data analysis helpful in the proposed project. Data summaries from similar studies may provide a basis by which the student can compare findings from the proposed research project.

Finally, the student may find a study that seems appropriate to replicate—a considerable saving in time and effort. Replication has the added virtue of increasing the depth of research in a particular area of nursing.

SUMMARY

Review of the literature refers to an extensive, thorough, and systematic examination of publications relevant to the research project. Critical review refers to the process by which the student examines the strengths and weaknesses of appropriate publications. The student must first locate important publications and must then review these critically.

Review of the literature is necessary for the following reasons: to determine how well theory and research are developed in the field of study; to define concepts; to examine research designs, methods, scales, instruments, measures, and techniques of data analysis used by others; to identify a study for replication or comparison; to examine difficulties reported by others; to define ethical implications of similar studies; and to identify a guide to use in writing the research report.

The preliminary review consists of three steps: (1) to identify and obtain important publications; (2) to summarize and record relevant contents; and (3) to compare what is reported in publications.

Identification of important publications begins with the most recent publication in journals. The most rapid access to journal citations is by computer search, such as *MEDLARS* or *MEDLINE*. Other acronyms, such as *CATLINE*, refer to specific subject areas in published articles. Manual search of card catalogs, indices, abstracts, and reference sources is necessary to obtain other literature, such as books.

The researcher must devise an orderly system to summarize and record contents of the literature. Bibliographical cards are essential and may be supplemented by various systems of color coding by which to identify direct quotes, the researcher's own words and insights, and criticisms of the publications.

Comparison of the recorded summaries of the literature enables the researcher to: contrast definitions of concepts, uncover competing theories used to explain the same phenomenon, consider the various designs that have been utilized to study the same problem, examine different methods of data collection, and find valid instruments already developed.

EXAMPLE FROM NURSING RESEARCH

A Review of the Literature From a Research Report

Margaret Miles (1985): Emotional symptoms and physical health in bereaved parents. Nursing Research, 34, 76–81.

The author's purpose for this study was "to compare the emotional symptoms and physical health of parents whose children had died suddenly in an accident, parents whose children had died following a chronic disease, and nonbereaved parents." She begins by stating that the death of a family member is a major life-stress event and that the death of a child is one of the greatest stresses that it is possible to experience. Miles makes no explicit reference to theory, although she implicitly refers to "stress" theories. She notes that few studies have evaluated the physical or emotional symptomatology in bereaved parents, since much of the research has centered on widows and widowers.

Miles first reviews five publications of research that included adults who had lost a parent, spouse, or child. These concluded that parents whose child has died experience more somatization, depression, anger, guilt, and despair than those who lost a parent or spouse. A retrospective study found that a number of depressed psychiatric patients were parents of children who had died. Miles reports that much of the literature about parental grief following the death of an older child has focused on families of children who died of cancer. She cites three studies that indicate that the parents experienced a long period of mourning leading to individual and family problems. Four additional studies referred to coping patterns used during grief, but only one dealt with parental grief following accidental death, in spite of the fact that accidents are the leading cause of death in children. One interview was cited that studied parents following a child's death by drowning.

Next, the author reviews literature dealing with anticipatory grief, which occurs in cases of expected death. Seven publications were cited. One other study dealt with the length of grieving. Few studies apparently dealt with the sudden death of a child. Miles notes at the conclusion of the review of literature that the grief process of parents in the case of sudden death may be intense due to the type of death, suddenness of loss, resultant guilt feelings, and shattered expectations for the child. The grief process after a long-term chronic disease may be intensified because of factors such as the long course of the disease, the increasing amount of parental energy required, and stresses experienced during the terminal phase. Conclusions following the research project include the following: bereaved parents with higher concurrent life stresses and parents from a lower socioeconomic background were at higher risk of emotional symptomatology.

STUDY QUESTIONS

1. Discuss the reasons for beginning a research project with a review of the literature.
2. What is the meaning of a critical review of the literature?
3. What does *MEDLARS* mean? How is it used? If available, examine library resources.
4. Select two articles related to your research proposal or a nursing problem in which you are interested. Summarize the problem statement; the research proposal; objectives, if any; hypotheses, if any; methods of data collection; findings of the study; implications for nursing, and suggestions for further research. Does the article include a bibliography of current publications?
5. Visit your library and locate the card catalog, indexes, and abstracts in nursing, and discuss how to arrange interlibrary loans. Find out how to utilize other resources with the librarian.
6. Select an article from *Nursing Research* to criticize, noting both strengths and weaknesses.
7. Begin a bibliography of your own.

SELECTED SOURCES OF RESEARCH IN NURSING AND ALLIED FIELDS

I. Journals that publish reports of nursing and related research include:
   Administrative Science Quarterly
   Advances in Nursing Science
   American Journal of Public Health
   American Sociological Review
   Current Anthropology
   Hospitals (Journal of the American Hospital Association)
   Hospital Progress
   International Nursing Review
   Journal of Advanced Nursing
   Journal of Gerontologic Nursing
   Journal of Nurse-Midwifery
   Journal of Nursing Education
   Journal of Obstetric Gynecologic and Neonatal Nursing
   Medical Care
   Modern Hospital
   Nursing Clinics of North America
   Nursing Dimension
   Nursing Forum
   Nursing Outlook
   Nursing Research
   Nursing Science
   Public Health Reports
   Research in Nursing and Health
   The American Journal of Maternal Child Health
   The American Journal of Nursing
   Western Journal of Nursing Research

II. Abstracts and excerpts include the following:
   Abstracts on hospital management studies. *Quarterly Index*, University of
      Michigan. Available on request beginning with Vol. 1, No. 1, Sept. 1964.
   Abstracts of studies in public health nursing, 1924–1957. *Nursing Research*
      8:45–115, Spring 1959.
   Basic Reference Aids for Small Medical Libraries

III. Bibliographies useful in nursing research include:
   Bio-bibliography of Florence Nightingale; Bishop and Goldie, International
      Council of Nurses, 1962.
   Bibliographies of Nursing, prepared for and published by the National League
      for Nursing, 1957, 14 volumes; now out of print.
   Medical Behavioral Science, published and distributed by the University of
      Kentucky Press, Lexington, 1963. Contains a selected bibliography of
      cultural anthropology, social psychology, and sociology in medicine.
   Reference Tools for Nursing is a selected classified list of books, pamphlets,
      and periodicals prepared by the Interagency Council for Library Tools for
      Nursing, 1964.

IV. Dictionaries: *American Nurses' Dictionary.* Philadelphia: W. B. Saunders, 1949.

V. Encyclopedias: *The Encyclopedia of Nursing.* Philadelphia: W. B. Saunders, 1952, prepared under the supervision of Lucile Petry. Terms used in nursing tests analyzed.

VI. Guides to Library Resources: Strauch, K., and Brundage, D. *Guide to Library Resources for Nursing.* Norwalk, Conn.: Appleton-Century-Crofts, 1980. Includes annotated listings of publications in nursing, and library information.

VII. Handbooks: *Library Handbook for Schools of Nursing,* 1953; *National League for Nursing.* Makes recommendations on organizing and administering a nursing library.

VIII. Indexes
   American Journal of Nursing: Annual and Cumulative Indexes. Combined subject and author listings since 1900.
   Card catalog of the library books.
   Cumulative Index to Nursing Literature, subject and author guide to 54 periodicals in nursing and related fields since 1956.
   National Library of Medicine: nursing, hospital, books, studies, and technical reports.
   Nursing Outlook: Annual and Cumulative Indexes, combined subject and author listing since 1952.
   Nursing Research: Annual and Cumulative Indexes, combined subject and author listing.
   Nursing Studies Index, edited by Henderson, V. Philadelphia: J. B. Lippincott, 1963. Annotated guide to reported studies. Four volumes.
   Public Health Nursing, an index to ANA and NLN publications, government publications, pamphlets, and book reviews.
   Research Grants Index, yearly report by the Division of Research Grants describes current research projects being conducted under Public Health Service by subject matter, name and address, or principal investigator.
   International Nursing Index, includes world-wide nursing literature from 1966.

IX. Inventories and Lists
   Clearing House List of Studies in Nursing, since 1955 by ANA.
   The Nations's Nurses by Marshall and Moses. New York: ANA 1965.
   History of Nursing Source Book. New York: G. P. Putnam's Sons, 1957. Gives excerpts from writings on nursing from Biblical times.
   Nursing Research: A Survey and Assessment by Simmons, L. and Henderson, V. New York: Appleton-Century-Crofts, 1964. Describes the beginnings of nursing research, directions, and forces impeding or promoting development.
   Inventory of Social and Economic Research in Health, published annually by the Health Information Foundation, Chicago.

X. Statistical Guides
Facts About Nursing, published annually by the American Nurses' Association since 1935.
Statistical Abstract of the United States, published annually by the U.S. Government Printing Office, Washington, D.C.

XI. Yearbooks
The Yearbook of Modern Nursing, edited by Conway. New York: G. P. Putnam's Sons, 1959. Reviews literature on nursing trends, education, research, and practice.

REFERENCES AND SUGGESTED READINGS

Fox, D. (1976): Fundamentals of Research Nursing (3rd ed.). New York: Appleton-Century-Crofts, pp. 27–30.
Johnson, J. et al. (1977): Altering children's distress behavior during orthopedic cast removal. In Downs, F. and Newman, M. (eds.), A Sourcebook of Nursing Research (2nd ed.). Philadelphia: F. A. Davis, pp. 33–45.
Miles, M. (1985): Emotional symptoms and physical health in bereaved parents. Nursing Research, *34*, 76–81.
Polit, D. and Hungler, B. (1978): Nursing Research: Principles and Methods. Philadelphia: J. B. Lippincott. *Chapter 5 deals with locating and summarizing information.*
Stetler, C. and Marram, G. (1976): Evaluating research findings for applicability in practice. Nursing Outlook, *24*, 559–563.
Treece, E. and Treece, J. (1977): Elements of Research in Nursing (2nd ed.). St. Louis: C. V. Mosby, chap. 7, "The Library Search."
Walizer, M. and Wienir, P. (1978): Research Methods and Analysis. New York: Harper & Row, pp. 136–150.

9

How to Criticize a Research Report

As students complete their preliminary review of the literature, they become aware of differences among the research reports—both merits and shortcomings. Such evaluations, or critical reviews, allow the student to assess the strong and weak elements of others' research, thereby aiding a critical examination of her or his own.

While expertise in evaluation comes with experience, a number of scholars, such as Fleming and Hayter (1974), Fox (1982), Downs and Newman (1977), and Downs (1984), suggest guidelines that assist the beginning researcher's evaluation of research reports.

Evaluation is made of both the structure—how the report is put together and organized—and the content—the sum and substance of the research. Both the structure and the content of a research report depend, to some extent, upon the experience and qualifications of the author, as well as upon the nature of the research. For example, pioneering research differs from research that replicates an established study.

Upon completion of this chapter, the student should be able to: (1) evaluate the qualifications of an author; (2) assess the logic of a report's structure; (3) criticize the introduction to the research report; (4) evaluate the review of literature, the research design, and the research methods; (5) judge the analysis and interpretation of data; (6) evaluate the bibliography, abstract, and writing style demonstrated in the report; and (7) conduct a critical review of a selected research publication.

HOW TO CRITICIZE A RESEARCH REPORT

Evaluating the Qualifications of the Author

Brief biographical material often accompanies research reports and books. This information enables the student to judge the qualifications of the author. It is not realistic to expect the same kind of research from a beginner that one expects from an experienced professional engaged in a long-term research project. The reader, therefore, needs to evaluate the qualifications of the author and the nature of the research reported. A beginning researcher who designs a simple, yet important, project should receive higher marks than one who chooses a problem that is either too large or too complex.

The Structure of the Report

The way in which a report is organized may vary from one researcher to the next. However, in all cases, the organization should be logical. It should begin with a clear identification of what is to be studied and how and should end with a summary or conclusion recommending further study or application. Often, the report follows the sequence of steps taken in planning the research and in collecting and analyzing the data. The researcher adds the final steps (summary, conclusions, and recommendations) after interpreting the data analysis in light of the objectives, theoretical framework selected, and hypotheses. Therefore, the structure of the report is evaluated on the basis of its logical flow. Since the logic of the structure is intimately related to the content of the report, its content and structure are often evaluated together.

Criticizing the Introduction to the Research Report

The purpose of the introduction is to inform the reader what was studied and how, and why the topic is important to nursing. The statement describes who was studied—the target population—and how the sample was obtained from the population; and when and where the study took place. The purpose of the study—observation in order to know, predict, control, explain, or practice—often follows.

This statement should be evaluated on the basis of its clarity, conciseness, and comprehensiveness. The general area of the study should be focused on a specific problem that is feasible, related to available data, and ethically appropriate.

The introduction may also include definitions of concepts used in the research statement; the objectives of the study; and the hypotheses, assumptions, and limitations of the study. However, the author may place these separately, immediately following the introduction.

The reader evaluates the concepts on the basis of their definition.

The definition must be clear and appropriate and must be rooted in the literature. The definition of variables is judged on the basis of how clearly the dependent and independent variables, and the operational definitions, are defined. The researcher should make the variables observable and measurable.

The reader evaluates the objectives on the basis of their ability to communicate the intent of the researcher, whether to inform (define, identify, name); to analyze (compare, contrast, distinguish); to classify (organize, systematize); or to interpret (differentiate, discriminate, explain). The objectives are also judged on the basis of their ability to denote measurable attributes of the study, while the author is evaluated on the basis of how well he or she met the objectives or explained what prevented the objectives from being met.

Hypotheses are evaluated on the basis of: (1) a clear prediction of the relationship between variables; (2) the clarity and conciseness of each statement; (3) the identification of the independent and dependent variables; (4) the theory or previous research to which they were related; (5) their relationship with the author's research statement; and (6) whether the author reached definite conclusions on each.

The assumptions are evaluated on the basis of their stated source; whether the opinion of experts, previous research reports, or theory. The reader also evaluates the assumptions in terms of their foundations. Limitations, aspects of the research that were not studied, are evaluated on the ability of the author to recognize factors that limit the applicability of the research findings.

Evaluating the Review of the Literature

The review of the literature is judged on the basis of its organization, comprehensiveness, and summary of opposing theory and research findings. The reader should also judge the extent to which the author used primary sources. The author should also be evaluated on the basis of his or her grasp of the breadth and depth of the literature review pertinent to the problem under study.

Judging the Research Design

The research design is evaluated on the basis of both ethical aspects and appropriateness. An experimental design should include methods of sampling, control, and manipulation. The reader evaluates the survey design according to the method used to select the sample, the worth of the instruments used, and the quantity and quality of response. A study of records and documents (historical design) is evaluated on the basis of: (1) the accuracy of the records—whether the recorder was willing and able to write observations accurately; (2) the completeness of the records— whether any records were lost or destroyed; and (3) access to the records—the extent to which the author had full entrance to the records. Historical research is open to more interpretation than any other type of research. Therefore, the reputation and credentials of the author should be carefully evaluated.

Evaluating Research Methods

The research methods are the means by which the author collects research data from the study sample; they include observation, measurement, questioning, and sampling.

Observing. The author should make clear whether he or she was a participant observer or a nonparticipant observer and whether or not he or she was the sole observer. The author who relies upon personal observations must be judged on how well he or she defined what was to be observed, made objective rather than subjective observations, and related the observations to the research project. The author must reveal whether the subjects being studied were informed or whether concealment was used; the latter suggests ethical implications that must be judged. The author who was assisted by other observers must document how these were trained; the reader must also assess the adequacy of the training. Finally, a judgment of the biases introduced by the human observer must be made, including both the selective attention of the observer and the effect of observation on those observed.

Measuring. An evaluation of measurement is often a complex task, since the reader must judge whether the correct instrument was used in the measurement and whether the author measured what should have been measured in order to answer the research question. One group of researchers (Johnson et al., 1977, pp. 33–44), for example, wanted to measure children's distress behavior during orthopedic-cast removal. Johnson used pulse rate, and verbal and nonverbal behavior as measures of distress. The reader must judge whether these factors do indeed measure distress and if this is what should have been measured.

In addition, the reader must evaluate attitude scales, questionnaires, and interview schedules used by the author. Since these rarely accompany research reports, the reader must rely on the author to report how it was determined that these were good measures. Physiological instruments (such as the sphygmomanometer, thermometer, and scales that weigh pounds and ounces) are more familiar measures, but the author should report how it was determined that such measures were accurate. The reader should expect the author to give a clear description of the instrument, to report whether the instrument had been tested, and to describe how the instrument was used. The reader should also evaluate the use of the subject's time in conjunction with a particular instrument—both the merits of the instrument and the amount of time required from the subjects should be clearly reported. Failure of the author to describe instruments and to explain how and why each was used (and pretested) marks the study as ineffective.

Questioning. Asking questions directly by interview or indirectly by questionnaire are common ways to collect data. Questioning is evaluated in terms of the instruments used (the questionnaire and interview schedule), which should be described by the author if not included within the report. If interviews were used, the author should report how interviewers were trained. If questionnaires were used, the author should report the number returned and the extent to which all questions were answered. Subjects who refused to participate should also be noted.

Sampling. *Sampling* is the method by which the study subjects were selected from the target population. Sampling is a critical aspect of research determining the extent to which the study-sample data may be generalized to the larger population. The data-collection methods and the sample-selection methods must each be carefully evaluated. These procedures are critical for evaluating whether the research findings can be applied in general or only in reference to the small sample studied. The author must have chosen the sample by a scientific process, such as random sampling (each unit in the target population is given an equal chance of being chosen), in order to be assured that the sample represents the population. Therefore, the procedures for selecting the sample of study subjects should be carefully described, as should the size and characteristics of the sample. Failure to report sampling procedures greatly weakens any research report.

Criticism of the Analysis and Interpretation of Data

The analysis of data is dependent upon all that has gone on before: how the sample was drawn, the use of controls, the type of scale utilized, and whether hypotheses were supported and objectives were met. The reader judges whether the author has included: (1) a complete discussion of the data; (2) a thorough examination of each hypothesis, including the use of appropriate statistical analysis and the decision to accept or reject the hypothesis; (3) an explanation of how missing data were handled; (4) presentation of data in tables and graphs, together with a description of each; and (5) the use of experts where needed to assist in the analysis of data.

The reader must judge whether the author interpreted the data properly. Each hypothesis or objective should be discussed in light of the research findings reported in the review of the literature. Authors should make clear whether the findings of their studies agree or disagree with previous reports; should state which relationships have been illuminated by their studies, and should report to what extent their findings can be generalized.

In addition, the reader judges an author on the report's relevance to nursing. The significance of the study should be clear, and the author should likewise suggest what further research needs to be conducted.

Evaluation of the Bibliography, Abstract, and Writing Style

The bibliography reflects the review of the literature, the search for valid and reliable instruments, definitions of concepts, formulation of the research statement, the objectives, the hypotheses, and any other material used in the content. Each reference cited in the body of the report should be included in the bibliography. The bibliography should be presented in a consistent and acceptable form and, if time and space allow, annotations should be included. If appendices are used, these should be concise, complete, and well-organized.

The abstract, a brief summary of the research article, is often required for publication. The abstract should clearly describe what was studied, how it was studied, how the sample was drawn, how the data were analyzed, and the findings of the research—all in one concise paragraph.

The reader should also judge the writing style of the author. If the research has considerable merit but the writing style is poor, the labor and care of the project may be all but lost. However, criticism of the writing style should not be confused with criticism of the research itself. Effective communication of research depends upon the author's ability to organize and to write clearly and objectively.

SUMMARY

A criticism of research articles entails evaluating the following: the qualifications of the author to undertake the research; the logical structure of the entire report; the importance of its contents; and the kind of research that is being reported, whether descriptive, experimental, a survey, or other kind. In addition, each part of the report should be judged, including the extent to which the introduction informs the reader of what the author has studied and of its importance to nursing; the clarity and brevity of the problem statement; whether the author refers to the literature in the definition of concepts; the objectives of the researcher or, if hypotheses are used instead, the quality, clarity, and relevance of the statement of hypotheses.

Moreover, the critic judges the report on the basis of whether there is a clear explication of the variable; whether the operational definitions make the variables observable and measurable; whether the assumptions of the researcher are stated; and the theoretical perspective noted. The critic also judges how well the author has reviewed the literature—both the comprehensiveness and the types of publications used, whether primary or secondary sources. Criticisms also involve judging the research design, the research methods, and the method of sampling—whether it allows the researcher to generalize the findings. The critic must also judge the method of data collection—whether it was ethical and proper. The critic must judge the analysis and interpretation of data; and whether the author has completely discussed the data, tested the hypotheses, presented the data in tables and graphs, used experts to assist in statistical analysis where necessary, and explained how missing data were handled. An evaluation of the data interpretation involves a judgment of how the author compared the findings of the research with those of other studies reported in the literature. The critic must also judge whether the author generalized from the sample to the target population properly and reported the limitations, weaknesses, and strengths of the research. The critic must also note whether the author discussed implications for nursing, recommended further research, and noted possible applications for practice.

To criticize the bibliography, the reviewer must examine the extent and date of the publication and whether all works cited in the report were included in the bibliography. The critic must likewise judge whether the abstract is clear and succinct and whether the writing style is well-organized and objective.

EXAMPLES FROM NURSING LITERATURE

A Research Critique

Florence Downs (1984): Elements of a research critique. In Downs, F. (ed.), A Source Book of Nursing Research (3rd ed.). Philadelphia: F. A. Davis.

Downs divides the research critique into seven subtitles:

    I. The problem statement, terms, and hypotheses;
    II. The review of literature and theoretical rationale for the study;
    III. The population and sample;
    IV. Instrumentation;
    V. Procedure for data collection;
    VI. Analysis of data; and
    VII. Conclusions and implications.

She suggests that the reader/critic of a research report ask a number of questions under each of the seven parts as the article is being reviewed.

Part One: the problem statement, terms, and hypotheses. Downs asks six questions to evaluate the worth of this section:

1. Is the general problem introduced promptly?
2. Has the problem been substantiated with adequate background and need for the study?
3. Has the general problem been narrowed down to a specific research problem or to a problem with subproblems, as appropriate?
4. Are the terms of the problem defined both conceptually and operationally?
5. Do the hypotheses directly answer the research problems?
6. Are the hypotheses specific to one relationship, so that they can be either supported or not supported?

Part Two: the review of the literature and theoretical rationale. Downs asks three questions:

1. Was there a sufficient review of the literature or theoretical rationales so that the reader could be assured that the investigator had considered a broad spectrum of possibilities for investigating the problem?
2. Is the theoretical rationale for the hypotheses explicit?
3. Is it clear how the study will extend previous findings?

Part Three: population and sample. Downs asks seven questions to judge the worth of the population and sample selected by the researcher:

1. Are the parameters of the study population specific enough so that it is clear to what population the findings may be generalized?
2. Is the sample representative of the population as defined?
3. Would it be possible to replicate the study population?
4. Is the method of sample selection appropriate?
5. What bias, if any, is introduced by this method?
6. What evidence is presented that indicates that the rights of the study's subjects have been protected?
7. Is the sample size appropriate? How is it substantiated?

Part Four: instrumentation. Downs asks two questions here:

1. Are the methods of collecting data appropriate to the study? Do they actually obtain the data that the investigator seeks?
2. Is the investigator specific regarding the validity and reliability of the instruments used?

Part Five: procedure for data collection. Downs asks four questions:

1. What steps were taken to control for extraneous variables?
2. Were the treatment conditions distinctly different and replicable?
3. Is the strength of the independent variable sufficient to overcome concomitant influences?
4. In a laboratory study, is the manipulated variable a valid representation of reality?

Part Six: analysis of data. Downs asks three questions:

1. Are the analyses reported clearly related to each hypothesis?
2. Is it clear what statistical test was used and what values were obtained?
3. Is there a statement of whether or not the data support the hypotheses?

Part Seven: conclusions and implications. Downs asks five questions:

1. Did the investigator relate the findings to the theoretical position of the study?
2. Did the investigator identify methodological problems?
3. Did the investigator overgeneralize?
4. What are the implications of the findings for practice?
5. Are there suggestions for further research?

STUDY QUESTIONS

1. Select an article from *Nursing Research*, *Research in Nursing and Health*, the *Western Journal of Nursing Research*, or the *International Journal of Nursing Studies*. Utilizing the guides in this chapter, criticize the article, noting its strengths and weaknesses.
2. What part of the selected research report do you find the most interesting? The most important?
3. Why is it important to know the credentials of the author of a research report?
4. Why do you think Downs asked so many questions of some parts of the research report and so few of others?

REFERENCES AND SUGGESTED READINGS

Downs, F. (1984): Elements of a research critique. In Downs, F. and Newman, M. (eds.), A Sourcebook of Nursing Research (2nd ed.). Philadelphia: F. A. Davis, pp. 1–15.

Downs, F. and Newman, M. (1977): A Sourcebook of Nursing Research. Philadelphia: F. A. Davis.

Fleming, J. and Hayter, J. (1974) Reading research reports critically. Nursing Outlook, *22*, 172–176.

Fox, D. (1982): Fundamentals of Research in Nursing (4th ed.). Norwalk, Conn.: Appleton-Century-Crofts, Chap. 7.

Johnson, J. et al. (1977): Altering children's distress behavior during orthopedic cast removal. In Downs, F. and Newman, M. (eds.), A Sourcebook of Nursing Research (2nd ed.). Philadelphia: F. A. Davis, pp. 33–44.

Leininger, M. (1968): The research critique: Nature, function and art. In Batey,

M. (ed.), Communicating Nursing Research: The Research Critique. Boulder: WICHE, pp. 21–23.

Polit, D. and Hungler, B. (1983): Nursing Research. Philadelphia: J. B. Lippincott, Chap. 26.

Polit, D. and Hungler, B. (1985): Essentials of Nursing Research. Philadelphia: J. B. Lippincott, pp. 366–380. *Presents a fictitious research report for criticism.*

Stetler, C. and Marram, G. (1976): Evaluating research findings for applicability in practice. Nursing Outlook, *24,* 559–563.

Walizer, M. and Wienir, P. (1978): Research Methods and Analysis. New York: Harper & Row, pp. 136–150.

PART IV

Research Designs

10

Qualitative and Quantitative Research Designs

Research design refers to the way in which the researcher plans and structures the research process. The design provides flexible guideposts that keep the research headed in the right direction. There is no such thing as one correct design—designs vary from one study to another. Each researcher chooses the design that is most useful for her or his research purpose—whether to observe in order to know, to know in order to predict, or to predict in order to control or prescribe.

If the purpose of the research is to observe, describe, explore, and assemble new knowledge, a descriptive or exploratory design is used. The documentary, or historical, design is used to describe or compare data collected in the past. If the purpose is to predict a causal relationship between variables or to establish correlations, an experimental or correlational study design is used. The survey design is used to obtain information from the self-reports of people in the natural setting in order to provide either quantitative or qualitative descriptions or to discover relationships. Secondary analysis, the use of available research data, is used to obtain new information from data already scientifically collected for another study. A methodological research design is used to describe, develop, test, or evaluate research instrumentation. In addition, the overall approach of a research design may be classified as qualitative, quantitative, or a combination of the two.

This chapter begins with a comparison of the major levels and types of research designs used in the nursing literature. Next, qualitative and quantitative designs will be defined and examined. In the following three chapters, specific designs will be studied: Chapter 11 describes the descriptive and historical designs; Chapter 12 examines the experimental and quasi-experimental designs; and Chapter 13 recounts the survey, ex-post-facto, correlational, and other designs found in nursing research literature.

Upon completion of the chapter, students should be able to: (1) compare the major research designs and levels of research used in nursing research; (2) describe what distinguishes the experimental, descriptive, historical, and survey designs: (3) define major concepts used in the various research designs; (4) define and compare the qualitative and quantitative designs; and (5) analyze an example from nursing research so as to identify elements of both designs.

OVERVIEW OF RESEARCH DESIGNS

Levels of Research Designs Identified by Nursing Scholars

Levels refers to a hierarchy from the most basic to the most complex (Diers, 1979, p. 51). Use of "levels" in research designs is found in Diërs (1979) and in Brink and Wood (1978).

Diers, who worked with the philosophers Dickoff and James, draws on their four levels of theory to develop four levels of research designs with accompanying questions, as follows: At Level 1, the research asks the question "What is this?"; the research design is exploratory, formulative, descriptive, or factor-searching; and the theory is naming theory. At Level 2, the researcher asks "What's happening here?"; the research design is exploratory, descriptive, or relation-searching; and the theory is factor-relating or one that describes. At Level 3, the researcher asks "What will happen if . . .?"; the design is one that tests either associations or causal hypotheses, including: correlational designs, surveys, natural experiments, experiments, nonexperimental, explanatory, or predictive; and the theory is one from which predictions may be derived. At Level 4, the researcher asks "How can I make . . . happen?"; the design is one to test prescriptions; and the theory is prescriptive. Diers writes that the purpose or goal of nursing research is the improvement of patient care; therefore, the approach to nursing research is different from the conventional path of research, whose purpose is "only the discovery and testing of knowledge."

Brink and Wood (1983, pp. 91–95) identify three levels of research, with accompanying questions and designs: At Level 1, the researcher asks "What?" questions, and the research design is exploratory-descriptive. At Level 2, the researcher asks "What are the relationships?", and the research design is a descriptive survey. At Level 3, the researcher asks "Why?" questions, and the research design is experimental.

Levels (or stages) of research designs, questions, and theories are evolutionary or developmental approaches—each stage is thought to have evolved from the prior stage. This seems to be an organized and logical approach to research, especially in disciplines that are familiar with a developmental approach. However, Simon (1978, p. 120) sounds a warning about over-reliance on stages. Writing specifically about descriptive research, he notes that it is unsound to view descriptive research as only a stage in the research process, for two reasons: First, descriptive research is of important scientific value in itself. Putting it at the bottom level may suggest that it is of less importance (or is less developed, or evolved) than higher stages. Second, he notes that there is no solid evidence for an evolutionary view of research stages that suggests that one stage evolves out of another. This is a consideration worth keeping in mind— a research design is only a guide, not an imperative.

A Comparison of Selected Designs

Fox (1982, pp. 137ff) writes that research designs such as the experimental, the historical, and the survey, may be distinguished from one another on the basis of several characteristics. These include: (1) the control that the researcher has over the data; (2) the time framework used; (3) the setting; (4) how the sample is selected; and (5) how the data are collected. Each of these will be examined in turn.

Control is the ability to regulate and check each element of the research process. This includes the manipulation of the independent variable (the cause, the experimental treatment) and the use of random sampling, both to select study subjects or objects and to assign these to either an experimental group or a control group. Control is a crucial part of the experimental design. In contrast, control is not a significant factor in either the historical or the descriptive design, since neither has a set of clearly delineated variables to control. In the survey design, the researcher has less control than is found in the experiment but considerably more than is found in either the descriptive or historical design. For example, in survey designs, the researcher controls the construction of the instruments that generate data (the questionnaire and interview schedule) and can use techniques of random sampling to select the study subjects from whom the data are generated. Thus, the researcher usually exerts maximum control in the experimental design, minimum control in the historical and descriptive designs, and varying levels of control in the survey design.

The *time framework* refers to the orientation in time that various designs use. The experimental design utilizes hypotheses that predict what the researcher will find upon observation—a future orientation. In contrast, the historical design seeks to cast light upon the present by a study of the past. The survey may combine features of the present, the past, and the future. The survey collects data from contemporary populations—a present orientation—but study subjects may be asked to recall past behavior and attitudes and to predict what their future behavior will be. The descriptive design, on the whole, depends upon the collection of current observations.

Setting refers to the place where the research data are collected. The true experiment usually takes place in the laboratory or in a similar setting, where the greatest control can be maintained. In contrast, the survey design utilizes a natural setting, where the respondents behave in their usual ways. The setting for historical data is in the past, although data must be collected from existing repositories of documents. The setting for the collection of descriptive data is limited only by the researcher's interest.

Sampling is the process of selecting a portion of a target population for study. The target population is defined as the entire set of subjects or objects that have a characteristic in common. In the experimental design, careful random sampling is critical if the researcher is to ensure that the findings from the experimental sample apply to the population from which the sample was drawn; this is also true of the survey design. In contrast, researchers who utilize the historical design often attempt to utilize *all* pertinent materials; i.e., the total population or universe of data that describes what has happened in the past. Sampling may be impossible in the descriptive research design, which seeks new knowledge, since the nature of the population may not be known.

The *data-collection process* refers to the way in which the researcher collects data—whether by observation, questioning, measuring, or a combination of the three. The experimental design must ensure that standard procedures for observing, questioning, and measuring are rigorously used so that all data are collected under similar circumstances by trained personnel. In contrast, the historical and descriptive designs often use whatever method is the most fruitful for data collection, including structured and unstructured approaches, as well as any other ethical means that allow new knowledge to be documented. The researcher who uses the survey design seeks consistency in data collection, although both structured and unstructured questions may be used.

The relationship and relative worth of qualitative and quantitative designs have become topics of debate among nursing scholars. The *humanistic approach*, which utilizes a qualitative research design, stresses the study and understanding of the symbols and values of humankind. Those who hold this view are concerned about the difficulty of quantifying complex phenomena, such as the relationship of one human being to another, to nature, and to the supernatural. In contrast, those who take a *scientific approach* argue that most things can be quantified, that the scientific method of selecting a sample, observing, collecting data objectively, and analyzing data statistically is the only scientific way to ensure validity and reliability.

However, Goodwin and Goodwin (1984) write that several myths have evolved concerning the differences between qualitative and quantitative research. One myth suggests that qualitative and quantitative designs are mutually exclusive, but in actual practice, research designs may sometimes be qualitative, sometimes quantitative, and sometimes a combination of both. Other myths suggest that qualitative and quantitative designs differ in the place where the research occurs, the amount of control that the researcher has over the variables, how the data are observed— whether subjectively or objectively, obtrusively or unobtrusively—and in the analysis of data. However, in actual fact, research designs may often be mixed. The researcher who uses a qualitative design may include quantitative features, such as standardized formats, plans for the production of quantitative numerical data, and plans to enhance validity and reliability through the use of multiple methods of data collection and of multiple recorders of data. At the same time, Goodwin and Goodwin note that the researcher who utilizes a quantitative design, which (according to the myth) is always controlled, obtrusive, and objective, may be none of these things in actual fact.

However, it is possible for the student to define the characteristics of polar types of research—either qualitative or quantitative—and then to identify when particular characteristics may be mixed in a research design.

QUALITATIVE AND QUANTITATIVE DESIGNS

A *qualitative research design* is one in which the researcher plans to observe, discover, describe, compare, and analyze the characteristic attributes, themes, and underlying dimensions of a particular unit. The researcher may study a process (decision making); a subject (chronic disease); a group (a family); a community (the Twin Poplars community); or a culture (the Navaho). For example, Phillips and Rempusheski (1985), noting that there were no empirical data on the subject, conducted a study to describe how health-care providers conceptualize the abuse and neglect of the aged. Utilizing a method described by Glaser and Strauss (1967) and, more recently, by Stern (1980), the researchers collected the data through the use of an open-ended interview schedule, tape-recording the responses of 29 health-care providers. At the same time, the researchers concurrently coded and analyzed the data. The purpose of the study was to formulate a conceptual model that described the decision-making processes that health-care providers used to identify poor-quality relationships between the elderly and those who give them care.

A *quantitative design* is one concerned with measurement—measuring the magnitude, size, or extent of a phenomenon. The quantitative design counts, measures, and analyzes data statistically. For example, Farr et al. (1984) studied the relationship between hospital stress and the timing of circadian rhythms. The experimental group consisted of 11 consenting surgery patients and a control group of age- and sex-matched control subjects. Theories of stress and physiology were used to create hypotheses and to identify the variables that were to be measured by observation and by the use of laboratory testing. Statistical methods of analysis were used.

Qualitative and quantitative research designs may be depicted as polar types of research projects, with research designs that mix both qualitative and quantitative elements falling in between the two poles (see Fig. 10–1). Although most designs are mixed, features of the two designs may be examined with reference to: (1) methods of reasoning that are or can be used; (2) techniques for data collection; (3) types of designs that include more of either the qualitative or the quantitative features; and (4) types of data analysis frequently used by each.

Features of Qualitative Designs

The researcher who uses the qualitative design plans to examine the properties, traits, and features that distinguish the subjects of research from one another. The qualitative design is structured to look for what

Extreme Example of Qualitative Design	Mixture of both designs falls between the two extremes	Extreme Example of Quantitative Design
—Little information available		—Sufficient information to identify measures that will be used before or after observation
—Purely descriptive designs		—Designs that measure
—Setting selected by interest		—Setting where measurements can be best controlled
—Techniques often center on first-time participant observation		—Techniques center on all approaches that can be counted and/or measured
—Inductive reasoning from observations		—Deductive reasoning from theory
—Sample selected by availability		—Random sampling used
		—Hypotheses/variables stated
		—Variables to be measured, defined by operational definition before observation
—Data analyzed by content analysis and comparison		—Data analyzed by descriptive and inferential statistics
—Concepts invented after observation, classification, and naming		—Hypothesis accepted or rejected following statistical testing

Figure 10–1. Polar characteristics of qualitative and quantitative research designs.

is special and different—what distinguishes the case or group, what characterizes the community and its values. The design includes the following features: (1) methods of reasoning; (2) methods for data collection; (3) types of designs; and (4) methods of analysis of data. Each of these will be examined in turn.

1. *The method of reasoning in the qualitative design is usually inductive.* For example, the researcher who uses the descriptive case study design starts with observation and may end with a description of what has been observed; or, the researcher may continue with analysis so as to create one or more empirical generalizations and may then move to formulate a theory to explain what has been observed. However, Simon (1978) writes that deductive reasoning based on sound premises can be more accurate than the empirical research data from which inductive reasoning proceeds. A critical point in the use of deductive reasoning is that the researcher must be aware of the particular risk involved—the initial assumption or premise may be faulty. If the assumption is faulty, all subsequent reasoning is faulty. For example, a qualitative research design is faulty if it begins with the assumption that a patient views the world in the same way that the nurse-observer does. The view of the patient—the emic, or subjective, view—expresses what the situation means to the patient. The view of the nurse—the etic, or objective, view—expresses what the situation means to the observer. These may be, and usually are, two different views. Therefore, the researcher must be aware of the risks involved when assumptions are used to guide the deductions of the researcher. To help overcome the risks, the assumptions must be well-founded, well-documented, and well-established in the literature. Often, so little information may exist in a qualitative study that the researcher is forced to begin with observation, although the experience and education of the researcher precedes the observations and colors what is observed.

2. *Methods for data collection in the qualitative design include participant observation, the opinion of experts, content analysis, and simulation.*
   a. *Participant observation* is a method whereby the researcher becomes totally immersed in the study of a group or culture, participating while observing and faithfully recording what has been observed through the use of field notes, tape recorders, and filming. It is a technique long used by anthropologists and is useful for nurses who wish to combine research and practice (as long as ethical implications are resolved). Designs using this technique expect the researcher to spend months or years living and working with the group under study in order to observe and record new, rich, and varied data.

b. *The opinion of experts* is a technique used by the researcher to identify important patterns or features of the culture. Persons born or reared in the group or experts on the topic under study are valuable sources of clues and general guidance. Opinions of experts may be either a central part of the design or a possible shortcut to important material.

c. *Content analysis* is a method of both data collection and data analysis. The researcher first identifies the material to be analyzed—whether conversation, interview, or the content of the media (including advertisements, speeches, articles, magazines, or television shows)—and then classifies and summarizes the findings.

d. *Simulation* has a variety of definitions but basically manipulates a model of reality through the use of various artifacts, such as mannequins to simulate patients, or games or computers to "play like" reality. For example, Hamm & Brodt (1982) used simulation and gaming to teach male juvenile delinquents how to use assertiveness skills to cope with real-life interpersonal situations. Simulation can be an advantage in nursing research when real-life conditions do not permit ethical manipulation. However, the value of simulation is in direct proportion to the quality of the reality in the data used.

3. *Types of research designs that are purely qualitative include all those designs that seek to collect and describe new observations where little or no prior information exists.* The researcher creates a design that plans for observation, questioning, description, exploration, or all of these, in order to assemble new knowledge. Major examples of qualitative designs include: (1) the descriptive or exploratory design; (2) the historical or documentary design; and (3) survey designs which include qualitative data from unstructured questions on a questionnaire or interview schedule.

The descriptive or exploratory design may be either a case study design that plans to describe a single unit; a comparative design to compare and contrast several units or cases; a classification study design to put observations and descriptions into categories; or a design which plans to name or formulate new concepts. The historical-documentary design differs from the descriptive design in that the information already exists, but the researcher must plan to find the material in public or private documents, or in the mass media. Unstructured questions on a questionnaire or interview schedule are those which ask the respondent to answer a question in his or her own words.

4. *Methods of analyzing data obtained by a qualitative design center upon content analysis; cross-cultural comparison; the identifica-*

tion of new concepts; and, if possible, the use of inductive reasoning to create an empirical generalization that states the relationship between two concepts. Content analysis is a systematic method for analyzing both the written or spoken language, as well as visual materials. The researcher usually begins by a careful review of either his or her own documented data or, if a historical-documentary approach has been used, the observations of others found in the literature, public or private documents, or the media. Next, the researcher may focus on the messages that are being sent by subjects' behavior, and by the spoken or written language. The researcher describes and analyzes who sent and received the message; how the message was sent; the content of the message; the meaning or intent of the message; and the effects of the message. Then the researcher attempts to identify general patterns found in the data, such as themes, trends, attitudes, and needs of an individual, group or society. Next, the researcher either finds concepts in the literature which stand for the observed patterns, or in the absence of established concepts, the researcher formulates new concepts to stand for categories of observations. Finally, the researcher attempts to state a relationship between two of the concepts (an empirical generalization), and if possible, offer an explanation for the interrelationship between two or more empirical generalizations.

Cross-cultural analysis is a procedure in which the researcher uses data from one or more groups or cultures as a basis for comparative analysis. For example, Glittenberg (1978) studied two agrarian villages in highland Guatemala to examine patterns of child rearing.

Features of Quantitative Designs

The researcher who uses a quantitative design plans, from the beginning, to count and measure data. This requires both that the data be observable and measurable and that instruments exist (or can be invented) by which to measure the data.

1. *Methods of reasoning in quantitative designs include both deductive and inductive reasoning.* Commonly, *deductive reasoning* begins with a well-established theory from which hypotheses are deduced in order to predict what will be found on observation. The hypotheses identify the concepts or variables to be measured, and the operational definition transforms the unobservable concept into one that is observable and measurable. *Inductive reasoning* begins with observation. To introduce measurement into observations, the researcher must have some idea of what is to be observed, either from reading primary documents that describe

what others have observed or from the researcher's own experience. Where observations are totally new, the researcher may have to first go through a period of observation and reasoning before identifying what can be measured.

2. *Techniques for data collection include all approaches that can be quantified.* If deductive reasoning has been used, the researcher knows what is to be observed and must locate the specific instruments needed to measure. Instrumentation includes, not only the human sensory organs, but all technology that extends the senses and is capable of counting or measuring data (such as the sphygmomanometer, electronic counting devices, biochemical testing, and scales of all sorts, both mechanical and paper-and-pencil types).

3. *Types of quantitative designs include all designs that involve plans for the collection of numerical data.* This includes relationships such as quantities, degrees, and/or extent of observation. Counting is a basic component; comparison requires standard units of measurement and instruments by which to obtain the numerical data. Scales may include both those with equal intervals (such as a thermometer or a weight-and-height scale) or scales with "equal-appearing intervals" (such as attitude scales that seek to measure the number of objects that agree or disagree with statements). However, the only numerical data to be collected from attitude scales would be those that result from counting the frequency with which respondents either agree or disagree.

4. *Quantitative data analysis utilizes numerous statistical techniques to summarize and interpret quantitative data.* Techniques include the use of descriptive statistics and inferential statistics. *Descriptive statistics*—statistics that describe and summarize data—include counting frequencies; the use of percentages; measures of central tendency, such as averages; and measures of variability, such as the numerical range and standard deviation. These techniques are often the first steps that the researcher utilizes to describe, summarize, and organize the mass of numerical data. *Inferential statistics*—statistics that permit the researcher to judge or infer whether relationships found in a sample are likely to be found in the population from which the sample was drawn—are based on the data collected from samples that have been selected by random sampling (giving every unit in the population an equal chance of being chosen for the research sample). Procedures include techniques to test hypotheses. This enables the researcher to generalize findings from the sample studied to the population from which the sample was drawn.

SUMMARY

Research design refers to the way in which the researcher plans and structures the research process. It is a set of flexible guideposts designed to keep the research headed in the right direction. Levels of research designs identified in the nursing literature are structured by the type of questions asked. At Level 1, the researcher asks "What is this?", and the research design is exploratory, formulative, or descriptive. At Level 2, the researcher asks "What are the relations?", and the research design is exploratory, descriptive, or a descriptive survey. At Level 3, the researcher asks "How are dependent variables caused?", or "How are factors correlated?", or "Why?", and the research design is one that tests association or causal hypotheses, including correlational designs, surveys, natural experiments, experiments, nonexperiments, and designs that explain or predict. At Level 4, the researcher deals with application: "How can I apply research findings?", and the design is one that tests nursing prescriptions.

Research designs may be compared with one another on the basis of the extent to which control is exerted; the time framework (whether present, past, or future); the setting (whether in a laboratory or a natural setting); the sampling process (whether by random sampling or another type); and the data-collection process (whether by observation, questioning, measuring, or a combination of these).

The relationship between qualitative and quantitative designs has become a topic of debate in nursing but, according to some scholars, myths have evolved concerning the differences between the two that are refuted in actual practice.

Qualitative and quantitative research designs differ, in that qualitative designs are often developed when little information is available on a topic. The researcher plans to look for and describe attributes, themes, and underlying dimensions of a particular unit in order to discover what distinguishes the characteristics or attributes of the unit. The quantitative design aims to measure the magnitude, size, or extent of the units. Although polar types of qualitative and quantitative designs may be developed, many designs contain features of both.

Features of qualitative designs include the method of reasoning, which is usually inductive but which may include deduction; methods for data collection, such as participant observation or the opinions of experts; content analysis; and simulation. Features of quantitative designs include the use of both inductive and deductive reasoning—inductive reasoning to identify what has been observed that can be counted or measured; deductive reasoning to create hypotheses in order to predict what will be measured. Techniques for the collection of numerical data include all approaches that can be quantified, using instruments to supplement the human sense organs, such as machines, electronic counting devices, biochemical testing, and scales of all sorts. Types of quantitative designs include all those that collect numerical data. Quantitative data analysis utilizes both descriptive and inferential statistics. Descriptive statistics include statistics that describe and summarize data, such as percentages, averages, and standard deviations. Inferential statistics are those that permit the researcher to judge whether the relationships between variables found in a sample are likely to be found in the population from which the sample was drawn.

EXAMPLE FROM NURSING RESEARCH

A Qualitative-Quantitative Design

Pamela J. Brink (1984): Value orientations as an assessment tool in cultural diversity. Nursing Research, 33, 198–203.

Brink describes her use of value orientations as an assessment tool in cultural diversity in Nigeria. She describes the tools as extremely easy to administer, with possibilities of establishing the values and beliefs of both the individual nurse and the client. Brink (p. 198) writes that the tool can be used to indicate where the nurse and client will agree on values and whether the values may be in conflict. *Value orientation* is the name given to a theoretical construct developed by anthropologist Florence Kluckhohn more than 30 years ago. The construct, which has stood the test of time, centers upon problems faced by human beings and on the solutions to these problems, which create the distinctive profile of a culture. Kluckhohn identified five common human problems, each of which has three solutions, arranged in a preferential sequence. All three solutions are present in every society but are preferred to different degrees. The problems are:

1. *What is the character of innate human nature?* (human-nature orientation). This question was later dropped from the original interview, since construct validity was not established.

2. *What is the relation of humankind to nature and the supernatural?* (humankind–nature and supernatural).

3. *What is the temporal focus of human life?* (time orientation).

4. *What is the modality of human activity?* (activity orientation).

5. *What is the modality of human beings' relationships to other human beings?* (relational orientation).

The answers to questions 2, 3, 4, and 5 form the basis for the Value-Orientation Profile. These are as follows:

Three alternative solutions to the human being–nature question: (1) *subjugation to nature*—humankind is subjugated to nature; (2) *harmony with nature*—both nature and humankind live in harmony; or (3) *mastery over nature*—humankind masters nature and uses it to whatever purpose is considered useful or advantageous.

Three alternative solutions to time orientation: (1) *past-oriented*—the traditional approach; (2) *present-oriented*—the now approach; or (3) *future-oriented*—use information from past and present to plan for the future.

Three alternative solutions to activity orientation: (1) *being*—what a human being is; (2) *being-in-becoming*—what a human being can become, striving for growth, self-actualization; or (3) *doing*—what a human being can achieve by being active.

Three alternative solutions to relational orientation: (1) *individual*—autonomy of the person; individual goals dominate group goals; (2) *collaterality*—group goals, such as family goals, take precedence over individual goals; or (3) *lineality*—the individual, group, or class dominates the individual, and relations are hierarchical, as in dominance or submission by class, age, or sex.

Data analysis suggested by the Kluckhohn report (1961) includes three steps: The first step utilizes the Kendall S statistic to test for the degree of consensus for all choices and indicates whether the answers could have happened by chance. The second step uses binomial analysis to test the strength and direction of the pattern of responses for each item in the questionnaire. The third step uses the "t"-test to determine if there is a significant pattern for each value orientation. The final descriptive summary is the profile of what a people value at one moment in time.

The value orientation of Americans includes an emphasis on: (1) *doing and achieving*; (2) *individualism* (i.e., individual goals over group goals); (3) *the future* (i.e., planning for change); and (4) *mastery over nature* (i.e., the use of technology to solve all problems).

To determine the value orientation of another culture, Brink used a schedule developed for rural populations to study village life in Nigeria. A deliberative sample was selected for Brink by the speaker for the House of Representatives and by the local village representative. The sample was chosen to represent different geographical areas, levels of education, and seniority. Ten men, their senior wives, and a few others comprised the convenience sample of 28 persons (15 men and 13 women). Two Annang interpreters translated the interview schedule during the interviews. Upon completion of the analysis, Brink found that the value orientation of the Nigerian village contrasted sharply with that of Americans in emphasizing being over doing, group over individual, and present over future, and in indecision over whether humankind should master nature or live in harmony with it (pp. 199, 202). Brink attributes the indecision to cultural change occurring in Nigeria.

Brink writes that the value-orientation schedule is not limited to research on small groups, but can be administered as any other assessment tool. In her view, health-care givers should administer the schedule to themselves in order to assess their own value orientation prior to administering it to their patients to determine theirs.

STUDY QUESTIONS _____

1. Define "research design."
2. Select a level of nursing research that you would like to pursue.

What research question would you ask? Which design would you use?

3. Select a research design that you would like to use. State how your design would use the following: control; time framework; setting; sampling; and data collection.
4. Define qualitative and quantitative research.
5. What myths are associated with the differences between these two designs?
6. Name and define six methods suggested by Simon that are useful in qualitative designs. Select one method and describe how you would use it.
7. Read the research design utilized by Brink (summarized in this chapter), and discuss it in terms of its qualitative and quantitative features.

REFERENCES AND SUGGESTED READINGS

Bogdan, R. and Biklen, S. (1982): Qualitative Research for Education: An Introduction to Theory and Method. Boston: Allyn & Bacon. *Discussion of research helpful in qualitative nursing research.*

Bloch, D. (1980): Interrelated issues in evaluation and evaluation research. Nursing Research, *29*, 69–73. *Evaluation as a research design.*

Brink, D. and Wood, M. (1978): Basic Steps in Planning Nursing Research. North Scituate, Mass.: Duxbury Press.

Brink, P. (1984): Value orientations as an assessment tool in cultural diversity. Nursing Research, *33*, 198–203. Brink uses the tool in Nigeria.

Diers, D. (1979): Research in Nursing Practice. Philadelphia: J. B. Lippincott.

Downs, F. (1983): One dark and stormy night. Nursing Research, *32*, 259.

Farr, L. et al (1984): Alterations in circadian excretion or urinary variables and physiological indicators of stress following surgery. Nursing Research, *33*, 140–146. A quantitative design.

Fox, D. (1982): Fundamentals of Research in Nursing, 4th ed. Norwalk, Conn.: Appleton-Century-Crofts.

Glaser, B. and Strauss, A. (1967): The Discovery of Grounded Theory: Strategies for Qualitative Research. Chicago: Aldine. *Useful in qualitative designs.*

Glittenberg, J. (1978): Fertility patterns and child rearing of the Ladinos and Indians of Guatemala. In Leininger, M., Transcultural Nursing. New York: Wiley, pp. 417–432. *Example of qualitative approach.*

Goodwin, L. and Goodwin, W. (1984): Qualitative vs. quantitative research or qualitative and quantitative research? Nursing Research, *33*, 378–379. *Myths about the difference in qualitative and quantitative research.*

Gorenberg, B. (1983): The research tradition of nursing: An emerging issue. Nursing Research, *32*, 347–349. *Comments on qualitative, quantitative designs.*

Hamm, B. and Brodt, D. (1982): Guts: Teaching assertiveness skills by simulation and gaming. Nursing Research, *31*, 246–247. *Simulation.*

Ianni, F. and Orr, M. (1979): Toward a rapprochement of quantitative and qualitative methodologies. In T. Cook and C. Reichardt (eds.), Qualitative and Quantitative Methods in Evaluation Research. Beverly Hills, Calif.: Sage Publications, pp. 87–98. *Commonalities in the two perspectives discussed.*

Klenow, D. (1981): Qualitative methodology: A neglected resource in nursing research. Research in Nursing and Health, *4*, 281–282. *Qualitative designs.*

Knafl, D. and Howard, M. (1984): Interpreting and reporting qualitative research. Research in Nursing and Health, *7*, 17–24. *Qualitative research.*

Kovacs, A. (1985): The Research Process. Philadelphia, F. A. Davis., pp. 170–171. *Briefly discuss the appropriate and preferred statistic for qualitative research statistics, nominal (mode and range) and ordinal levels of measurement (mode, median, quartile range).*

LeCompte, M. and Goetz, J. (1982): Problems of reliability and validity in ethnographic research. Review of Educational Research, *52*, 31–60. *Problems in qualitative research.*

Leininger, M. (1978): Transcultural Nursing. New York: Wiley. *Various methods of analysis of qualitative research and analysis throughout book.*

Lofland, J. and Lofland, L. (1984): Analyzing Social Settings: A Guide to Qualitative Observation and Analysis (2nd ed.). Belmont, Calif.: Wadsworth. *Qualitative analysis.*

Lynch, K. (1983): Qualitative and quantitative evaluation: Two terms in search of meaning. Educational Evaluation and Policy Analysis, *5*, 461–464. *Concept evaluation.*

Mullen, P. and Iverson, D. (1982): Qualitative methods for evaluation research in health education programs. Health Education, *May/June*, 11–18. *Evaluation methods.*

Pelto, P. and Pelto, G. (1978): Anthropological Research: The Structure of Inquiry (2nd ed.). Cambridge: Cambridge University press. *Qualitative perspective discussed.*

Phillips, L. and Rempusheski, V. (1985): A decision-making model for diagnosing and intervening in elder abuse and neglect. Nursing Research, *34*, 134–139. *Research using Glaser's grounded-theory methodology.*

Polit, D. and Hungler, B. (1985): Essentials of Nursing Research. Philadelphia: F. A. Davis, *pp. 272–275. Discuss major purposes of qualitative analysis.*

Reichardt, C. and Cook, T. (1979): Beyond qualitative versus quantitative methods. In T. Cook and C. Reichardt (eds.), Qualitative and Quantitative Methods in Evaluation Research. Beverly Hills, Calif.: Sage Publications, pp. 7–32. *Qualitative and quantitative.*

Sieber, S. (1978): The integration of field-work and survey methods. In N. Denzin (ed.), Sociological Methods: A Sourcebook (2nd ed.). New York: McGraw-Hill, pp. 358–380. *Observation and methods in the field.*

Simon, J. (1978): Basic Research Methods in the Social Sciences. New York: Random House, Chap. 14, pp. 201–218. *Discusses deductive reasoning, the case study, participant observation, expert opinion, content analysis, simulation.*

Smith, J. (1983): Quantitative versus qualitative research: An attempt to clarify the issue. Educational Researcher, *12*, 6–13. *Examination of the two approaches to research.*

Spradley, J. (1979): The Ethnographic Interview. New York: Holt, Rinehart & Winston. *Qualitative methods discussed.*

Spradley, J. (1980): Participant Observation. New York: Holt, Rinehart & Winston. *A technique for qualitative research.*

Stern, P. (1980): Grounded theory methodology: Its uses and abuses. Images, *12*, 20–23. *A qualitative methodological approach.*

Swanson, J. and Chenitz, S. (1982): Why qualitative research in nursing? Nursing Outlook, *30*, 241–245. *Qualitative research in nursing.*

Zif, J. (1976): Optional vs. fixed information system in a simulation game. Simulation Games, *7*, 35–52. *Simulation.*

11

Descriptive and Historical Research Designs

The descriptive and historical research designs are basic, in that many researchers refer to these as essential for providing information upon which later studies may build. The designs are similar, in that neither is intended to generate control over data, and both designs use whatever method of data collection is the most helpful. They differ, in that the descriptive design usually purposes to describe current data, while the historical design is a study of the past.

Upon completion of this chapter, the student should be able to: (1) discuss descriptive research designs and the advantages and disadvantages of each; and (2) describe the historical research design and its advantages and disadvantages.

THE DESCRIPTIVE/EXPLORATORY DESIGN

With the descriptive/exploratory design, the researcher plans either to assemble new information about an unstudied phenomenon or to take a new look at old data or old nursing routines. The purpose is to obtain new knowledge by describing, comparing, and classifying observations and by inventing concepts to stand for what previously may have been unorganized or unrelated observations or data. These designs tend to be more qualitative than quantitative.

Exploratory designs differ from purely descriptive designs, in that exploratory designs may be more focused upon specific areas. This assists the researcher to use the data collected either to formulate nursing questions or problems for investigation later or to develop hypotheses for subsequent testing.

The *descriptive design*, on the other hand, seeks to describe accurately the characteristics of an individual, a situation, or a group and then may determine the frequency with which the event occurs or the frequency with which one event is associated with another.

Diers (1979, pp. 100–123) calls descriptive studies "factor-searching studies," which the researcher uses in the clinical area when the nursing problem is to describe or name the part of a given event. In her view, descriptive studies include historical studies and ethnoscience, a type of anthropological study that attempts to understand how natives look at their culture rather than how the observer sees it–or, in nursing terms, how the patient views his or her sickness and health rather than how the nurse views it. Dividing designs into levels of inquiry, Diers places the descriptive design into the first level of inquiry, which asks the question "What is this?" To analyze data, the researcher compares the data, puts them into categories, and names the categories. Diers considers descriptive studies to be basic but also to be both sophisticated and difficult. However, the studies may lead to new ways of thinking about important clinical problems and may possibly lead to changes in nursing practice.

The descriptive research design includes four different approaches: (1) the descriptive case study; (2) the comparative study; (3) the classification study; and (4) the concept-formulation study.

1. *The* descriptive case study *is used in nursing to examine and describe a single unit, such as an individual, group, community, culture, situation, problem, or process.* Case studies are often used in practicing professions such as nursing, law, social work, and medicine. Nurses use the descriptive case study design to conduct intensive and lengthy investigations.

   There are several advantages to the descriptive case study design. First, the case study is often a source of stimulating insights. At times, the researcher is able to create a *Gestalt*—a whole—from diverse bits of information. The researcher thus brings life to the individuals or groups, portraying them as human beings rather than as study objects. Second, particular diagnoses (such as a mental illness) may be studied to illustrate patterns of both illness and health, thereby casting light on what is "normal," or on what is considered "wellness." Third, the case study is useful to describe processes of development—pregnant women becoming nursing mothers, infants becoming children, patients going through stages of an illness or stages of dealing with loss or grief. Fourth, the design is helpful to study adjustment—it illuminates the experience of adjusting to handicaps or chronic disease for both the patient and the nurse. And fifth, the case-study design has the advantage of being flexible. The researcher may structure the research in terms of available time, materials, study subjects, and money.

The most serious disadvantage of the case study is the question of representativeness. There is no way of knowing whether the study represents a population. And for all intents and purposes, replication is impossible.

EXAMPLES FROM NURSING RESEARCH

Resio and Verhonick (1973) used the design to analyze the characteristics of patients who had developed decubitus ulcers, collecting data from 96 patients on 375 characteristics. Leininger (ed., 1978) published a number of case studies from field work in which nurses described different cultures within the United States and other parts of the world. These included studies that traced specific roles (such as that of the aged black) through history and space and those that described the culture, history, values, and social structure of a people (such as the Japanese).

2. *The* comparative-descriptive design *is structured to describe and compare several units or cases.* The researcher looks for reasons why things are similar or different. In addition to comparing concepts, the researcher may compare customs or behaviors of health care utilized by different cultural groups. For example, research is needed to describe how recent immigrants to the United States—the Vietnamese, Koreans, Cubans, Mexicans, and Haitians, among others—use health-care facilities in this country, as compared to their former countries.

Comparisons may be made on one dimension. For example, the frequency of high blood pressure among recent black immigrants from the West Indies or Africa may be compared with that of native-born blacks. Or comparisons may be made of several characteristics. For example, an index to measure social class on the basis of education, occupation, and income may be used to compare the frequency of high blood pressure among recent immigrants and the native-born by the various social classes found among each.

EXAMPLE FROM NURSING RESEARCH

Norris (1975, p. 107) was interested in comparing the concept "restlessness" in several groups of patients, including the dying, those suffering from coronary problems, patients with hyperinsulinism, and those who were simply bored.

3. Classification studies *put observations into categories and name the categories.* To put observations into categories, the researcher first describes the facts observed, puts those characteristics that are alike in the same category, and then names the category.

Classification research is useful to summarize, compare, clarify, and explain. To summarize, the researcher puts data into categories and counts the frequency. To compare, the frequency of patients in one category (such as ongoing pain) can be compared with the frequency with which patients fall into the "inflicted-pain" category. Classification leads to clarification through the understanding of the phenomena being classified. Finally, classification leads to explanation when the researcher is able to establish the relationships among categories or when the categories, taken together, explain the total situation or process under investigation.

EXAMPLES FROM NURSING RESEARCH

Brill and Kilts (1980) classified nursing diagnoses as "immediate," "foreseeable," and "possible," based on descriptions of present behavior, previous health responses, and similar descriptions of potential diagnoses.

4. Concept formulation studies *organize observations and descriptions into a meaningful and coherent whole,* expressed by the concept, which stands for the category of related data that are not yet named. However, concept formulation is a difficult task. The concept is not a simple and directly observable item but is a complex combination of interrelated observations and descriptions. For example, to make a concept observable and measurable, the researcher must develop an operational definition. Descriptions of persons crying, weeping, sobbing, and lamenting may be ordered into one concept—grieving. Concept formulation is somewhat like an operational definition in reverse: the researcher observes, describes, and measures the frequency of complex behavior and then invents a name to stand for it. The name is the concept. Concept formulation arises from inductive reasoning—beginning with observation, the researcher organizes descriptions by logical thought into categories, and then into concepts. The researcher who is able to name the concepts and to state a relationship between two concepts has formulated an empirical generalization and has thus taken a significant step toward the formulation of a theory.

EXAMPLE FROM NURSING RESEARCH

King (1971) invented a construct (which is like a concept but which is generally inferred indirectly from observation or is invented from a number of other concepts) called "personal system." This construct stood for a number of other concepts, such as the ways in which an individual uses perceptions, self, body image, growth and development, and time and space to form a system. She used "personal system" and other constructs to form a *conceptual framework*, an organization of common elements that can lead to theory formulation once the interrelations among the concepts and constructs are found in research and are formally stated.

Advantages and Disadvantages of Descriptive Designs

Descriptive and exploratory designs have a number of advantages. First, the researcher assembles a broad range of data with a richness of detail that has not been available before. Second, by describing, comparing, and classifying data, the researcher gains a holistic view—the patterns and processes may be comprehended as a whole. Third, the researcher may be able to move from observation and description to classification and then to conceptualization. Fourth, in the process of analyzing the descriptive data, the researcher may be able to telescope the stages of research, moving from description of data to an *empirical generalization*— a statement of a purposive relationship between two concepts.

Disadvantages of the descriptive design include, first, its difficulty. It is not easy either to observe objectively or to organize a mass of observations that may have taken months to collect into an organized, succinct account. Second, one is seldom able to generalize the findings from the study of one case or community to a broader population; thus, findings are limited to the unit studied. Third, because the procedure is not standardized, descriptive studies cannot be replicated or evaluated. Even the same researcher may not be able to repeat precisely what was done before. Finally, descriptive studies may not always be accurate; the observer's view may be biased in various ways (that is, observations may differ consistently from what a "true" accurate observation actually is).

However, if the views of Diers and Brink and of Wood are accurate, unless sound descriptive studies are completed at Level 1, studies that seek to establish associations or to predict will not be possible. In addition, descriptive studies have lasting value. Theories may fall out of use or may be modified, but a good descriptive account of an important process in nursing never goes out of date and should be taken into account when the researcher conducts a review of the literature on that subject, if only to show changes that have occurred.

THE HISTORICAL/DOCUMENTARY DESIGN

The historical research design is structured to collect and interpret data by examining material that already exists. The eight steps in the design are to: (1) identify the major sources of material relevant to the research problem or hypothesis; (2) ascertain the location of pertinent materials and documents; (3) ascertain the accessibility of documents; (4) obtain permission to use the materials; (5) examine the data thoroughly; (6) establish categories for the data; (7) review current interpretations of the data; and (8) examine the data for new perspectives and explanations.

The major sources of data are public records and documents, private records, and the mass media. These may include *primary sources*, first-hand descriptions of observation, or *secondary sources*, publications that refer to or that analyze primary sources.

Public Documents

Public documents include official governmental reports, such as statistical data (census data, birth rates, death rates, morbidity rates, etc.); police records (suicides, violence, drug use, child abuse); production data (agricultural production, industrial output, etc.); and health data (immunizations, life expectancy, etc.). Such data afford an economical approach to research and may be found in many libraries. Courthouse documents (such as court cases, wills, deeds, and taxation data) are also useful.

Records of hospitals and health departments are official confidential documents that require special permission to study. Nurses who have open access to patients' records during clinical practice should obtain permission to use the same records for research studies.

Private Documents

Private documents include diaries, notes, letters, journals, and autobiographies, which give glimpses of the private worlds of the authors. The problems associated with using private documents are considerable, including questions of validity. Moreover, personal documents are often inaccessible, although the researcher may use records from her or his own family and friends that would not be available to other scientists.

The Mass Media

Books, magazines, movies, plays, and innumerable other popular sources may be worthwhile records for the researcher who seeks to examine what is being communicated about nursing, sickness, health, living, and dying. For example, television shows use the dramatic potential of the hospital to portray nurses, doctors, and patients in particular roles. Such depictions may have an impact on the public's view of nurses and nursing. This impact may subsequently be reflected in support for or against health agencies or personnel.

Folk beliefs concerning health and disease may likewise be examined by analyzing advertisements for products designed to cure ills or prevent disability. Magazines, newspapers, billboards, and television commercials help to sell millions of dollars' worth of drugs, palliatives, and cures. Little work has been done in this area, although a method of data collection related to records (content analysis) is well-known.

To assess the validity of archival sources, the researcher may apply both external and internal criticism. *External criticism* is concerned with the document itself: Are letters purported to be from patients in mental institutions actually written by the patients themselves? Is the diary of the child in the rehabilitation center a fake? *Internal criticism* is concerned with the content of the document: Was the primary witness able to tell the truth? Is the primary witness accurately reporting in the document, as compared to other sources?

The comparatively low cost of acquiring such data makes historical analysis and records review attractive. However, there are risks of error implicit in archival and historical sources, such as errors arising from selective deposit, selective survival, and selective editing. The competence of the person who collected and recorded the data may determine the usefulness of the material. Official sources tend to be more reliable than nonofficial records, but the researcher must carefully evaluate all documents. In using historical materials, the researcher must also distinguish between primary sources and secondary sources. Primary sources include first-hand descriptions of observations, such as minutes of a meeting, interview schedules or questionnaires used in a survey, research reports, hospital records, diaries, films, newspaper eyewitness accounts, or ethnographies and case studies. Secondary sources include books, articles, speeches, or publications that refer to, describe, compare, or analyze primary sources. Each of these has its use in historical designs, but it must be clear which the researcher is using.

EXAMPLE FROM NURSING RESEARCH

Using records from two state hospitals in Washington State, Nakagawa et al. (1972) present an historical epidemiological investigation that extends over a 26-year span. The sample was chosen by systematic selection: every 15th name on the roster of 9,257 names of patients who were admitted to the hospital for the first time. A detailed system to code the data at the time of record review was developed and was used together with content analysis, a method of data collection (see Part V). In order to examine the items and categories for change over time, the researcher compiled the 617 cases into groups. The trends over the 26-year span were shown by changes in proportions of an item or category among the intervals.

Advantages and Disadvantages of the Documentary Design

The major advantage of historical research designs is that data collection may be less expensive, because the observations are already collected and documented. However, the researcher must assemble, classify, and analyze the documents. Private and public documents may cover a long period of time. In addition, they may have been collected for purposes other than the research and may, therefore, be biased. However, the disadvantages of the historical design are considerable: The data may have gaps—they may be incomplete in the very areas crucial to the research problem. Records may also be lost, damaged, or otherwise inaccessible. The recorder may have been unwilling or unable to observe and record accurately. Bias may have intruded into the data-collection process, or records may be inaccurate in other ways. Yet, if critically examined, the historical/documentary approach provides nursing with a source of knowledge helpful in understanding the nursing process.

SUMMARY

The descriptive-exploratory design proposes to observe, describe, explore, and assemble new knowledge. Four types of descriptive design include the descriptive case study, the comparative-descriptive study, the classificatory study, and the concept-formulation study. The descriptive case study examines a single unit in depth, often providing stimulating insights, as well as data, to study change and adjustment. The greatest disadvantage of the case study is the researcher's inability to generalize from only one case, or to replicate the original study. The comparative-descriptive design allows the researcher to describe how the units under study are alike and how they differ. Comparisons may be made on one dimension, or an index of several dimensions may be useful. In classification studies, observations are put into categories and the categories are named—classification follows description and is derived from it. Classification aids in summarization and in comparison and clarifies description. It leads to explanation if and when the researcher is able to establish relationships among the categories of data. Concept-formulation studies seek to organize description into a coherent whole, expressed by a concept. Conceptualization is the process of ordering observation by means of appropriate concepts. Formulating concepts from descriptive data is difficult but provides the basis for an empirical generalization that states the relationship between two or more concepts. The primary objective of descriptive or exploratory research is not to generalize but to provide new information.

With the documentary-historical design, the researcher examines records and documents already in existence. Major sources of data include official and unofficial documents, statistics, audiovisual media, and general historical data. To assess the validity of archival sources, the researcher uses external criticism, which is concerned with the document itself, while internal criticism is used to judge the writer's ability and willingness either to tell the truth or to report accurately. The researcher must distinguish between primary sources, or first-hand descriptions of observations, and secondary sources, such as books, articles, speeches, or publications based on primary sources. The major advantage of documentary or historical designs is that the data have already been collected. But therein lies its weakness: the data may have gaps or be incomplete, lost, damaged, or inaccessible; or, the recorder may not have been willing or able to observe and record accurately and without bias.

EXAMPLE FROM NURSING RESEARCH

A Descriptive Research Design

Raphella Sohier (1978): Gaining awareness of cultural difference: A case example. In Madeleine Leininger (ed.), Transcultural Nursing. New York: Wiley pp. 433–448.

A descriptive account of a Presbyterian Scottish nurse who went to live and work (participant observation) in Belgium in a large Jewish community. Most of the members were of Eastern European origin, and most displayed the customs of the traditional Shtetl communities of Russia, Poland, and Hungary. For 19 months, she was the private-duty nurse in the home of a Jewish man suffering from severe myocardial infarction and an aortic aneurysm. She describes how, in the beginning, her lack of knowledge of Jewish background, values, and attitudes interfered with her attempt to deliver total nursing care. In the early months, her patient's frustrations were directed (at times) toward her, and he would shake his head and say "Vreemd goyish meidl"—"strange non-Jewish woman." As Sohier's lack of knowledge about Jewish culture limited the quality of health care that she might provide, she made a formal request to the family to be instructed about their culture, learning the dietary laws and their relationship to the patient's peace of mind; the traditional roles of men and women in the Jewish culture; the importance of the family; and the difference between the physical pain and the emotional anguish that her patient experienced. As the therapeutic process between nurse and patient developed, the patient explained the traditional dying practices of the Jews in the Shtetl communities and asked the nurse to arrange for him to die in the traditional manner, "namely, lying on the floor, covered but naked." The patient's transfer to the hospital brought a deep inner conflict between the nurse's cultural values, which made it seem cruel to have her patient die on a hard terrazzo floor; the subcultural values of nursing, which valued supporting the dying with physical comfort measures; and the values of the traditional Jewish culture. However, when the patient's time of death came, Sohier, with the help of the physician, laid the patient on the floor, as he had trusted her to do.

In recapping the phases and themes of the nurse–patient relationship, Sohier noted several general themes: (1) the mutual sharing of knowledge about each other; (2) the testing of the nurse by the patient; and (3) the emergence of a helping modality. In a transcultural situation, the first theme takes longer: " . . . it is necessary for the nurse to gain knowledge which will enable her to understand the patient by putting herself in his place." However, without a realization of the cultural values, attitudes, beliefs, and lifestyles of different cultures, she writes, a therapeutic relationship is difficult to develop.

EXAMPLE FROM NURSING RESEARCH

A Documentary/Historical Research Design

Elen Baer (1985): Nursing's divided house—an historical view. Nursing Research, 34, 32–38.

Baer uses historical analysis to examine the nature and scope of the divisions in nursing in America in the last third of the 19th century. The upheaval of the Civil War, developing industrialization, and the growth of class factors led to social turbulence. Nursing reflected these changes. Baer used historical analysis, distinct from historical chronology, to interpret and explain these events. She identified three models of nursing, which competed with one another for support within nursing and recognition and acceptance in society. (1) The Nightingale model was adapted by American schools in 1873. It kept nursing separate from hospital and medical domination but left it supervised by boards of lady managers. (2) The Linda Richards model, initiated at Boston City Hospital in 1878, subjected nursing to medical control. (3) The professional model espoused by Isabel Hampton toward the end of the 19th century sought self-determination and regulation for nursing. The competition among these models produced divisions within nursing that have never been resolved.

The documents utilized by Baer include: (1) the Hunter-Bellevue Archives, Hunter College Library Administration, including Bellevue Hospital records and reports of the Bellevue Hospital Visiting Committee, and a student diary from the class of 1890; (2) the Alan Mason Chesney Medical Archives at Johns Hopkins Medical Institution, including student application letters from 1888 to 1889; (3) the Historic Library of the Pennsylvania Hospital, papers of nursing school dismissal from 1899 to 1901; (4) magazine articles from the 19th century, including "Hospital Nursing" in the *English Illustrated Magazine*, 1891; (5) bylaws of the 19th century, such as Nurses' Associated Alumnae of the United States and Canada, Bylaws, 1897; (6) papers and discussions from the International Congress of Charities, Correction and Philanthropy, 1893; (7) publications from the 19th century such as Woolsey, A., *A Century of Nursing with Hints towards the Organization of a Training School*, first published in 1876; (8) publications of the 20th century, including Clara Barton's *A Story of the Red Cross* (1904); (9) unpublished doctoral dissertations, including Noel, N. (1979), "Isabel Hampton Robb: Architect of American Nursing," and Reverby, S. (1982), "The Nursing Disorder: A Critical History of the Hospital–Nursing Relationship, 1860–1945"; and various nursing histories.

STUDY QUESTIONS

1. What is an exploratory design or descriptive design?
2. Describe a nursing problem that you have observed. What descriptive design would you use to study it: the case study design, the comparative study design, or another?
3. What is a descriptive case study design? What are its disadvantages?
4. Think of a concept in nursing (similar to "restlessness") that you can describe and compare in some way.
5. Classify into at least two different categories the complaints that you have heard from a particular group of patients (such as surgical, obstetrical, medical, or psychiatric). Examples may in-

clude kinds of pain, kinds of discomfort from specific nursing procedures, kinds of nurses or nursing care, etc.

6. Nurses sometimes classify co-workers by a particular concept (at times, by a slang term such as "eager beaver," "goof-off," etc.). Can you identify any names invented to describe categories of patients—other than diagnosis?

7. Concept formulation is a difficult task. However, concepts are sometimes invented in the process of nursing practice and research. Can you think of behaviors that you have observed over and over in nursing that have no names?

8. "Nursing care" is a construct comprised of a number of concepts. Can you name the concepts? What is the difference between a construct and a concept? Is "social class" a construct? Why or why not?

9. Distinguish between primary sources and secondary sources. What primary sources can you identify in nursing research? What secondary sources?

10. What are major sources for the collection of historical or documentary data?

11. How do external and internal criticism assess the validity of archival sources?

12. What are the advantages and disadvantages of descriptive and historical-documentary research?

REFERENCES AND SUGGESTED READINGS

Amborn, S. (1976): Clinical signs associated with the amount of tracheobronchial secretions. Nursing Research, *25*, 121–126. *An exploratory correlation design.*

Austin, A. (1957): History of Nursing Source Book. New York: G. P. Putnam's Sons. *Excerpts from author's writings on nursing from historical perspective.*

Austin, A. (1958): The historical method in nursing. Nursing Research, *7*, 4–10. *Means used in the historical design.*

Baer, E. (1985): Nursing's divided house—An historical view. Nursing Research, *34*, 32–38.

Branch, H. (1979): Women in pain. In Kjervik, D. and Martinson, I. (eds), Women in Stress: A Nursing Perspective. New York: Appleton-Century-Crofts, pp. 237–255. *Includes use of the case study.*

Brill, E. and Kilts, D. (1980): Foundations for Nursing. New York: Appleton-Century-Crofts.

Christy, T. (1975): The methodology of historical research. Nursing Research, *24*, 189–192. *The use of the historical design.*

Diers, D. (1979): Research in Nursing Practice. Philadelphia: J. B. Lippincott, Chap. 4 and 5.

Fox, D. (1982): Fundamentals of Research in Nursing (4th ed.) Norwalk, Conn.: Appleton-Century-Crofts, Chap. 9, "Research Approaches: An Overview."

Goode, W. and Hatt, P. (1952): Methods in Social Research. New York: McGraw-Hill, Chap. 7.

Holaday, B. (1980): Implementing the Johnson model for nursing practice. In Riehl, J. and Roy, C. (eds.), Conceptual Models for Nursing Practice (2nd ed.). New York: Appleton-Century-Crofts, pp. 266–263. *Case study design used.*

Josten, L. (1979): Child abuse. In Jervik, D. and Martinson, I., Women in Stress: A Nursing Perspective. New York: Appleton-Century-Crofts, pp. 218–236. *Case reports.*

Kerlinger, F. (1973): Foundations of Behavioral Research (2nd ed.) New York: Holt, Rinehart, & Winston, Part 6, "Designs of Research," pp. 300–423.

King, I. (1971): Towards a Theory for Nursing. New York: Wiley.

Kjervik, D., and Martinson, I. (eds.)(1979): Women in Stress: A Nursing Perspective. New York: Appleton-Century-Crofts. *Twenty articles survey various stressful situations.*

Kovacs, A. (1985): The Research Process: Essentials of Skills Development. Philadelphia: F. A. Davis.

Leininger, M. (ed.) (1978): Transcultural Nursing. New York: Wiley. *Twenty-six articles, a number of case studies.*

Mill, J. (1930): A System of Logic (8th ed.). New York: Longmans.

Nakagawa, H., et al. (1972): An epidemiological study of psychiatric symptom pattern change: Pilot study findings. In Batey, M. (ed), Communicating Nursing Research. Boulder, Colo.: WICHE. *An historical epidemiological approach.*

Norris, C. (1975): Restlessness: A nursing phenomenon in search of meaning. Nursing Outlook, *23*, 103–107. *Illustration of description of nursing phenomena in the clinical area.*

Notter, L. (1972): The case for historical research in nursing. Nursing Research, *21*, 483. *Historical design.*

Polit, P. and Hungler, B. (1985): Essentials of Nursing Research. Philadelphia: J. B. Lippincott.

Resio, D. and Verhonick, P. (1973): On the measurement of analysis of clinical data nursing. Nursing Research, *22*, 388–393. *Case study analysis of characteristics of decubitus ulcer data.*

Sellitz, C. et al. (1976): Research Methods in Social Relations (3rd ed.). New York: Holt, Rinehart, & Winston. *Chapters 4 and 5.*

Sohier, R. (1978): Gaining awareness of cultural difference: A case study. In Leininger, M. (ed.), Transcultural Nursing. New York: Wiley, pp. 433–448.

Verhonick, P. (ed.) (1975): Nursing Research I. Boston: Little, Brown. *Six articles.*

Verhonick, P. (ed.) (1977): Nursing Research II. Boston: Little, Brown. *Seven articles.*

12

Experimental and Quasi-Experimental Research Designs

Experimental designs and variations fall into two major categories: the "true," or classical, experimental design, and the "quasi-experimental" design. A third subtype, the "pre-experimental design," is described by Campbell and Stanley (1966, p. 6), but only as a minimum reference, since pre-experimental studies have a total absence of control, which takes them out of the category of true or even quasi-experimental designs.

The *true experimental design* maintains maximum and rigorous control through the use of both random sampling to select subjects and manipulation to manage the independent variable. The *quasi-experimental design* lacks full experimental control over the scheduling of experimental stimuli (the experimental treatment or cause), but does have the ability to introduce random exposure into data-collection procedures. For example, the researcher can control when measurements occur and which study subjects (or objects) are measured. The use of the quasi-experimental design is encouraged but, at the same time, the researcher must become aware of the kinds of settings in which the quasi-experiment should occur.

This chapter begins by defining "control" in research and then turns to the major processes that the researcher uses to achieve control: (1) random sampling and randomization; (2) the use of matched pairs or groups, extraneous variables as independent variables, and successive experimental groups; (3) manipulation of independent variables; (4) identification and control of extraneous variables, including personal variables, environmental variables, and others that threaten internal validity of the research design; and (5) sampling controls to achieve external validity of the research design.

The chapter then examines the characteristic steps to be taken in the true experimental design, and describes the Solomon Four-Group True design and the Two After-Groups design, with examples from nursing. Third, the chapter describes quasi-experimental designs, including the Time Series and Multiple Times Series designs. Fourth, the chapter examines pre-experimental and quasi-experimental designs, with several examples of each.

Finally, the advantages and disadvantages of the various experimental designs will be described.

Upon completion of this chapter, the student should be able to: (1) define concepts, including control, random sampling, randomization, matched pairs, matched groups, multiple independent variables, manipulation, independent variables, dependent variables, extraneous variables, environmental and personal variables, variables that threaten internal validity of the research design, external validity, and the "Hawthorne effect"; (2) describe the use of these concepts; (3) discuss the steps in the true experimental design; (4) describe and compare the true experimental design and the quasi-experimental design; (5) contrast features of the pre-experimental design with those of the experimental design; and (6) discuss the advantages and disadvantages of experimental and quasi-experimental designs.

CONTROL

Control has several meanings in research. Broadly speaking, *control* is the researcher's ability to regulate and check all possible elements of the research. The purpose of control is to limit sources of error in research to the greatest extent possible. For example, a researcher, such as Wells (1982), who studied the effect of relaxation on postoperative muscle tension and pain, wants to be sure that only the independent variable (which, in this case, is "relaxation") is producing the observed effect—the extent of "postoperative pain and muscle tension." To do so, she used an experimental design with an experimental group and a control group. The researcher should be aware of how to control as many elements of the research design as possible.

Major means of control include the use of random-sampling techniques and the manipulation of independent variables by the researcher. Each of these will be examined in turn.

Control Through the Use of Random Sampling and Randomization

Random sampling is the selection of a sample in a manner that ensures each member or unit of a target population the equal probability or chance of being selected for the study sample. The *target population*, sometimes called the *universe*, is the set of persons, things, or measurements having an observable characteristic in common. Sometimes the researcher refers to the *accessible populations*—the population of subjects available for sampling, often a nonrandom subset of the target population whose characteristics are well-known.

Random sampling is a powerful tool to use, since it ensures samples that are free of bias—the subjects to be studied will be representative of the population that the researcher wishes to study. This allows the researcher to generalize what is found in the smaller sample to the larger population from which the sample was drawn. However, in reality, the selected sample will not always coincide exactly with the target population. For example, the target population may be all of those persons who share the characteristic of being diabetic. But even if the researcher had the time and money to identify every person with diabetes in the world, the sample would be totally representative of that population only at the very instant that it was drawn. Later, some members of that population could be dead, while others who had just become diabetics could be added to the population, and so on. Nonetheless, random sampling of the target population is a potent means of controlling elements of the research process and allows the researcher to generalize what is found in the small sample to the larger population.

Randomization, also called *random assignment* or *random allocation*, is the assignment of study subjects to the experimental group or to the control group from an available pool of study subjects. It aims to equalize the composition of the experimental and control groups so that they are as identical as possible with regard to as many characteristics as possible. Randomization creates comparable pretreatment groups, thereby eliminating systematic bias or distortion in the experimental and control groups. Randomization differs from random sampling, in that it is concerned with the equalization of the study groups rather than with the selection of units or persons from a target or accessible population. For example, Wells (1982), for obvious reasons, could not first select study subjects from a population by random sampling, then divide the study subjects into an experimental and a control group, and then subject them to surgery so that she could generalize from the sample to the population. However, she could take patients as they appeared in the hospital (the subjects available in one pool), and use randomization—random assignment—to randomly divide the patients who were to have surgery into two groups, one to receive training in relaxation techniques (the experimental group), and one to receive the usual preoperative instruction, which did not include relaxation techniques. While randomization is no guarantee that the two groups will be equal in every respect (same age, same sex, same weight, same race, same lifestyle, etc.), randomization is the most effective method of equalizing the experimental and control groups, since it controls possible sources of individual variation. It is random sampling applied to a nonrandom pool of subjects so as to divide the subjects into experimental and control groups.

Control Through the Use of Matched Pairs or Groups, Use of Extraneous Variables as Independent Variables, and Successive Experimental Groups

Matched pairs, or *matching,* is the process of finding study subjects with the same characteristics—such as age, sex, race, marital status, etc.— in order to divide them up between the two research groups. When it is not feasible to use randomization, the researcher sometimes uses matching to try to equalize the experimental and control groups. This is not easy, since it is difficult to find persons with identical characteristics in any small sample; even identical twins differ in some respects. In addition, while the researcher may match for a few common variables (such as sex, age, and race), the process gets more difficult after a few variables.

EXAMPLE FROM NURSING RESEARCH

Floyd (1984) used two groups of matched subjects, 35 hospitalized patients matched with 35 outpatient controls, to study the interaction between personal sleep–wake rhythms and psychiatric hospital rest–activity schedules. The inclusion criteria aimed to equate the two groups with regard to general health status and degree of psychiatric impairment. The hospitalized subjects were inpatients who agreed to participate in the study, 18 years of age or older, mentally able to participate in the study, free from chronic illness (other than psychiatric illness), and hospitalized a minimum of two weeks. The outpatient control subjects consisted of the first 35 outpatients who could be matched to inpatient subjects on gender and diagnosis, 18 years of age or older, mentally able to participate in the study, free from chronic illness (other than psychiatric illness), living in the present environment a minimum of two weeks, and free from a change in the timing of waking activities during the previous two weeks. However, there is no way to know beyond doubt that such characteristics should be matched to ensure that these are not affecting the dependent variable.

    Matched groups, or *homogeneous groups,* are those that are alike— homogeneous—in terms of one or more extraneous variables, such as sex (all male or all female), race (all white, all black, or all Oriental), marital status (all married, all single, all divorced, or all widowed), and age (all between 40 and 41). This process is not difficult and controls these extraneous variables, but its usefulness in terms of other samples is limited. For example, the findings for an all-male group would not be relevant to groups that are female. Comparability in this design is by the group rather than by the individual. The researcher can report the differences found between the control and experimental groups, and this can be compared with differences found in other groups of white men who are married and are between 40 and 41; however, like research that utilizes nonrandom pools of study subjects, ability to generalize is limited to the pool of study subjects.

Extraneous variables used as independent variables is a means of controlling an extraneous variable. The inclusion in the research design of an extraneous varible that is expected to be a factor in the research as an independent variable assists in control. For example, if sex is expected to influence the outcome of the study, then sex is included as an independent variable, and the assignment of subjects to either the experimental or the control group is accomplished through the use of randomization, separately performed for males and females. This ensures control over sex as a variable.

Successive experimental groups are those in which the same study subjects make up successive experimental groups. It is rarely used because of the problem of internal validity. Successive experiments can sensitize the study subjects and can influence the change in the dependent variable. Therefore, randomization remains the most practical and trustworthy way of control.

Control Through Manipulation of the Independent Variable

Manipulation is the introduction of a stimulus, a treatment, or a causal element—called the *independent variable*—into the experimental group in order to measure what the independent variable does to the dependent variable (which is also called the effect, the response, the outcome, or the criterion measure). For example, Wells (1982) used a structured program to teach relaxation to the patients in the experimental group to see if it had an effect on the dependent variable: postoperative muscle tension and pain. Manipulation and the use of random sampling are two powerful sources of control.

Control of Extraneous Variables

The third type of control that the researcher can use is control of the extraneous variables. *Extraneous variables* are those variables present in large numbers in the environment that are not of interest to the researcher but which may act along with, and confuse the effect of, the independent variables upon the dependent variables. An extraneous variable is a form of independent variable itself, but is one that the researcher has no interest in and does not want to use at the time of the experiment. Numerous extraneous variables exist, including the following categories, which may overlap: (1) personal variables; (2) environmental variables; and (3) other variables that threaten the internal validity of the research design.

Personal variables are individual characteristics, such as: (1) the individual's physiological variables, including anatomy, physiology, history of organic sickness-wellness, and genetic make-up; (2) psychological variables, such as motivation, attitudes, and self-image; and (3) demographic and social variables, including age, sex, race, marital status, occupation, education, income, and social class. These are sometimes called *organismic variables*.

Environmental variables include, among others, the setting and time factors. The *setting* for experimental research may be: (1) a highly controlled laboratory, or (2) a partially controlled experiment in the field—the natural setting. The most highly controlled setting, which is also the most artificial, is the experimental laboratory, where the researcher designs the setting to control as many extraneous variables as possible. However, the artificial setting itself may prove to be an extraneous variable that may affect behavior. People do not behave naturally in an artificial setting or in any setting where they know that they are being watched. For example, the *"Hawthorne effect"* is a concept that describes the changes in behavior that occur when individuals know that they are being observed or treated in a new way as part of a study.* The process of being observed, of being in the study, itself acts as an unwanted extraneous independent variable that can change behavior, thereby confusing the effect of the chosen independent variable. Techniques such as two-way mirrors, which allow the researcher to observe the subjects unaware, are unethical unless the researcher obtains the consent of the subjects, which makes the subjects aware that they are being observed! One solution to extraneous variables that arise from the setting is to combine a randomly selected sample with a consistent environment. The research design must include, as nearly as possible, the same features in the same setting for every subject.

A partially controlled experiment in the field is one in which the research design includes observations in the natural environment. The researcher exerts some control over management of the setting without destroying natural behavior. For example, the researcher learns to observe as unobtrusively as possible; or the researcher who plans to use an interview arranges to use the same quiet, private, comfortable room for every interview. In every case, the researcher must learn the art of putting the study subjects at ease whatever the setting.

The *time factors* include the time of season, the month and the time of the month, the day and the time of the day, the time of the shift (if applicable), and the pressures of time on the researcher and subjects. Again, control is maintained by a thoughtful analysis of the times available and of the times that are pertinent, and by consistence in the use of time.

Internal validity of the research design refers to its ability to measure what it purports to measure. The researcher must control extraneous variables that have been identified as a threat to internal validity, including history, maturation, testing, instrumentation, selection, and mor-

---

*The name "Hawthorne effect" is derived from the Hawthorne Works of the Western Electric Company, where researchers were conducting a study on the relationship between workers' production and various environmental conditions. One of the findings was that the subjects (the workers) responded to the researcher's attentions, to being observed, to being part of a study, as much as, or more than, they did to changes in the environment.

tality. For example, a researcher may want to know the effectiveness of an experimental instructional program that teaches diabetics about diet, medication, and exercise. One way to measure the effectiveness of the program is to assign the study subjects randomly to two groups: the experimental group, which is to be taught the experimental instructional program, and the control group, which is to be taught the traditional program. The researcher gives both groups a "pretest" before the program starts in order to assess what they already know about diabetes. The researcher then introduces the independent variable, the instructional program, into the experimental group. At the end of the teaching program, the researcher gives both groups a "post-test," the same test as the "pretest," to determine if the experimental group now knows more about diabetes than does the control group. After evaluating the tests, the researcher found that the experimental group did have a higher grade than the control group. The question is, did the experimental treatment (the experimental instructional program) make the difference? Did the research design have internal validity? Did it measure what it purported to measure—increased knowledge of diabetes?

Campbell and Stanley (1966) identify a number of extraneous variables that, if not controlled, may confuse the effects of the independent variables. These include:

1. *History*, which may have caused the difference in the scores. History includes events that occur concurrently with the independent variable and that affect the dependent variable (the test scores). For example, an event such as a television show on diabetes, which the experimental group saw, may have occurred between the first and second tests in addition to the experimental instructional program, and may have influenced the higher test scores.
2. *Maturation* may have taken place: the passage of time may have affected both groups of patients as they grew more tired, or not as well, or better.
3. *Testing* may have affected subjects' scores on the second test: the patients may have remembered the questions/answers from the first test differently.
4. *Instrumentation* may have been involved: different teachers may have graded the first and second tests differently.
5. *Selection* may have produced a control group and an experimental group that were not equivalent, in ways that influenced the scores on the second test.
6. *Mortality*, the differential loss of subjects from either the control or the experimental group—also called *attrition*—may have caused the groups that were once equivalent to lose their equivalence.

The researcher controls such extraneous variables through the use of random sampling, random assignment, and manipulation of the independent variable.

Control of Sampling: the External Validity of the Research Design

External validity of the research design is the extent to which the researcher is able to generalize from the sample studied to the larger population from which the sample was drawn. If the sample has been randomly selected from a target or accessible population, the findings of the study of the sample *can* be generalized to the entire target or accessible population. However, the use of random assignment or selection alone means that the findings of the research can be generalized only to those study subjects who were in the pool before it was randomly divided into the experimental and control groups. Researchers who select patients or subjects as they come into the hospital, clinic, or other setting, and who then divide the pool of patients into experimental and control groups, can generalize their findings only to that group of patients and no other. However, as Wooldridge et al. (1978, p. 144–146) point out, " when the purpose is to develop a causal theory, the most important thing is to use random assignment to reach a valid conclusion about effectiveness for the subjects studied. A firm causal inference about an atypical sample is more useful to the clinician. This point is made by Campbell and Stanley (1966) when they say internal validity is logically prior to external validity."

DESIGNS

The Classic, or True, Experimental Design

The *classic*, or *true, experimental design* (Fig. 12–1) is a four-cell design in which study subjects or objects are randomly selected from the total population, are randomly assigned to either the experimental or the control group, and are measured both before and after the researcher introduces the independent variable into the experimental group only, withholding it from the control group.

The characteristic steps to take in the true experimental design are:

1. Delineate the population or universe to be studied (i.e., the set of subjects or objects that share a common observable characteristic).
2. Select a sample from the population by random sampling.
3. By random assignment, subdivide the sample into two subsamples.
4. Specify one subsample as the experimental group and the other as the control group.
5. Before introducing the independent variable, observe and record all important characteristics of the two groups.
6. Introduce the independent variable into the experimental group but withhold it from the control group.

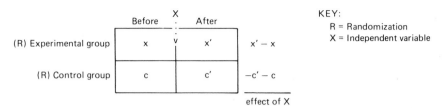

Figure 12–1. The true experimental design.

7. After introducing the independent variable, observe the dependent variable in both the experimental and the control groups.
8. Compare the changes that occur in the experimental group with those that may have occurred in the control group.
9. Record the difference.
10. Compare these values with statistically computed values that judge the significance of the difference, and indicate whether or not the observed differences could have occurred by chance.

The degree to which the findings are significantly greater than would be expected to occur by chance alone indicates the degree to which it is probable that a causal connection has been established.

At times, the researcher may supplement random sampling with other processes, such as the use of homogeneous populations.

The Solomon Four-Group True Experimental Design

The Solomon four-group true experimental design includes the four-cell classic experimental design plus two additional after-groups, an experimental after-group and a control after-group (Fig. 12–2). The two after-groups assist in controlling whatever effects of testing or measurement the before-groups may have experienced. For example, if the researcher wishes to measure the effect of teaching a diabetic patient about diet, the researcher may give a test before the teaching, introduce teaching as the

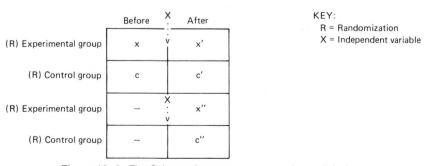

Figure 12–2. The Solomon four-group true experimental design.

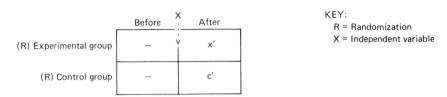

Figure 12–3. The after-groups control design.

independent variable X, and then give the same test after the teaching to measure the effect that the teaching has had. But the researcher cannot be sure that the first test in the before period did not influence the effect and cloud the action of the independent variable, the teaching. The use of two groups, neither of which was tested in the before period, helps control the effect of the testing. This design enables greater comparison. If all comparisons are in agreement, the ability to generalize increases. However, more work is involved.

Two After-Groups Control Design

The two after-groups control design is comprised of two randomly selected groups, neither of which is pretested or premeasured in the before period of time. The independent variable is introduced into the experimental group and is withheld from the control group. These two groups are identical to the last two groups of the Solomon four-group design. The process of random sampling is sufficient in itself to assure a lack of bias (Campbell and Stanley, 1966, p. 25). In situations where pretesting or premeasuring is not feasible, this design is appropriate (Fig. 12–3).

EXAMPLES FROM NURSING RESEARCH

Numerous examples of experimental designs from the clinical area are reported in the nursing research literature. However, the researcher often cannot use random sampling, since the study subjects must be taken as they arrive in the clinic or hospital, rather than being drawn from a target population by random sampling. In such cases, randomization takes the form of random assignment: the existing sample of patients is randomly subdivided into the experimental group and the control group. The resulting groups should be equivalent: the design should ensure the collection of verifiable data (i.e., it has internal validity), but the loss of random sampling weakens the ability to generalize to a target population (i.e., it does not have external validity). In such cases, a basic strategy is to run a series of small-sample experiments, whose cumulative results enable the researcher to generalize with more confidence (Wooldridge et al., 1968). This suggests the need to replicate studies, an invitation to nurses and students, whose cumulative replications will add to the ability to generalize from the original study.

Various hospital settings, such as the operating room, premature nursery, and recovery room, contain fairly well-controlled environments and have been used by researchers, such as Hasselmeyer, and Dumas and Leonard. Hasselmeyer (1961) conducted an experiment in the premature nursery to determine the effect of continually supporting the backs of premature infants with a diaper roll. She randomly assigned 59 infants to either the experimental group or the control group, introducing the diaper roll into the experimental group only. All other conditions were kept constant, including the amount of feeding, clothing, and handling. Each of the 59 infants was observed for definite periods of time by trained observers, using a scale developed to measure the dependent variable, the behavior of the infants.

Dumas and Leonard (1963) studied the effect of nursing on the incidence of postoperative vomiting. Patients on the operating schedule were randomly assigned membership in an experimental group (which received interaction with an experimental nurse) or a control group (which did not receive the experimental interaction). Vomiting in the recovery room was used as the dependent variable to indicate stress.

Other experimental studies in nursing include Cleland's (1977) investigation of the prevention of bacteriuria in hospitalized female patients with indwelling catheters; and Brown and Grunfeld's (1980) examination of infants' taste preferences for sweetened or unsweetened foods.

QUASI-EXPERIMENTAL DESIGNS

A quasi-experimental design is one in which full experimental control—usually random sampling—is not possible. The use of quasi-experimental designs requires that the researcher be aware of the points on which the results are questionable. If neither random sampling nor random assignment is used, it is not possible to generalize from the findings. And judging whether the independent variable (experimental manipulation) resulted in the observed differences between the experimental group and the control group requires more careful evaluation. Three examples of the quasi-experimental design follow:

The Four-Cell Design Without the Use of Random Sampling

The study subjects in this design are not randomly selected or randomly assigned. Instead, the groups are naturally assembled collectives, such as those found in classrooms or clinics. The researcher chooses the study subjects to be as similar as availability permits. To judge the similarity of the two groups, a pretest or premeasurement is made in the "before" time period. The more similar the scores on the pretest, the more effective this control becomes (Fig. 12–4). The independent variable is introduced into the experimental group only, after which, both the experimental and control groups are tested or measured (the "after" period). Even though the researcher is not able to use random selection or assignment of study subjects, the use of a control group helps the researcher to determine

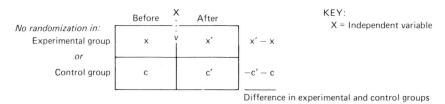

Figure 12–4. Four-cell design without randomization.

whether or not the independent variable actually made a difference in the experiment.

McGillicuddy (1977) used a somewhat similar design. She studied two groups of hospitalized children: one group had the mother rooming-in with the child, and the other group did not. Each group had prehospitalization and posthospitalization tests to measure changes in the children's behavior.

Huckabay (1978) used two samples of students to study the effect of an innovative teaching program. One group of students was taught with an innovative teaching program, while the other group was taught with lecture and discussion methods. Both groups were tested before and after the teaching programs in order to determine any differences in the students' learning behavior.

The Time Series Experimental Design

The time series experimental design, a single-group experiment, is comprised of a series of observations in the "before" time period so as to establish a baseline. The experimental (independent) variable is then introduced, followed by another series of observations designed to examine the effect of the independent variable (Fig. 12–5). For example, Hanson (1973) studied the effects of administering cold and warm tube feedings on the temperatures and heart rates of five volunteer subjects. The variables—temperature and heart rates—were established during the feedings and compared with those recorded when the feedings reached the stomach.

DeWalt and Haines (1977) used a similar design. The researchers studied the effect of stressors (oral breathing, continuous flow of oxygen, and intermittent mechanical suctioning) on the healthy oral mucosa of a volunteer. Observations of the subject took place in a laboratory setting,

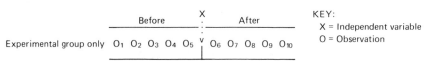

Figure 12–5. The time-series experiment.

at 15-minute intervals over a five-hour period, to determine both the effects of the stressors on healthy oral mucosa and the effectiveness of nursing interventions designed to minimize the effects of the stressors.

The Multiple Time Series Design

Considered an excellent quasi-experimental design (Campbell and Stanley, 1963, p. 55), the multiple time series design is similar to the one-group time series experimental design, except that a control group is added. The independent variable is introduced into a series of observations on the experimental group but is withheld from the series of observations made on the control group. The use of the control group, and the manipulation of the independent variable in the experimental group, increase the certainty with which the researcher can generalize findings.

PRE-EXPERIMENTAL DESIGNS

Pre-experimental designs is the name given to three designs that are considered weak experimental designs (Campbell and Stanley, 1963, pp. 6–13). The weakest of the three is the single-group, or single-case, study, which is studied only once following a treatment or an agent presumed to cause change (Fig. 12–6). Because the study design has a total absence of control, it is considered to be of little value as an experiment. At least one comparison is needed before scientific evidence is possible. However, many variations of this design exist, including the *ex-post-facto* design, in which the researcher attempts to explain a phenomenon that has already occurred.

Before-and-After Experimental Group: One-Group Design

The second pre-experimental design is one in which the top two cells of the experimental design are used without a control group. That is, only one group is observed before and after the independent variable is introduced (Fig. 12–7). Loss of the control groups decreases the usefulness of the study but may be necessary in cases where it is not possible or feasible to have control groups. For example, Fieve et al. (1971) used the design to measure the effects of lithium in treating manic psychosis. Six psychotic patients diagnosed as manic were tested by using the Psychiatric Evaluation form. The patients were then put on a regimen of lithium and

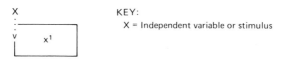

Figure 12–6. One-group studied once after stimulus.

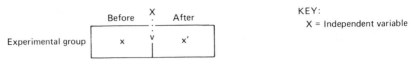

Figure 12–7. The experimental group only, before and after.

were tested again later. The before scores served as a control group. The differences in the before and after scores were considered a measure of the effectiveness of lithium.

The Static Group Comparison Design

With this pre-experimental design, a group that has experienced the independent variable is compared with one that has not (Fig. 12–8). Lindeman and Van Aernam (1977, p. 49) used this design to study the effects of structured and unstructured preoperative teaching on the postoperative behavior of study subjects. The experimental group was comprised of subjects admitted during a specified time period, while the control group consisted of subjects admitted during a different time period. The experimental group received the independent variable, structured preoperative teaching, while the control group did not. The weakness in such a design is that the groups may not have been equivalent.

Advantages and Disadvantages of the Experimental Designs

The advantages of the experimental design follow from three of its major characteristics—control, randomization, and manipulation. When the variables are narrow, well-defined, and controlled, it may be possible to establish a causal relationship, the process in which the independent variable or stimulus invariably precedes the effect. This is most clearly seen in the classical experimental design. Used when better designs are not feasible, quasi-experimental designs introduce a design that is similar to the classical experimental design, although randomization is often lacking. Experimentation is important in the task of theory testing and adds to the accumulating body of knowledge.

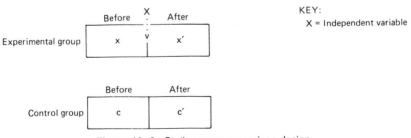

Figure 12–8. Static group comparison design.

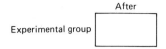

Figure 12–9. Ex-post-facto design.

However, there are many disadvantages to be found in the use of the experimental approach. First, neither may work well with the study of human subjects, a complex and complicated group. There are few, if any, valid criterion measures, or measures of the dependent variable, available to indicate the effects of independent variables upon human subjects. In addition, the experimental setting may not accommodate the variables, some of which are too broad for the laboratory or for any artificial setting. Moreover, the independent variable may take years to manifest itself. The correlation between smoking and cancer is an example of the long time span necessary in some cases. Likewise, cooperation may be difficult when the researcher wishes to use the experimental method on human subjects who have full knowledge of the nature of the experiment. Finally, the widespread use of random assignment alone, rather than in conjunction with random sampling, interferes with the researcher's ability to generalize from the sample to a broader population without a large number of studies to bolster the claim.

SUMMARY

With the experimental design, the researcher has maximum control over the independent variable and over the selection and assignment of subjects to different experimental conditions. A major means of control is random sampling—the process that ensures every unit in the target population an equal chance of being chosen for the study sample and each unit in the study sample an equal chance of being assigned to either the experimental or the control group. A second means of control is manipulation—the process by which the researcher treats or manages the independent variable in order to study its effect upon the dependent variable. The researcher must also control extraneous variables, those factors present in large numbers in the environment that are not interesting to the researcher but that may act upon the dependent variable and confuse the effect of the independent variable.

Three types of true experimental designs include: (1) the classic experimental design, comprised of both a randomly chosen and assigned experimental group and a control group, which is measured before and after the independent variable is introduced into the experimental group; (2) the Solomon four-group, which adds two after-groups to the classic experimental design (an additional after-experimental group and an additional after-control group); and (3) two after-groups, an experimental and a control group. All groups of the true experimental design are randomly chosen from a target population, with the subjects randomly assigned to either the experimental or the control group. All groups enable the researcher to manipulate the independent variable in order to study its effect.

With quasi-experimental designs, full experimental control, usually randomization, is not possible. If neither random sampling nor random assignment is used, the researcher cannot generalize from the findings of the sample to the population. And the researcher must carefully judge whether the independent variable resulted in observed differences between the experimental and control groups. There are many quasi-experimental designs, including a four-cell experimental group, which is similar to the true classical experiment except for the lack of randomization. Other designs include the time series experimental design, in which one group is observed several times before and after the introduction of the independent variable; and the multiple time series design, which is similar to the time series design, except that a control group is added.

Pre-experimental designs include: (1) the single-group design, which is studied only once following a treatment or an agent presumed to cause change; (2) one group, studied before and after a stimulus is introduced; and (3) the static-group design, in which a group that has experienced the independent variable is compared with one that has not. Although none is strong, the weakest of these three is the single-group design.

EXAMPLE FROM NURSING RESEARCH

Jane Dixon (1984): Effect of nursing interventions on nutritional and performance status in cancer patients. Nursing Research, 33, 330–335.

Dixon writes that nutritional complications are among the most serious manifestations of cancer and its treatments. Efforts to improve the nutritional status of such patients include dietary maneuvers, patient education, oral supplementation, and behavioral techniques. Dixon developed an experiment to examine the effects of nutritional supplementation and relaxation training on weight loss in cancer patients.

The sample consisted of persons with various cancers, most with either colorectal cancer (27 percent) or lymphoma (16 percent). Subjects were recruited from a variety of sources, including a medical center, a community hospital, and four oncology practices. They were informed about the study and were asked to participate in a screening procedure. The participating sample consisted of 50 males and 38 females who were at risk nutritionally. Fifty-eight percent of the subjects were receiving chemotherapy. Nutritional risk was based on at least one of three categories of evidence: a weight loss of more than 5 percent over a two-month period; persistent changes in patterns of eating since one year prior to diagnosis, or persistent problems (such as fatigue) that interfered with eating.

The 88 subjects were randomly assigned to a control group or to one of four intervention groups. One experimental group received nutritional supplementation; one received relaxation training; one received both, and one received neither. Fifty-five of the original 88 received a complete four-month intervention period, during which all except the control group were visited biweekly by a nurse. Twenty-three subjects (26 percent) died during the four months, while ten subjects (11 percent) chose to withdraw.

A considerable amount of data was collected, but the present analysis focused on: (1) anthropometric characteristics, including weight, height, triceps and skinfold taken at the midpoint of the upper arm; (2) performance status, measured by the five-point Eastern Cooperative Oncology Group Performance Status Scale, which focuses on ambulation, self-care, and ability to work; and (3) subject perception of intervention effectiveness, measured by questionnaires after completion of all other data collection.

The result for all three variables included greatest gain for the relaxation group and the most severe loss in the control group. Dixon believes that these findings suggest that the cachexia of cancer may be slowed or reversed through noninvasive nursing interventions.

STUDY QUESTIONS

1. What is control? How does the researcher exert control?
2. Define random sampling.
3. Define randomization, random assignment, and random allocation. How do they differ from random sampling?
4. What are matching, matched pairs, and matched groups?
5. Discuss the use of extraneous variables as independent variables.
6. What are successive experimental groups? What is the weakness inherent in these?
7. Define manipulation.
8. Why do you think that random sampling and manipulation are two of the most powerful sources of control?
9. Discuss the control of extraneous variables, such as environmental variables.
10. What is the Hawthorne effect?
11. To what does internal validity of the research design refer?
12. Discuss several classes of extraneous variables that may confuse the effect of the independent variable if not controlled.
13. What is meant by the term external validity of the research design?
14. Discuss the classic, or true, experimental design.
15. How does the Solomon four-group design differ from the classic design?

16. What is the two after-groups control design? How is it like the Solomon four-group design?
17. What is a quasi-experimental design?
18. Discuss a time series design.
19. Name and define a pre-experimental design.
20. What are the advantages and disadvantages of the experimental design?

REFERENCES AND SUGGESTED READINGS

Brown, M. and Grunfeld, C. (1980): Taste preferences of infants for sweetened or unsweetened food. Research in Nursing and Health, *3*, 11–17. *Experimental design using random assignment.*

Campbell, D. and Stanley, J (1966): Experimental and Quasi-experimental Designs for Research. Chicago: Rand McNally. *Includes experimental, quasi-experimental, and pre-experimental designs, and factors jeopardizing validity.*

Cleland, V. (1977): Investigations in the clinical setting. In Verhonick, P. (ed.), Nursing Research II. Boston: Little, Brown, pp. 33–76. *Experimental design in the clinical setting.*

DeWalt, E. and Haines, A. (1977): The effects of specified stressors on healthy oral mucosa. In Downs, F. and Newman, M. (eds.), A Sourcebook of Nursing Research (2nd ed.). Philadelphia: F. A. Davis, 24–32. *Experimental research.*

Dixon, J. (1984): Effect of nursing interventions on nutritional and performance status in cancer patients. Nursing Research, *33*, 330–335.

Downs, F. and Newman, M. (eds.) (1977): A Sourcebook of Nursing Research (2nd ed.). Philadelphia: F. A. Davis. *Fifteen articles on research identify research designs.*

Dumas, R. and Leonard, R. (1963): The effect of nursing and the incidence of postoperative vomiting: A clinical experiment. Nursing Research, *12*, 12–15.

Fieve, R. et al. (1971): A critical trial of methysergate and lithium in mania. In Kuper, D. (ed.), Lithium and Psychiatry Journal Articles. New Hyde Park, N.Y.: Medical Examination Publishers. *An experimental study.*

Floyd, J. (1984): Interaction between personal sleep–wake rhythms and psychiatric hospital rest–activity schedule. Nursing Research, *33*, 255–259.

Hanson, R. (1973): Effects of administering cold and warmed tube feedings. In Batey, M. (ed.), Communicating Nursing Research. Boulder: WICHE. *Time series experimental design.*

Hasselmeyer, E. (1961): Behavior Patterns of Premature Infants. Washington, D.C.: Government Printing Office. *Experimental design.*

Huckabay, L. (1978): Cognitive and affective consequences of formative evaluation in graduate nursing students. Nursing Research, *27*, 190–194. *Quasi-experimental design.*

Lindeman, C. and Van Aernam, B. (1977): Nursing intervention with the presurgical patient—The effects of structured and unstructured preoperative teaching. In Downs, F. and Newman, M. (eds.), A Sourcebook of Nursing Research (2nd ed.). Philadelphia: F. A. Davis, pp. 45–63. *Pretest/post-test static group design.*

McGillicuddy, M. (1977): A study of the relationship between mothers rooming-in during their children's hospitalization and changes in selected areas of children's behavior. In Downs, F. and Newman, M. (eds.), A Sourcebook of Nursing Research (2nd ed.). Philadelphia: F. A. Davis.

Stouffer, S. (1950): Some observations on study design. American Journal of Sociology, *55,* pp. 356–359. *Models for experimental designs.*

Wells, N. (1982): The effect of relaxation on postoperative muscle tension and pain. Nursing Research, *31,* 236–238.

Wooldridge, P. et al. (1978): Behavioral Science, Social Practice and the Nursing Profession. Cleveland: The Press of Case Western Reserve University. *Discusses the use of small samples with high internal validity to claim external validity.*

13

Additional Research Designs

The *survey* is a research design that relies heavily upon the validity of verbal reports. One of the most widely utilized research designs, it combines a distinct method of data collection—interviews and questionnaires—with a special form of statistical data analysis.

The *ex-post-facto* ("after the fact") *design* is one in which the researcher examines the effect of an event that happened in the past. For example, the drug thalidomide was taken by a group of women during pregnancy and was subsequently thought to be the cause of birth defects in the children of these pregnancies. The researcher studies the drug as the independent variable believed to cause birth defects (the dependent variable).

A *correlational design*, also called a *concomitant-variation* or *associational design*, is one that looks for patterns of variation between two or more phenomena, such as smoking and cancer. The distinction between ex-post-facto and correlational designs is that the ex-post-facto design looks for the cause of an event in the past in order to describe its effect in the present, whereas a correlational design analyzes how two variables are associated with each other, positively or negatively.

Secondary analysis of data is a research design that uses large sets of data, such as census material, for a re-analysis from a new perspective.

The *needs-assessment design* is less a design in itself than it is an objective of a design. It determines what needs a category of persons requires in the way of services or policy.

In like manner, the *evaluation design* is as much an objective as a design. The researcher evaluates or judges the success of a nursing practice, policy, or program in terms of intended outcomes or in terms of the consequences of practices, policies, or programs.

The *methodological design* is a plan to study the methods and instruments used in research. The researcher focuses on methods such as observing, questioning, and measuring or upon the various instruments used in nursing research.

Upon completion of this chapter, the student should be able to: (1) define, describe, and distinguish the following designs: the survey, the ex-post-facto study, the correlational design, the secondary analysis of data, the needs-assessment design, the evaluational study, and the methodological design; (2) define the time factors used in research designs, including the static, the cross-sectional, the longitudinal, the retrospective, the prospective, the trend study, the cohort study, the panel study, and the follow-up study; (3) describe how each design is used in nursing research; and (4) describe the weaknesses and strengths of each design.

THE SURVEY

Survey research is a mode of inquiry that relies heavily upon the validity of verbal reports. A well-known example of a survey is the United States Census. It combines a distinct method of data collection (interviews and questionnaires) with a special form of data analysis by statistical means. Surveys tend to study the effect of social forces in the field that are not under the researcher's control. In this case, the major controls are statistical rather than experimental, the critical factors being the use of random sampling to select a representative sample from the target population, and the statistical analysis and interpretation of data.

Modern survey research is not old, dating back only to the 1930s, when Gallup and Roper brought the mode of inquiry and the form of statistical analysis together. It requires that standardized information be collected from or about subjects selected from a larger population by random sampling. The size of the sample is often quite large, although some studies have used fewer than 100 cases. The units of analysis range from individuals to groups, communities, or organizations. Common methods of data collection include the interview, the mailed questionnaire, the telephone interview, and the survey that retrieves data from existing records or archival material.

Aims of the Survey Design

The survey may be either descriptive or explanatory. The aim of the descriptive survey is to look for data about the distribution and frequency of a particular datum in a population or subgroup. For example, the descriptive survey may seek to learn how respondents answer a question on abortion in order to compare the responses of different groups, such as married and single, males and females, or Catholics and Protestants. Or, the descriptive survey may seek to determine how one or more characteristics are distributed in a population; for example, who has diabetes, high blood pressure, or malnutrition, and where do they live in a particular community?

On the other hand, explanatory surveys seek to discover why the distribution takes the form that it does. Why does malnutrition occur among the poor, teenagers, or the elderly? Why does it occur in one sector of the community more often than it does in another?

Time Factors in the Survey

The survey may be *static*; that is, a *cross-section* of the population is examined at one point in time; or the survey may be *longitudinal*, including elements of change over a period of time. Longitudinal studies may be either *retrospective*, beginning at one point in time and tracing a phenomenon backward, or they may be *prospective*, beginning in the present and following a group or phenomenon forward over a period of time.

Longitudinal studies of change also include trend studies, cohort studies, panel studies, and follow-up studies. A *trend study* repeatedly asks the same question of equivalent samples of different individuals, while a *panel study* interviews the same subjects at two or more points in time. A *cohort study* examines a category of persons born during a particular time period. For example, a cohort of women born in 1940 may be studied in 1990 to determine the number of children ever born to them. At 50 years of age, the women are presumably past the childbearing period and may be considered as having completed families. *Follow-up studies* seek to determine any change or development in individuals or groups that have been previously studied.

In all of these cases, two or more groups may be used, one exposed to an independent variable and one not. The absence of random assignment of the sample to either experimental or control groups distinguishes the survey form from the classic experimental design. The location of the research also differs, surveys being conducted more often in the field than in the laboratory.

Advantages and Disadvantages of the Survey Design

A major advantage of the survey is that data are gathered from a more natural setting. The variables are examined as they are found in the existing social milieu. A large amount of data can also be gathered at a fairly reasonable price. Surveys using the questionnaire are likely to cover a wide geographical area, reach many people, ensure respondents' anonymity, and require less skill to administer. With careful pretesting of the instruments used, and with the use of random sampling techniques, the survey has a considerable degree of representativeness. No other method can reach as large a population as rapidly and be as accurate.

A major weakness of the survey design is that it only collects self-reports. This means that recall may be selective or that the respondent may not be willing to express attitudes or beliefs on sensitive topics. Standardization of the questionnaire also means that the least common denominator is represented. In addition, the response rate may be low, thereby introducing a bias. Finally, unless the researcher uses the interview, which is more expensive, he or she is not able to observe the study subjects directly, thereby losing the "feel" of the situation.

EXAMPLES FROM NURSING RESEARCH

The survey is widely used in nursing research to collect data by questionnaire or interview. At times it may be combined with other research methods, or it may be used alone. Hash et al. (1985) used a telephone survey with a standardized schedule to assess the educational needs of nurses, completing between three and thirty calls per hour from a wide geographic sample. McKeever and Galloway (1984) used the Menstrual Cycle Information Questionnaire, a structured interview guide in two parts, to determine the effect of nongynecological surgery on the menstrual cycle. Subjects were interviewed in the hospital 72 hours or more following surgery and again about 6 weeks later by telephone.

Hurwitz and Eadie (1977) used both the survey and dream analysis to study the psychological impact on nursing students of participating in abortion procedures. Using a series of questionnaires, together with dream reports written at the same time, data were collected over a four-week period, during which the students were assigned to various clinical experiences. The first week, the clinical experience took place in abortion units, and the questionnaire included a question on the students' feelings about abortion. Four basic questions were asked on the students' dreams, which were included each week. The following weeks did not include abortion experiences, but did have other surgical experiences. Questionnaire data were analyzed using the chi-square statistic, while dream data were analyzed by content analysis.

Stillman (1977) used a questionnaire to investigate the nature of women's health beliefs about breast cancer and breast self-examination, and the extent of breast self-examination. A convenience sample of 122 women members of an organization filled out a five-part questionnaire. Data were analyzed using descriptive statistics.

Ford (1973) studied the cultural criteria and determinants for the acceptance of modern medicine among reservation Indians of South Dakota. Several designs, including unstructured interviews, focused on beliefs, attitudes, and interpersonal relations. The sample included Yuwipi and herbal medicine men and women and their clients, Peyote leaders and their clients, and persons using modern medicine (Ford, 1973, p. 45). Analysis of data was descriptive, with case-study presentations.

THE EX-POST-FACTO DESIGN

The ex-post-facto study is one that occurs "after the fact." The researcher attempts to explain a phenomenon that has already occurred. Something has happened in the life of an individual or group of individuals that the researcher wishes to explain or describe. For example, birth defects can only be studied after the fact. The birth of the so-called thalidomide babies was presumed to be a result of the use of the drug thalidomide during pregnancy. The researcher could not manipulate the independent variable, the drug thalidomide, for ethical reasons. However, once the appearance of the birth defects was documented, researchers could look for preceding factors that may have been the presumed cause or that may be correlated with the effect.

The ex-post-facto study design is similar to the pre-experimental design described earlier. Goode and Hatt (1952, p. 85) suggest its similarity to the single-cell design (see Fig. 12–9). The basic logic of the experiment and of the ex-post-facto design is the same: the researcher wishes to establish the relationship between the independent variable and the dependent variable (Kerlinger, 1973, p. 379). The difference between the experiment and the ex-post-facto design is that control is lost in the ex-post-facto design. The independent variable cannot be manipulated, and the subjects cannot be randomly selected from the target population or randomly assigned to the experimental group or control group. Accompanying these differences is an associated problem: proper interpretation of data. Therefore, interpretation of ex-post-facto findings should be tentative, even when hypotheses are carefully selected and tested.

The value of ex-post-facto studies lies in the fact that many important research problems cannot be studied by experimentation. Ethical research prohibits the researcher from introducing a variable that may harm the study subjects. Certain variables cannot be manipulated, such as environmental, economic, and social factors, or personal characteristics of individuals, including sex, age, or diagnosis. The ex-post-facto study investigates cases in which these variables have been manipulated by life events: the environment has become polluted, jobs have been lost, or sex changes have been attempted. A second value of the ex-post-facto study is the relative "naturalness" of the design. Study subjects are not studied in a laboratory, but at home, at work, or in a situation where they have been placed by life.

EXAMPLE FROM NURSING RESEARCH

Burkhardt (1985) utilized an ex-post-facto design to study the impact of arthritis—pain and functional impairment—on the quality of life. The researcher sought to describe and explain how past physical, psychological, and social factors influenced the perception of the quality of life experienced by people with arthritis. The researcher developed a model that related the variables of the disease to demographic and social factors. To collect the data, Burkhardt interviewed 94 adults in their homes, using instruments such as the Quality of Life Index, the Severity of Pain Index, and others.

THE CORRELATION DESIGN

Correlation and Causation

Correlation is the pattern of variation in two phenomena. Correlation, sometimes called concomitant variation or association, is a process that examines how a change in the amount of one variable is accompanied by a comparable change in the amount of another variable.

A causal relationship is also an association, but one that is strong enough to have predictive powers. To infer that one variable is the cause of another, the researcher must have three types of evidence: (1) the cause X and the effect Y must vary together in the way predicted by a specific hypothesis: (2) Y must not precede X in time; and (3) other factors must not determine Y (Selltiz et al, 1976, p. 489). As Mill (1930) puts it: when two or more cases of a given phenomenon have one and only one condition in common, then that condition is regarded as the cause of the phenomenon. When the researcher is unable to determine with certainty that the effect was directly caused by the stimulus, then the change is said to be associated, or correlated, with the stimulus rather than caused by the stimulus. Some researchers are wary of causality. Kerlinger (1973, p. 393) warns that the study of cause and causation is an endless maze. Particularly in the study of human subjects, causal relationships should be regarded as difficult to establish.

Correlational designs are similar to ex-post-facto studies, in that neither expects to determine causality. However, correlational designs differ form ex-post-facto designs, in that correlational designs may examine past events but may likewise include other time frameworks.

EXAMPLE FROM NURSING RESEARCH

Heineken (1982) studied disconfirmation in dysfunctional communication in order to examine the correlation between mental illness and a decline in an individual's links with others. Disconfirmation was defined, following Laing (*The Self and Others*, 1961, p. 83), as subtle but persistent negation and discounting toward the impaired person. Psychiatric-patient groups from four treatment facilities who agreed to participate in the study comprised the sample. Five hundred and fifteen interpersonal interactions were scored and analyzed. Following the study, the author proposed hypotheses with the following correlations: There is a positive correlation between the degree of psychopathology and the frequency of disconfirming responses; in acutely psychotic individuals, the frequency of disconfirming responses will decrease as the severity of the psychosis subsides.

EXAMPLES FROM NURSING RESEARCH

Time Frameworks

Correlational designs may include either prospective studies or cross-sectional studies. A well-known prospective study, the Framingham Heart Study, followed 5,209 persons for over two decades. Gibbs et al. (1974) utilized a record review of 15 months, and interviews during a three-month period, to study reproductive health care patterns among the poor of San Antonio.

Amborn (1976) conducted a brief cross-sectional correlational study to examine the clinical signs associated with the amount of suctioned tracheobronchial secretions. Data were collected from 35 study subjects over a one-hour period.

Elder (1976) used a predictive correlational study to explain variables that may influence a dependent variable. A large number of variables (education, religion, sexual experience, age, etc.) were used to predict the willingness that nursing students demonstrated to participate in the provision of contraceptives.

Advantages and Disadvantages of Ex-Post-Facto and Correlational Designs

Both designs have the advantage of examining the results of factors that could not be studied because of ethical restraints. In the ex-post-facto design, life has introduced the presumed independent variable. The researcher examines the effect, searching among the processes of the past so as to identify a possible agent whose presence is correlated with the effect. The disadvantage of the ex-post-facto design is the loss of control—both manipulation and randomization.

Correlational designs are useful to examine the extent to which changes in one factor vary with changes in one or more other factors. The disadvantage of the correlational design is the researcher's tendency to attribute causality to descriptive relationships. However, carefully designed, with valid hypotheses, correlational studies provide information that may be used to predict.

SECONDARY ANALYSIS OF DATA: A DESIGN TO USE DATA PREVIOUSLY COLLECTED BY OTHERS

The researcher who plans a secondary analysis of data intends to search for new relationships in existing data previously collected either by the researcher or by some other agency for some other purpose. These data are usually from surveys of large dimensions.

For example, the 1980 world population data sheet (prepared by the Population Reference Bureau in Washington, D.C.) lists all geopolitical entities in the world with a population larger than 200,000 and all members of the United Nations. It includes information on birth rates, death rates, infant mortality rates, fertility rate, life expectancy at birth, urban populations, and projected ultimate population size. The United States Census collects massive data every 10 years, with intermediate collections in between. Private and public agencies, such as insurance companies and health departments, collect and publish numerous vital statistics reports, including reports on birth, death, marriage, divorce, and disease. Every public school board or board of education conducts its own census on local populations of school-age children every two years or so in order to plan for the assessment of educational needs and funding.

Hospitals and clinics keep extensive data, many of which use specific guidelines for data collection designed for planning and reporting. Data from public survey agencies, such as the Gallup and Roper polls, are often available, while data banks funded by agencies, such as the National Science Foundation, are appearing. In addition, cross-cultural data on childrearing and other facts of interest to nursing are available for analysis from Yale University's Human Area Relations File, which contains nearly 500,000 pages of source materials taken from several hundred cultures. A sophisticated system of coding allows the researcher to locate quickly the specific data needed.

Use of collected data is a considerable advantage, since the sampling, development of instruments, and collection of data have been completed. However, the use of someone else's data is not without problems. Massive collections can be overwhelming, even when considerable analysis is already complete. In addition, even official data often contain frustrating omissions and errors. Finally, the data are not always published in a convenient form—there is no guarantee that relevant data can always be found.

In spite of these handicaps, secondary analysis of existing data is a fertile area worth exploring. The researcher can discuss or analyze the data using a number of research designs, including the descriptive, correlational, or ex-post-facto.

EXAMPLE FROM NURSING RESEARCH

Secondary analysis of data is not widely reported as yet in nursing research, no doubt awaiting increasing expertise and easier access to both the data and the computer. Munro (1980) used a national sample to study dropouts from nursing education, while Deardorff, Denner, and Miller (1976) utilized State Board Examination scores and scores on the National League for Nursing tests as the criterion variable and predictor variables in a correlational study. Woods (1985) utilized data from the United States Department of Labor reports (*Handbook on Women Workers,* 1975; and *Women in the Labor*

Force, 1977) to examine employment, family roles, and mental ill health in young married women.

RESEARCH DESIGNS THAT USE ONE OR MORE DIFFERENT DESIGNS

Needs Assessment: Use of One or More Designs to Assess Needs

The *needs-assessment design* is less a particular design in and of itself than it is a combination of a number of different designs. For example, the researchers may use one design or a combination of several research designs, including (among others) the survey, the correlational, the ex-post-facto, the descriptive, and the historical/documentary design. The needs-assessment design is utilized to obtain, document, and summarize information needed by organizations, categories of persons, or a specific community. The researcher examines the needs, provides referrals for services, or recommends policies.

EXAMPLES FROM NURSING RESEARCH

Hain and Chen (1976) used a survey to assess the health conditions and needs of the elderly. The researchers used an interview schedule comprised of 20 questions in order to obtain data from 128 persons aged 65 years and over who were living in high-rise apartments. The researchers assessed the health needs of the sample, including access to, and cost of, health care, and the subjects' own health condition and physical functioning.

Steffen and Francis (1978, pp. 287–288) used screening, a type of descriptive design, to assess the health status of migrant children, including Chicanos and Kickapoo children, at six locations throughout northern Utah, in order to provide referrals for further services. The assessment was part of a larger study concerned with transcultural nursing experiences and care of migrant children. One of the primary needs assessed was that of "sensitivity"—the need for physicians and other health-care providers to be sensitive to the cultural values and beliefs of the Kickapoo Indians.

The needs assessment design may be structured to collect data from: (1) *a sample* drawn from the target population whose needs are being assessed through the use of interviews and questionnaires; (2) *selected key individuals,* considered to be either a key to the understanding of the community or experts in the needs of the group or community. The researcher interviews these persons, and then uses the responses to assess needs; and (3) *existing records,* from which the researchers can conduct a secondary analysis of data in order to infer "indicators of needs."

Programs and policies of federal agencies such as the National Cancer Institute, the National Institute of Mental Health, and the U. S. Public Health Service are based on what the available data say about need. Therefore, researchers interested in policies of health care are interested in research designs concerned with needs assessment.

Evaluation-Research Designs: Use of One or More Designs to Evaluate Nursing Programs, Policies, and Practice

The researcher structures the evaluation-research design so as to judge how well a designated process, such as a nursing program, policy, or practice, is working. Without knowing the stated objectives, a judgment may be made either on how well the program meets its stated objectives or goal or on its outcome or impact. Like the needs-assessment design, evaluation research may be either one design or a combination of many designs, including experimental, ex-post-facto, survey, and descriptive. Evaluation research may utilize different time perspectives, either evaluating material while the program, policy, process, or practice is being developed (the *formative time framework*) or evaluating an ongoing program, one already in operation, in order to assess the worth of its continued use (a *summative time framework*).

The traditional approach to evaluation is a judgment of how well the objectives of a program or policy are being met. The researcher first determines the objectives of the program, policy, or practice, and then locates an instrument that will measure the extent to which these objectives were met. If the objectives are not clearly stated, observable, or measurable, the researcher's first task may be to determine the intended objectives implied in the program, policy, or practice and to create definitions that will make each objective observable and measurable. Objectives stated as behavioral objectives concerned with intended consequences (or outcomes) should be both observable and measurable. The traditional approach is useful to determine whether the objectives of the program, policy, or practice are being met.

An approach to evaluation that differs from the traditional evaluation of how well objectives are being met is the "goal-free" approach. In this case, the objectives are deliberately left unknown by the researcher in order to avoid potential bias. Instead, the researcher evaluates the consequences or outcome of various policies, programs, and practices without knowing the objectives that the outcomes were intended to meet. It is believed that both the manifest aspects of the program (associated with the intended consequences, or outcomes) and the latent aspects of the program (associated with unintended consequences, or outcomes) can be judged without knowledge of objectives. However, this is an unstructured approach, which may take more time and money. In addition, it may not be useful to those who make decisions on the basis of evaluation.

Evaluation is part of a political process—decisions may be made on the basis of the findings to create funding, implement new programs, continue or discontinue policies and programs, expand or contract services, employ or "destaff" positions, and so on. For this reason, it can be threatening to those who are concerned with their positions and reputations, thereby decreasing cooperation. In addition, evaluation of a program or procedure with more than one objective creates the problem of overall evaluation. How is the total program, policy, or practice to be judged if the researcher discovers that some objectives are met and some are not?

In Diers's view (1979, pp. 205–207), evaluation research neither leads to theory, nor is based on theory, nor does it create knowledge that will explain relationships among concepts. However, evaluation is a contemporary issue that affects applied aspects of the professions. The extensive literature on evaluation invites a summary and description with an emphasis on the nursing perspective.

EXAMPLES FROM NURSING RESEARCH

In the clinical area, Ventura et al. (1982) used the Risser Patient Satisfaction Scale to evaluate the effectiveness of implementing key concepts of primary nursing on an orthopedic unit. The objective was patient satisfaction. Vincent and Price (1977) report the evaluation of a VNA mental-health project, and Griggs (1977) reports an evaluation of instructional material—a systems approach to the development and evaluation of a minicourse for nurses. In addition, Santopietro (1980) reports an evaluation of the effectiveness of a self-instructional module for counseling in human sexuality.

Methodological Designs: Use of Several Designs to Invent and Evaluate Methods and Instruments

The researcher who uses a methodological design plans for the invention, development, and evaluation of methods and tools used in research. The researcher investigates the methods of data collecting, such as observing, questioning, and measuring, and the instruments, scales, and tests used in selected methods. A number of research designs may be used by the researcher, including the survey, the experimental, the historical, and the descriptive.

The steps in the methodological design differ from the phases and steps generally used in research. The methodological design involves invention and evaluation rather than sampling, data collection, and analysis.

EXAMPLES FROM NURSING RESEARCH

Ailinger (1982) modified an instrument used in a national survey to reflect Hispanic cultural beliefs and practices (see research example at end of chapter). Stevenson (1982) began with a conceptual model developed by McClusky (1963) to study the life of adults in process, and then translated a construct from the model into an instrument for research and clinical use. The process was not easy, but an examination of her account reveals some of the steps involved in the development and evaluation of a complex instrument.

The first step was to define the concepts. Second, Stevenson developed a list of "discrete dimensions of adult life," including physiological functioning, intellectual development, self-concept, spiritual-religious domain, family, work, and community.

Third, using the categories of the discrete dimensions of adult life as the basis, Stevenson developed six subscales to cover the "totality of human experience," which included religiosity-spirituality, self-concept, body (physical functioning), family, extrafamilial human relationships, and nonperson environment.

Fourth, Stevenson developed "Form 1" of the instrument. She utilized a sample of healthy adult volunteers to answer a questionnaire that included the scale, and she later interviewed 10 percent of the respondents.

Fifth, Stevenson utilized the responses and comments of the subjects to revise the scale, developing "Form 2." She then gave "Form 2" to 103 normal adult volunteers, including 66 subjects who had taken Form 1 four months earlier.

Sixth, Stevenson used statistical tests to compare test-retest reliability, test-effect bias, and other factors. She revised the scales and tested them before producing "Form 3."

Finally, in order to compare the answers of the healthy with those of the sick, Stevenson gave the scale to 63 persons with chronic illness, such as multiple sclerosis, diabetes, cardiac problems, or chronic mental-health problems.

The author concluded that, while continued validity and reliability testing were still needed, the first test showed positive results and could be useful in measuring the whole human being as an interactant in his or her life space.

SUMMARY

The survey is a mode of inquiry that relies heavily upon verbal self-reports. The national census is an example of a survey research design. The method of data collection by questionnaire and interview is combined with a special form of data analysis by statistical means. Random sampling is used to select a representative sample from the target population or, in the case of the national census, the total population is studied. Units of study thus range from individuals to national populations. The survey may be either descriptive or explanatory. The descriptive survey collects data about the study subjects or objects in order to describe selected characteristics, attitudes, or behavior. The explanatory survey seeks to discover the relationship between variables. A survey may examine a population at one point in time (the cross-section) or it may study changes over a period of time (the longitudinal study). The longitudinal study may be retrospective (beginning at one point in time and tracing a phenomenon backward) or it may be prospective (following a group or phenomenon forward over a period of time). The trend study repeatedly asks the same question of equivalent samples of the population, while the panel study interviews the same subjects at two or more points in time. The cohort study examines a group of persons who were born at the same time (and thus experienced similar events), while the follow-up study examines changes in or development of those who have been previously studied.

A major advantage of the survey is that data are gathered from a natural setting. In addition, large amounts of data may be collected from a broad geographical area. The major weakness of the survey design is the reliance on respondents' self-reports, which may be selective or incorrect. In the case of the questionnaire, lack of response is also a disadvantage, because the returns may not be sufficient to represent the population.

Ex-post-facto designs examine the data after life (or nature) has introduced the independent variable. The researcher does not have direct control, either because the effect has already been manifested or because it is not possible to manipulate the independent variable; however, in cases where it has been introduced, the researcher can try to study its presumed effect.

Correlational studies examine how variables change in terms of one another. Correlational designs may be prospective (beginning at one point in time and following study subjects forward) or they may be cross-sectional (studying the changes in the amount of one variable in relation to changes in another, in a concurrent time framework). Correlational studies are useful for providing information about the extent of changes between associated variables.

Secondary analysis of data is a search for new descriptions or relationships in existing data, usually from large surveys. Data sets available include world population data, United States Census data, and data from private and public agencies (such as insurance companies, health departments, hospitals and clinics, disease-control centers, Gallup and Roper polls, and the Human Area Relations File). Use of collected data is a saving in time and money, since sampling, development of instruments, and data collection are completed. However, there are problems associated with the use of someone else's data, including omissions and errors.

Needs assessment is a combination of a number of different designs, including the survey, correlational, ex-post-facto, descriptive, and historical. The object is to collect, document, and summarize information by various organizations, persons, and communities. Data may be collected from a sample, selected key individuals, and existing records, from which indicators of need may be inferred.

Evaluation designs are structured to judge how well a process (such as a nursing program, policy, or practice) is working. A number of research designs are useful in evaluation research, including experimental, survey, and descriptive. Without a knowledge of the objectives, the data collected may judge either how well a program, policy, or practice meets its stated objectives or the consequences of such programs. A formative time framework is one in which evaluation research is conducted while the program, policy, or practice is being developed. A summative time framework is one that evaluates a program, policy, or practice already in operation. Evaluation is part of a political process involved with decision making and, as such, may be considered threatening, thereby decreasing the level of cooperation obtainable from those involved with the programs, policies, or practices.

Methodological designs are plans for the invention, development, and evaluation of the methods and tools used in research. Many types of research designs are incorporated into the methodological design, including the survey, experiment, historical, and descriptive. Development of adequate research tools is indispensable in nursing research, although the process is challenging. Statistical methods are used to evaluate the validity and reliability of the method or instrument invented.

EXAMPLE FROM NURSING RESEARCH

A Survey/Methodological Design

Rita L. Ailinger (1982): Hypertension knowledge in a Hispanic community. Nursing Research, 31, 207–210.

Ailinger's research focuses on two research designs: (1) the development and evaluation of an instrument to assess the level of knowledge of hypertension, and (2) a survey by interview to determine the level of knowledge of hypertension found in an Hispanic community in Virginia.

Methodological Portion of Research: Ailinger developed the Hypertension Knowledge Interview Schedule from an existing instrument that had not been validated or tested for reliability. She modified the instrument by adding items to reflect Hispanic cultural beliefs and practices. She evaluated content validity, discriminant validity, and reliability of the instrument in several ways: (1) three nurses and one physician, all nationally known for their work in hypertension, evaluated the content validity, concerned with the instrument's sampling adequacy; (2) two student groups, including nursing students who had just completed a study unit on hypertension and sociology students who had little knowledge about hypertension, took the test, the difference in the scores of these two groups establishing discriminant validity; and (3) the reliability of the instrument was tested using Cronback's alpha (a reliability index that estimates internal consistency of a measure with several subparts).

Survey Design: Four bilingual interviewers were trained and instructed in methods for assuring uniformity in interviewing, coding reliability, confidentiality, and securing informed consent. The target population was an Hispanic community in Virginia that included 6,315 persons. To identify the sample of study subjects, the researchers: (1) obtained ten census tracts with the highest concentration of Hispanics from the 1970 census data; (2) noted all streets within the ten tracts; (3) identified 330 households from the phone directory whose addresses were listed on these streets and whose surnames were Hispanic; and (4) selected one adult in each household for study. Interviewers made telephone contact with each household in order to secure an appointment for a home interview with an adult. Four unsuccessful contacts caused the name to be deleted from the study. Most interviews were on Saturday or Sunday or between 4 and 8 P.M. during the week. The Hollingshead Index of social class was used to compute socioeconomic class. Findings indicated that 36 percent of the respondents did not have adequate knowledge about hypertension. Hispanics were more informed about some areas but, in comparison with other studies, showed deficits in other areas.

STUDY QUESTIONS

1. What is a survey? What are the aims of the survey design?
2. How does a descriptive survey design differ from an explanatory survey design?
3. Describe a cross-sectional survey design and a longitudinal survey design.
4. Distinguish a retrospective survey design from a prospective survey design.
5. Compare survey designs that include trend, cohort, panel, and follow-up studies.
6. What distinguishes a survey design from an experimental design?
7. What are the advantages and disadvantages of the survey design?
8. What is the ex-post-facto design? How does it differ from the experiment? What is its value?
9. What is the difference between causation and correlation?
10. How does a correlational design differ from an ex-post-facto design?
11. What time frameworks are used in correlational designs?
12. What are the advantages and disadvantages of the ex-post-facto and correlational designs?
13. Define "secondary analysis of data." What are possible sources of primary data?
14. What are the advantages and disadvantages of the secondary analysis of data design?
15. Name three research designs that utilize a number of designs in their research plan.
16. How does a study of "needs assessment" differ from a research design?
17. What is the source of data in a needs-assessment study?
18. What does an evaluation research design structure do? How does the traditional approach differ from the "goal-free" approach?
19. What are methodological designs? What do the phases and steps of a methodological design involve?
20. Describe Stevenson's steps in the development of an instrument.

REFERENCES AND SUGGESTED READING

Ailinger, R. (1982): Hypertension knowledge in a Hispanic community. Nursing Research, *31*, 207–210. *A survey and instrument development.*

Amborn, S. (1976): Clinical signs associated with the amount of tracheobronchial secretions. Nursing Research, *25*, 121–126. *An exploratory correlations design.*

Backstrom, C. and Hursh, G. (1980): Survey Research (2nd ed.). Evanston, Ill.: Northwestern University Press. *The Survey.*

Boruck, R. (ed.) (1978): Secondary Analysis. San Francisco: Jossey-Bass. *Using data collected by others for new analysis.*

Brink, P. (1984): Value orientations as an assessment tool in cultural diversity. Nursing Research, *33*, 198–203. *The use of the Kluckhohn and Strodtbeck instrument in an interview schedule.*

Brown, J., et al. (1984): Nursing's search for scientific knowledge. Nursing Research, *33*, 26–32.

Burkhardt, C. (1985): The impact of arthritis on quality of life. Nursing Research, *34*, 11–16. *Example of ex-post-facto design.*

Caldwell, R. et al. (1983): Sex differences in separation and divorce. Issues in Mental Health Nursing, *5*, 103–120. *Longitudinal study using interviews.*

Cornell, S. (1974): Development of an instrument for measurement of the quality of nursing care. Nursing Research, *23*, 108–117. *Methodological design to develop a research tool.*

Cornell Medical College (1956): Cornell Medical Index–Health Questionnaire, rev. ed. Ithaca, N.Y.: The College. *Questionnaire.*

Cowan, M. and Murphy, S. (1985): Identification of postdisaster bereavement-risk predictors. Nursing Research, *34*, 71–75. *Correlation study.*

Cox, C. (1985): The health self-determinism index. Nursing Research, *34*, 177–183. *A psychometric evaluation of a new measure of motivation in health behavior.*

Deardorff, M., Denner, P., and Miller, C. (1976): Selected National League for Nursing achievement test scores as predictors of state board examination scores. Nursing Research, *25, Secondary analysis of data.*

Derdiarian, A. and Clough, D. (1976): Patients' dependence and independence levels on prehospitalization–postdischarge continuum. Nursing Research, *25*, 27–34. *Longitudinal study.*

Diers, D. (1979): Research in Nursing Practice. Philadelphia: J. B. Lippincott. *Example of research in the clinical area.*

Downs, F. and Fitzpatrick, J. (1976): Preliminary investigation of the reliability and validity of a tool for the assessment of body position and motor activity. Nursing Research, *25*, 404–408. *Methodological design.*

Downs, F. and Newman, M. (eds.) (1977): A Sourcebook of Nursing Research. Philadelphia: F. A. Davis. *Fifteen articles on research identify research design used.*

Elder, R. (1976): Orientation of senior nursing students toward access to contraception. Nursing Research, *25*, 338–345. *Correlational study.*

Fink, A. and Kosecoff, J. (1980): An Evaluation Primer Workbook: Practical Exercises for Health Professionals. Beverly Hills: Sage. *Evaluation discussed.*

Fitts, W. (1964): Tennessee Self-Concept Scale. Nashville, Tenn.: Counselor Recordings and Tests. *Scale.*

Flaskerud, J. (1980): A tool for comparing the perceptions of problematic behavior by psychiatric professionals and minority groups. Nursing Research, *29*, 4–9. *Comparative study.*

Flaskerud, J. (1984): A comparison of perceptions of problematic behavior by six minority groups and mental health professionals. Nursing Research, *33*, 190–197. *Twelve nurse–investigators in different parts of the country sampled and interviewed each minority and professional group.*

Flynn, B. (1984): An action research framework for primary health care. Nursing Outlook, *32*, 316–318. *Interviews, record reviews, vital statistics, community assessment.*

Ford, V. (1973): Medicine among the Teton Dakota, Rosebud Indian Reservation, South Dakota. In Batey, M. (ed.), Communicating Nursing Research. Boulder: WICHE. *Research using the survey and other designs.*

Franck, P. (1979): A survey of health needs of older adults in north west Johnson County, Iowa. Nursing Research, *28*, 360–368. *Survey.*

Gibbs, et al. (1974): Patterns of reproductive health care among the poor of San Antonio, Texas. American Journal of Public Health, *64*, 37–40. *Longitudinal study.*

Goode, W. and Hatt, P. (1952): Methods in Social Research. New York: McGraw-Hill. *An old but good approach.*

Griggs, V. (1977): A systems approach to the development and evaluation of a minicourse for nurses. Nursing Research, *26*, 34–41. *Evaluation.*

Hain, M. and Chen, S. (1976): Health needs of the elderly. Nursing Research, *25*, 433–439. *Needs assessment.*

Hash, V., Donlea, J., and Walljasper, D. (1985): The telephone survey: A procedure for assessing educational needs of nurses. Nursing Research, 126–128. *Survey; needs assessment.*

Heineken, J. (1982): Disconfirmation in dysfunctional communication. Nursing Research, *31*, 211–213.

Hubbard, P., Muhlenkamp, A., and Brown, N. (1984): The relationship between social support and self-care practices. Nursing Research, *33*, 277–270. *Descriptive survey; nonrandom sample with hypotheses.*

Hurwitz, F. and Eadie, F. (1977): Psychologic impact on nursing students of participation in abortion. Nursing Research, *26*, 112–120. *Questionnaire and dream collection.*

Kerlinger, F. (1973): Foundations of Behavioral Research (2nd ed.). New York: Holt, Rinehart, & Winston. *Useful in general.*

La Rocco, S. and Polit, D. (1980): Women's knowledge about the menopause. Nursing Research, *29*, 10–13. *Survey of 500 women in greater Boston.*

Magilvy, J. (1985): Quality of life of hearing-impaired older women. Nursing Research, *34*, 140–144. *A survey, interview; causal model specified.*

McClusky, H. (1963): The course of the adult life span. In Hallenbeck, W. (ed.), Psychology of Adults. Washington, D.C.: Adult Education of the USA, pp. 10–19.

McGillicuddy, M. (1977): A study of the relationship between mothers' rooming-in during their children's hospitalization and changes in selected areas of children's behavior. In Downs, F. and Newman, M. (eds.), A Sourcebook of Nursing Research (2nd ed.) Philadelphia: F. A. Davis, pp. 64–77. *Use of interviews, questionnaires, comparative groups.*

McKeever, P. and Galloway, S. (1984): Effects of nongynecological surgery on the menstrual cycle. Nursing Research, *33*, 42–46. *Structured interview; methodology—menstrual cycle information questionnaire designed by the investigators.*

Meleis, A. (1985): International nursing: A force for knowledge development. Nursing Outlook, *May/June*, 144–147.

Miles, M. (1985): Emotional symptoms and physical health in bereaved parents. Nursing Research, *34*, 76–81. Survey; mailed questionnaires.

Mill, J. (1930): A System of Logic (8th ed.). New York: Longmans. *The logic of causation and correlation.*

Munro, B. (1980): Dropouts from nursing education: Path analysis of a national sample. Nursing Research, *29*. *Secondary analysis.*

Neugarten, B. et al. (1961): Measurement of life satisfaction. Journal of Gerontology, *16*, 134–143. *Measurement.*

Nolan, J. (1985): Work patterns of mid-life female nurses. Nursing Research, *34*, 150–154. *Use of interview.*

O'Brien, M. (1980): Hemodialysis regimen compliance and social environment. Nursing Research, *29*, 250–255. *Panel study.*

Olade, R. (1984): Evaluation of the Denver developmental screening test as applied to African children. Nursing Research, *33*, 204–207. *Evaluation of instrument for cross-cultural studies, needs assessment.*

Phillips, L. and Rempusheski, V. (1985): A decision-making model for diagnosing and intervening in elder abuse and neglect. Nursing Research, *34*, 134–139. *Interview; evaluation.*

Rotter, J. (1966): Generalized expectancies for internal versus external control of reinforcement. Psychological Monographs, *80*, 1–28. *Locus of control.*

Santopietro, M. (1980): Effectiveness of a self-instructional module in human sexuality counseling. Nursing Research, *29*, 14–19. *Evaluation research.*

Schoen, D. (1975): Comparing the body systems and conceptual approaches to nursing education. Nursing Research, *24*, 383–387. *Trend study.*

Selltiz, C., et al. (1976): Research Methods in Social Relations. New York: Holt, Rinehart & Winston. *Correlation and causation.*

Shaw, E. (1985): Female circumcision. American Journal of Nursing, *June*, 685 ff. *Informal interviews with 11 circumcised women from various cultures living in the U.S.*

Steffen, M. and Francis, F. (1978): Transcultural nursing experience and care with migrant children. In Leininger, M. (ed.), Transcultural Nursing. New York: Wiley, pp. 283–297.

Stevenson, J. (1982): Construction of a scale to measure load, power, and margin in life. Nursing Research, *31*, 222–225. *Methodological study.*

Stillman, M. (1977): Women's health beliefs about breast cancer and breast self-examination. Nursing Research, *26*, 121–127. *Survey design using questionnaire.*

Ventura, M., Fox, R., Corley, M., and Mercurio, S. (1982): A patient satisfaction measure as a criterion to evaluate primary nursing. Nursing Research, *31*, 226–230. *Evaluation of primary nursing.*

Vincent, P. and Price, J. (1977): Evaluation of a VNA mental health project. Nursing Research, *26*, 361–367. *Evaluation research.*

Woods, N. (1985): Employment, family roles, and mental ill health in young married women. Nursing Research, *34*, 4–9. *Use of interview.*

PART V

Collecting the Data

14

Sampling

Sampling is the process by which the study subjects or objects are chosen from a larger population. Sampling is a crucial part of the research process, since the method of sampling determines whether or not the study sample represents the entire population from which it was drawn. If the sample does represent the entire population, the findings from the sample can be generalized to the population. If not, the findings apply only to the sample studied.

This chapter is designed to introduce the student to the complex topic of sampling. Upon completion of the chapter, the student should be able to: (1) define basic terms used in sampling; (2) state advantages of sampling; (3) discuss the theory of probability that underlies scientific sampling; (4) distinguish between probability sampling and nonprobability sampling; (5) identify and describe methods of probability sampling and nonprobability sampling; (6) describe steps to select particular samples; and (7) discuss sample size and biases in sampling.

BASIC TERMS USED IN SAMPLING

Basic terms encountered in sampling include the following: population, universe, sample, generalization, probability sampling, nonprobability sampling, and strata. Each of these will be briefly examined.

1. Population *is the total group of persons or objects that meets the designated set of criteria established by the researcher.* If the researcher is interested in female patients in the United States, the population consists of all females who are presently patients (or

who have ever been patients, if this is what interests the researcher). Thus, the population is all cases that conform to the researcher's established criteria. A list of all cases, objects, or groups of cases or objects in the population is called a *sampling frame*. The total population is also called the *universe* or *target population*—for example, the total number of female patients to whom the results of the research could be generalized. The enormous task of obtaining a list of all female patients in the population of the United States is obvious. If the list were obtainable from some central computer, the task would only just have begun. The sample drawn from the population would have to be contacted and studied, a formidable undertaking reserved for long-term, well-funded projects. Therefore, the *accessible population* is the population of subjects who are available to the researcher—for example, the population of female patients in a hospital at one time, or the female patients attending a weight-loss, prenatal, or hypertensive clinic. The list of all such patients would be more easily obtainable, and the sample drawn from the list would be easier to study. At times, all of the accessible population may be studied. However, the findings of a study sample apply only to the accessible population from which the study sample was drawn, and then only if certain sampling techniques—random sampling —ensure that each female in the accessible population had an equal chance of being chosen for the sample. Otherwise, the findings apply only to the sample studied, and the researcher is not able to generalize to the accessible population or to any other.

2. Sample *is the subset of cases drawn from the target, or accessible, population.* A single member of the population, or sample, is called an *element*, the basic unit from which data are collected. At times, several elements (or a set of elements) form a *sampling unit*. For example, if the researcher wished to study females attending all of the hypertensive clinics in a city, each clinic would be a sampling unit, and each patient would be an element.

3. Generalization *is the ability to apply the conclusion reached from studying the elements in a sample to the population from which the study sample was drawn.* The researcher concludes that the results of the study sample are the same as would have been reached if every element in the entire population had been studied. Every researcher wants to be able to generalize the results obtained from the sample, and this may be done if the sample is selected by probability sampling.

4. Probability sampling *is a process in which each element of the*

population has an equal chance of being chosen for the sample. Methods of probability sampling include simple random sampling, stratified random sampling, systematic sampling, and cluster sampling. (Each of these is examined in this chapter.)

5. Nonprobability sampling *is a process for selecting samples without using probability sampling.* Methods used include accidental sampling, quota sampling, and purposive sampling.

6. Strata *are two or more subpopulations.* Strata are comprised of mutually exclusive portions of the population, each of which is called a *stratum.* For example, a researcher studying female patients could divide the population into strata. Each stratum could consist of women of a particular socioeconomic class: upper class, middle class, and lower class. Each stratum would be as homogeneous as possible, with the same education, occupation, and income. A sample could then be drawn from each stratum to examine the influence of social class on female patients.

ADVANTAGES OF SAMPLING

The advantages of sampling include adequate time, money, efficiency, and safety. If a sample of the population will provide reasonably accurate data, it is not necessary to use the time and resources that would be needed to study an entire population. In addition, the study of certain populations could destroy the elements. For example, if the researcher wishes to test the contents of bottles of infusion solution, it is not necessary to open every bottle, which would destroy the usefulness of all. A scientifically chosen sample should give data from which it is possible to generalize. It is not necessary to examine all of the blood in a human body to study its contents—a small sample will do. The accuracy gained by including a total population is not enough to warrant the additional expense or risk sometimes involved. For example, advantages of sampling are apparent in experiments with drugs or treatments. In order to study the effects of an experimental drug or treatment, it is not feasible to include every patient who has cancer. Unpleasant or unknown side effects should be limited to as few persons as possible. In cases where dangers are suspected, a sample of animal subjects is usually tested. At times, it is not possible to examine or measure all members of a population. For example, studies of autistic children or those with Down's syndrome require long periods of intensive observation. To study a total population would rarely be possible. In such cases, the advantage of a small sample is apparent.

SCIENTIFIC SAMPLING

There are two basic methods of choosing a sample: probability sampling and nonprobability sampling. Based on probability theory, *probability sampling* is a method whereby each element in the population has an equal chance of being chosen for study. Probability sampling reduces the possibility of selecting a biased sample; that is, one in which all members of the population are not represented and the researcher is not aware of it. (For example, *The Literary Digest* conducted a study to predict the results of the election of 1936 between Roosevelt and Landon. By polling people whose names were selected from telephone directories or lists of automobile owners, Landon was predicted to win. The sample was biased by being limited to those who had telephones or owned automobiles and by neglecting poorer persons who had neither. Since it was based on a biased sample, the prediction of a Landon victory was wrong.) In addition, the data summaries based on randomly selected samples may be analyzed, using statistical techniques that can compute sampling error—the measure of how much sample findings differ from population values. An examination of probability sampling and the theory upon which it is based enables the student to understand the process of scientific sampling.

PROBABILITY THEORY

The theory of probability deals with the possibility of events occurring by chance. It establishes the rules for calculating the risks associated with predicting future events. Soon after its inception, probability theory began to be used to solve problems related to the study of populations. The concept of probability may be defined in three ways: (1) a subjective determination of fair odds; (2) relative frequencies expected to occur in a *series of events;* and (3) an equally likely *set of events* mathematically calculated (Dixon and Massey, 1957, Chap. 20).

1. Subjective probability *is a process by which an individual assesses the odds that some hypothesis may be true, based upon what is known.* This type of probability is used every day to make practical decisions; for example, whether or not to cross the street against a traffic light. If emergency circumstances warrant it, if it is early in the morning, or if there is no traffic on the street, then one may decide that he or she has enough knowledge to assess the odds of whether or not he or she will be hit while crossing the street against a light.

    Betting odds are another example of subjective probability; gamblers may estimate that they have enough information on a boxer, football team, or horse to give 2 to 1 odds that a particular one will win. Likewise, scientists may make statements such as, "Based on the present state of knowledge, the odds against life on the planet Venus are 10,000,000 to 1." As scientists learn more about Venus, the odds may rise or fall.

Much of nursing practice depends upon subjectively experienced, anticipated probabilities. For example, the decision to give one type of nursing care may be based upon the nurse's present experience and knowledge of the probability that the patient will benefit from this type of nursing care. In general, diagnosis and therapy in the health sciences presently rely heavily upon such subjective internal mental processes, although current medical research is seeking to formalize these probabilities in order to make more accurate diagnoses by using computers. As yet, however, people have not been able to supply the computer with as much information to use systematically as the experienced clinician has available in memory to use less systematically. Health care still has strong subjective elements.

2. Mathematical probability, *the second conception of probability into which both the "equally likely set of events" and "relative frequency" fall, is a mathematical one.* The probability of relative frequency expresses the notion that the frequency of the occurrence of a given event is relative to the nonoccurrence of that event, in any series of events that could produce either occurrence or nonoccurrence. For example, a nickel tossed into the air has an equal chance of turning up heads relative to the chance of not turning up heads; that is, of turning up tails. The probability equals the number of ways the coin can fall divided by the total number of possible outcomes. The relative frequency is simply a proportion: if an event is sure to happen, it has a probability equal to 1; if an event cannot happen, it has a probability equal to 0. Thus, the probability of any event must be a number between 0 and 1. In the case of tossing the nickel, probability may be expressed by the following formula:

$$\text{Probability} = \frac{\text{the number of ways the coin can fall}}{\text{the total number of possible outcomes}}$$

$$\text{Probability of heads} = \frac{1 \ (\text{heads } or \text{ tails})}{2 \ (\text{heads } plus \text{ tails})}$$

$$\text{Probability } P = 50\% \ (\text{or } 0.5, \text{ or } \frac{1}{2}, \text{ or } 50/100)$$

Therefore, if a coin is tossed into the air 100 times, heads would probably turn up 50 times. This definition of probability, called the *frequency definition*, is based on the classical theory of probability. The basic definition of classical probability is very simple:

the probability, symbolized as P, of a coin tossed in the air coming up heads is 1 in 2, or ½, or 50/100, or 0.5—four different ways of writing the same thing; that is, the frequency definition of probability.

3. Equally-likely probability, *a second mathematical approach, is related to a set of events (rather than a series, as above) that is possible or likely to occur.* For example, if we select one person from a well-mixed group of 50 persons, we may consider any of the 50 equally likely to be chosen; or, if we draw a card from a well-shuffled deck of 52, we would expect to have an equal chance of selecting any particular one of the 52 cards; or, if we draw a name written on a slip of paper from a box containing 100 identical (except for the names), well-mixed slips, we expect that any one of the slips is equally likely to be chosen. A comparable situation may occur when a sample of individuals has been scientifically drawn from a population for a public-opinion poll or when a group of patients has been scientifically chosen to estimate the characteristics of a population.

Probability enters into the very issues of what is knowledge and evidence. It is basic to the process of setting up and carrying out experimental questions and measurement procedures, and it is the foundation of the mathematical techniques used for both evaluating research and formulating what the results mean.

PROBABILITY SAMPLING

Probability sampling includes the following four methods of data collection: (1) simple random sampling; (2) systematic sampling; (3) stratified sampling; and (4) cluster sampling. The essential characteristic of all of these methods is that the researcher can specify for each element of the population the probability that it will be included in the sample. However, the most carefully selected sample will contain some degree of sampling error (random variation from the truly accurate sample) but, if probability sampling is used, it is possible to estimate the amount of sampling error. In addition, the researcher who uses probability sampling can specify the size of the sample needed in order to have a degree of certainty that sample findings do not differ by more than a specified amount from those of the total population. Each method of random sampling will now be examined.

1. Simple random sampling *is the basic probability design that gives each element in the population an equal chance of being chosen.* The first step in random sampling is to define the population: to specify all of the cases that conform to some designated charac-

teristic. Theoretically, this could be all of the people who reside in the United States. The survey of accessible population is that from which the survey sample is actually selected as a practical matter: for example, all nurses who work in a certain state or in selected states. In order not to mislead those who read the research report, it is essential that the researcher record precisely what the population was and how the sample was selected.

Once the population is defined, a number is assigned to each unit or element in the population. A simple random sample is then chosen by using a table of random numbers, which may be found in any statistics textbook. The researcher enters the table of random numbers at some random starting point; for example, making a blind stab. Once the starting point is identified, the researcher goes up, down, or diagonally in a systematic manner, noting the numbers and selecting those that correspond from the total population, until the previously selected sample size has been obtained (Table 14–1).

EXAMPLES FROM NURSING RESEARCH

To study the smoking behavior of nurses in western New York State, Wagner (1985) used random sampling to select 5 percent of the mailing list of R.N.s

TABLE 14–1. A SAMPLE TABLE OF RANDOM NUMBERS

25	19	64	82	84	28	31
23	02	41	46	04	97	19
55	85	66	96	28	82	80
68	45	19	69	59	03	68
69	31	46	29	85	65	16
37	31	61	28	98	24	65
66	42	19	24	94	02	72
33	65	78	12	35	79	16
76	32	06	19	35	04	75
43	33	42	02	59	40	64

To select a random sample of 20 cases from a target population of 90 cases, take the following steps:

1. Assign a number to each case, from 01 to 90; or use the last two digits of the Social Security number or patient number; or arbitrarily assign a number.
2. On the table of random numbers, arbitrarily pick a two-digit column.
3. With closed eyes, select a random start in that column.
4. Beginning with the starting number, continue to sequentially select every two-digit number in that column and in the next, if necessary, until 20 cases have been selected.
5. In the event that a random number not included in the sequence 01 to 90 occurs (i.e., 96), skip that number and proceed to the next one listed.

in western New York State, provided by the American Lung Association of Western New York.

To compare the professional activities of nurse doctorates with other women academics, Lia-Hoagberg (1985) used a sample of 346 faculty women. She obtained the sample of 173 nurse doctorates from lists of all nurse doctorates in eight university faculty directories. She then obtained a sample of equal numbers of nonnurse academic women by the use of random sampling to select nonnurse academic women in the social sciences, physical sciences, education, and languages/humanities from the eight institutions.

2. Systematic sampling *is the process by which every nth element is drawn from a list of the entire survey population.* For example, a survey population that lists 10,000 units may be used to select a systematic sample of 1,000 by selecting every tenth unit on the list. The researcher enters the list at a random point (by making a blind stab, or selecting a number from one to ten by simple random sampling) and selects that unit plus every tenth element that follows.

   If certain precautions are taken to ensure that the list arrangement does not introduce a bias, systematic sampling is considered superior to simple random sampling (see Babbie, 1973, p. 155). A study conducted during World War II (Babbie, 1973) used unit rosters to select a systematic sample: every 10th soldier was selected. However, the rosters reflected the table of organization in each military unit: in each squad of ten soldiers, sergeants first, then corporals, then privates. When the researchers chose every 10th person on the roster, they ended up with a sample that contained only sergeants. However, had they entered the list at another point, no sergeants would have been represented. The list introduced a systematic bias. Therefore, the researcher should carefully examine the nature of a list before using it.

EXAMPLE FROM NURSING RESEARCH

To obtain the subjects for a psychometric evaluation of a new measure of motivation in health behavior, Cox (1985) used systematic random sampling to obtain 345 names and addresses from a telephone directory. The sample was from a moderate-sized, stable community with a current and comprehensive listing of 95 percent of the total population of the county. Sample size was based on the analytic procedures to be performed and on the estimated response rate to mail surveys (p. 179).

3. Stratified random sampling *is possible when the composition of the total population is known, with respect to some significant characteristic.* Stratification involves grouping the units of a population into homogeneous strata prior to sampling, and then using simple, systematic, or cluster (see no. 4) sampling to select the

study sample. For example, a study of nurses can begin by dividing the population into nurses with an R.N. degree, those with a B.S.N. degree, those with an L.P.N. degree, and so on. Each stratum is homogeneous and ensures that appropriate numbers of each element will be drawn in a random sampling of each stratum. While there will be heterogeneity in the sample as a whole, each homogeneous subset or stratum will be better represented, thereby ensuring a sample with smaller sampling errors. The general principle is that, if stratification will result in homogeneous strata, then it is desirable to stratify. Stratification may take place either before or after a random sample is drawn from the population.

4. Cluster sampling *is the process in which the population is first divided into existing categories, or clusters, and then the elements or units to be included in the study samples are selected by random sampling from each cluster.* When research deals with a large, spatially scattered population, this approach is helpful. In such cases, obtaining a list of every element in the population may be expensive, if not impossible. For example, a study of the populaton of nursing students in the United States would require a list of every student nurse in every nursing school in order to draw a random sample. A cluster-sampling method would first require that nursing schools be placed in clusters; for example, all schools in each state or geographical region. A sample of the nursing schools could then be drawn by random sampling—simple, systematic, or stratified. Then a list of the student population of the randomly selected nursing schools could be requested, from which a sample of the students themselves may be randomly drawn. It is clear that a 10 percent sample of the schools that represented the total population of schools is a more manageable and realistic number with which to work.

Likewise, cluster sampling is helpful in obtaining permission to conduct research. For example, administering an interview in schools, hospitals, or factories would require disrupting activities in general in order to utilize a random sample of the entire population. If the population were divided into clusters (all surgical wards, all medical wards, etc.) from which the study subjects were then drawn, disruption, work, and expense would be minimum.

NONPROBABILITY SAMPLING

The major advantages of nonprobability sampling are convenience, economy, and time, although these must be balanced against the risks involved in not using probability sampling.

EXAMPLE FROM NURSING RESEARCH

Brown, J., Tanner, C., and Padrick, K. (1984): Nursing's search for scientific knowledge. Nursing Research, 33, 26–32.

Brown et al., assessing the reports of sampling in researcher publications since 1952, found that, in 90 percent of the studies, units were persons— students, nurses, or patients. Few studies sampled events or organizations, and none sampled families. Research of the health-care system, health agencies, and nursing administration was generally lacking. The settings in which samples were selected were mainly hospitals, clinics, and schools of nursing. Original sample sizes were frequently unreported; the median sample size of those reported varied from 84 in the 1950s to 60 in 1980.

Nonprobability sampling, usually convenience sampling, was almost always used. In the 15 cases in which random sampling was claimed, it was usually from a pool of readily accessible subjects meeting the criteria for inclusion. The authors note that it is questionable whether such sampling increases the generalizability of research results to the broader populations. However, they comment that the fact that small samples were selected by nonprobability means is doubtless due to the clinical nature of much nursing research, where it is difficult to obtain random samples of ample size. They cite the comments of Wooldridge et al. (1978) and O'Connell and Duffey (1978), who comment on the difficulty of adhering to sampling rules in clinical research and who stress the need for replication to permit generalizability of clinical results. However, the authors note that this advice has not been followed.

The major forms of nonprobability samples include: (1) accidental sampling, (2) quota sampling, and (3) purposive sampling.

1. Accidental, *or* convenience, sampling *is a process in which samples are fortuitously chosen; for example, the first 500 people in a shopping center, on a college campus, or on the street.* There is no known way of ascertaining the biases introduced in such samples; therefore, the findings may be misleading, since there is no control whatsoever.

EXAMPLES FROM NURSING RESEARCH

Magilvy (1985) sought to examine the major influences on the quality of life of women with hearing impairment. She selected a convenience sample of 66 women from a variety of sources, including a center on deafness, audiology practices, speech and hearing centers, and senior residences. Flaskerud (1984) and her investigators used convenience sampling to select 227 respondents for her study of the perceptions of problematic behavior by six minority groups and selected mental-health professionals. Twelve nurse-investigators in different parts of the country sampled and interviewed each of the minority groups and professional groups, each making independent decisions on sampling methods and sample size. The minority groups were represented by 159 subjects, and the mental-health professionals by 68 professionals, including psychiatrists, psychologists, psychiatric social workers, and psychiatric nurses.

2. Quota sampling *is a means by which samples reflect certain characteristics of the population being studied, without the use of random selection.* For example, a study of attitudes toward abortion in New Orleans used quota sampling to reflect as nearly as possible the composition of the New Orleans population. Since the population of New Orleans is 70 percent Catholic and 30 percent Protestant, the sample reflected these proportions. Since New Orleans is 40 percent black and 50 percent white, the sample likewise reflected these percentages. Finally, since 5 percent of New Orleans' residents live in area A (the rich), 25 percent in area B (the middle class), 50 percent in area C (the working class), and 20 percent in the slums (the lower class), similar percentages were drawn from these areas.

Other identifying characteristics could also have been used, such as education or occupation. The more carefully the quota sample is drawn, the more likely it is that the sample reflects the characteristics of the total population. Therefore, the study of attitudes toward abortion in New Orleans is more representative of the population as a whole. Demographic characteristics of an area are generally available from census material or from the local health department. Quota sampling does entail certain risks. Unless trained, interviewers tend to interview their friends in excessive proportion and tend to concentrate on areas where there are large numbers of potential respondents, such as college campuses and business districts, which are then over-represented. Where home visits are required, interviewers may concentrate on particular times of the day, when only certain people are at home, or on particular housing types; for example, avoiding housing of the very poor and the very rich.

EXAMPLE FROM NURSING RESEARCH

Pamela Brink (1984): Value orientations as an assessment tool in cultural diversity. Nursing Research, 33, 198–203.

To test an assessment tool identifying the dominant and variant values and beliefs that characterized the Annang of Nigeria, Brink sought a stratified sample believed to be representative of the population by having the speaker for the House of Representatives of the Cross River State and the Afaha Obong representative to the Abak local government area council select the sample. The sample represented men from different geographical areas, levels of education, and seniority. The rest of the sample was collected by convenience sampling: the women were the senior wives whom the men brought along, while some people asked to be interviewed, and were included.

3. Purposive sampling *is the process of picking cases that are judged to be typical of the population, restricting observations to subgroups.* For example, in light of the results of past elections, the researcher may choose a state or county as a barometer of an election outcome. Sampling errors and biases cannot be computed, and such sampling should not be used when the possible errors are serious or if probability sampling is at all practical.

EXAMPLE FROM NURSING RESEARCH

Rita Ailinger (1982): Hypertension knowledge in a Hispanic community. Nursing Research, 31, 207–210.

To test the knowledge of hypertension in a Hispanic community, Ailinger obtained a sample of 330 study subjects in the following manner: First, she selected the target population, the Hispanic community in Arlington County, Virginia. Then she obtained the 1970 census, which indicated that there were 6,315 Hispanics in the community. Next, the ten census tracts with the highest concentration of Hispanics were selected from the 1970 census data. All streets within the ten tracts were noted, and all Hispanic surnames of people living on those streets were identified from the phone directory, until a total of 330 households was obtained. Finally, one subject from each household was included in the study. However, a telephone contact was attempted to arrange for the interviews. If four unsuccessful telephone contacts were made to a household, the name was deleted from the study. Nonetheless, subjects were judged to be typical of the population.

SAMPLE SIZE

The size of the sample depends upon the size and nature of the population and the type of question asked. However, larger samples are better than smaller ones, regardless of the size of the target population. The more variable the characteristic being measured, the larger the population should be. If one were measuring different kinds of schizophrenia in the general population, one would need a very large sample to arrive at a stable estimate of how schizophrenia is distributed in the population. However, if the target population consisted of those persons in mental institutions, one would need a much smaller population, since a mental institution is a self-selected population that presumably includes a number of schizophrenics. The size of the sample may be smaller if the population is known to be homogeneous: in this case, the sample may be expected to represent the population.

Probability theory and random sampling are the basis of all statistical analysis and of research inference in general. Without the use of random sampling, the ability to generalize from a sample is greatly weakened.

BIAS IN SAMPLING

Bias may be defined as a systematic difference between a population, or *true value*, and the corresponding value taken from that population. Bias can occur for the following reasons: (1) the entire population is not included (for example, the *Literary Digest* telephone survey excluded persons without telephones); (2) faulty measurement was used; that is, the specific item to be measured is not measured (for example, nursing attitudes, rather than nursing behavior, are measured); (3) nonresponse; that is, self-selection of those who do not answer on the basis of some factor, such as health; (4) faulty design or schedule; (5) faulty interviewing and poor questions on the survey, which lead to incorrect information from the response; and (6) faulty tabulation and interpretation of analysis. Bias may be reduced by carefully identifying the target population; by using valid and reliable measures, including scales, questionnaires, interview schedules, and trained interviewers; and by using meticulous care in tabulating and analyzing data. (Bias is further discussed in Chapter 17.)

SUMMARY

Sampling is the process by which study subjects or objects are chosen from a larger population. A critical element of the research process, sampling determines the extent to which research findings from the study sample can be generalized to the larger population from which the sample was drawn.

Basic terms used in the study of sampling include population or universe, sample, generalization, probability sampling, nonprobability sampling, and strata. Population, or universe, is the total category of persons or objects that meet the criteria established by the researcher. The accessible population is the category that is available to the researcher for study. A sample is a subset of cases drawn from a population. An element is one unit of the sample from which data are collected. A sampling unit is comprised of several elements. Generalization is the ability to apply the conclusions reached from the study of a sample to the population from which the sample was drawn. Probability sampling is a process in which each element of the population has an equal chance of being chosen for the study sample, while nonprobability sampling does not use probability methods. Strata refers to two or more subpopulations comprised of individual, mutually exclusive layers, each of which is called a stratum.

The advantages of sampling include time, money, efficiency, and safety. When the study of a small sample will provide reasonably accurate data, it is not practical to study a population. At times, such as in testing drugs, it is unwise to study more subjects than necessary. Studies that require long and intensive observation and interpretation require a limited number of subjects. In such cases, the study of populations is rarely feasible.

There are two methods of choosing a sample—probability sampling and nonprobability sampling. Probability sampling reduces the possibility of bias, that is, selecting a sample, without the researcher's knowledge, in which all members of the population are not represented. Probability sampling also allows the researcher to compute sampling error, a measure of the extent to which sample findings differ from the true value of the population.

Probability theory, from which probability sampling is drawn, deals with the possibility of events occurring by chance. Probability may be subjective—that is, a determination of fair odds based on individual experience—or it may be mathematically calculated as the relative frequencies expected to occur in a series of events or in an equally likely set of events.

Probability sampling includes simple random sampling, systematic sampling, stratified sampling, and cluster sampling. Simple random sampling involves obtaining a list of the total population and selecting a sample by any method that gives each unit in the population an equal chance of being chosen. A common way is to assign numbers to each element in the sample, then to select numbers to be used in the sample by using a table of random numbers. A systematic sampling begins with a list and selects every nth element. However, precautions must be taken to ensure that the list does not introduce a bias. Stratified random sampling involves grouping the elements of a population into homogeneous strata prior to sampling, then using any method of probability sampling to select the correct percentage of subjects from each stratum. Cluster sampling is used to consolidate large groupings from which samples are selected by a method of probability sampling.

Nonprobability sampling involves selecting a sample without using a method of probability sampling. Major forms of nonprobability sampling include accidental sampling, or choosing the sample by convenience; quota sampling, or choosing the sample to represent the same percentage of characteristics found in the population; and purposive sampling, or selecting typical cases for the study example.

The size of the sample depends upon a number of factors, such as the size and nature of the population and the kind of question that the researcher wishes to answer. In general, larger samples are better than small samples. The more heterogeneous the population, the larger the sample should be, while the more homogeneous the population, the smaller the sample may be.

Bias is defined as the systematic difference between the true value of the population and the corresponding value taken as a sample from that population. Bias can be caused by not including the entire population in the sampling process or by faulty measurement of the sample. Bias may be reduced by carefully defining the population and by using random sampling to select a study sample.

EXAMPLES FROM NURSING RESEARCH

JoAnn Glittenberg (1977): Fertility patterns and child rearing of the Ladinos and Indians of Guatemala. In Leininger, M. (ed.) Transcultural Nursing, Chap. 23. Use of random sampling in the field.

Glittenberg investigated the importance of cultural influences on fertility with the goal of finding some causal relationships. The research design was a controlled, comparative one. Methods used included participant observation, key informant interviews, case studies, and a questionnaire. Glittenberg lived in two highland villages in Guatemala, one a Ladino village, the other Indian. Glittenberg reports that a "random sample of 82 fecund women between the ages of 15 and 49 years of age in each village was the population used in completing the 204-item questionnaire. The sample size, 82 in each village, was large enough to make statistically significant statements at the 95 percent level of confidence with a standard deviation multiplier of 0.25 and allowing for a 35 percent sampling error."

Susan Gortner, Mark Hudes, and Stephen Zyzanski (1984): Appraisal of values in the choice of treatment. Nursing Research, 33, 319–324. Use of convenience sampling.

Gortner et al. conducted research to determine the values that predominated in medical and surgical treatment situations, and to determine the relation of individual/patient values to those of family values, primarily represented by the spouse. The research instrument was the Gortner Values in the Choice of Treatment Inventory. The Inventory was administered to a convenience sample of 15 surgical-bypass patients who had undergone surgical treatment during 1980. A second trial was part of a larger study in June 1981–April 1982 of 100 families, of whom 70 had a member undergoing coronary-artery-bypass surgery, and 30 had a member undergoing medical treatment for coronary-artery disease. The two samples were selected as follows:

Sample 1, Surgical Treatment Group: Gortner obtained a convenience sample of 70 surgical patients and families from inpatients on the faculty surgical services of two university medical centers. Faculty surgeons at both sites allowed access to the patients and families who met Gortner's criteria.

Sample 2, Medical Treatment Group: Gortner obtained a convenience sample of 30 medical patients and families from the caseloads of five cooperating faculty cardiologists who had private practices. This allowed the sample to include a diversity of medical regimens and a range of severity of illness.

STUDY QUESTIONS _____

1. Identify a target population from which you wish to draw a sample for research. Define how to identify units of the population.

2. Use the units above to draw the following: (a) a simple random sample; (b) a systematic random sample
3. What is the theory of probability? What does it have to do with sampling?
4. Give three definitions of probability. How do they differ? How are they the same?
5. How would you use quota sampling to study abortion in your town?
6. If you wished to study blood pressure among blacks or an ethnic group of your town, how would you get a sample that was representative?

REFERENCES AND SUGGESTED READINGS

Ailinger, R. (1982): Hypertension knowledge in a Hispanic community. Nursing Research, *31*, 207–210. *Purposive sampling.*

Babbie, E. (1973): Survey Research Methods. Belmont, Calif.: Wadsworth. *Chapters 6 and 7 include the logic of sampling and examples of sample designs.*

Brink, P. (1984): Value orientations as an assessment tool in cultural diversity. Nursing Research, *33*, 198–203.

Brink, P. and Wood, M. (1983): Basic Steps in Planning Nursing Research. Monterey, Calif.: Wadsworth Health Sciences Division, Chap. 10, "Selecting the Sample."

Brown, J., Tanner, C., and Padrick, K. (1984): Nursing's search for scientific knowledge. Nursing Research, *33*, 26–32.

Cox, C. (1985): The health self-determination index. Nursing Research, *34*, 177–183. *Systematic random sampling used.*

Dixon, W. and Massey, F. (1957): Introduction to Statistical Analysis. New York: McGraw-Hill, Chap. 4, "Universe and Sample."

Flaskerud, J. (1984): A comparison of perceptions of problematic behavior by six minority groups and health professionals. Nursing Research, *33*, 190–197. *Accidental or convenience sampling used.*

Fox, D. (1982): Fundamentals of Research in Nursing (4th ed.). Norwalk, Conn.: Appleton-Century-Crofts. *Chapter 18 deals with sampling.*

Glittenberg, J. (1977): Fertility patterns and childrearing of the Ladinos and Indians of Guatemala. In Leininger, M. (ed.): Transcultural Nursing, Chap. 23. *Use of random sampling in a field study.*

Gortner, S., Hudes, M., and Zyzanski, S. (1984): Appraisal of values in the choice of treatment. Nursing Research, *33*, 319–324. *Use of accidental or convenience sampling.*

Johnson, A. (1977): Social Statistics Without Tears. New York: McGraw-Hill, Chap. 9, "Taking Samples."

Knapp, R. (1978): Basic Statistics for Nurses. New York: Wiley, Chap. 4.

Kovacs, A. (1985): *The Research Process.* Philadelphia: F. A. Davis, Chap. 9.

Lia-Hoagberg, B. (1985): Comparison of professional activities of nurse doctorates and other women academics. Nursing Research, *34*, 155–159. *Use of random sampling.*

Lin, N. (1976): Foundations of Social Research. New York: McGraw-Hill, Chap. 9.

Magilvy, J. (1985): Quality of life of hearing-impaired older women. Nursing Research, *34*, 140–144. *Accidental or convenience sampling.*

Messick, D. (1968): Mathematical Thinking in Behavioral Sciences. San Francisco: W. H. Freeman, Part 1.

Phillips, B. (1966): Social Research. New York: Macmillan, Chap. 16, "Sampling."

Phillips, H. and Thompson, R. (1967): Statistics for Nurses. New York, Macmillan, Part II.

Polit, D. and Hungler, B. (1985): Essentials of Nursing Research. Philadelphia: J. B. Lippincott, Chap. 9.

Selltiz, C., Wrightsman, L., and Cook, S. (1976): Research Methods in Social Relations (3rd ed.). New York: Holt, Rinehart, & Winston, Appendix A, "An Introduction to Sampling."

Trussell, P., Brandt, A., and Knapp, S. (1981): Using Nursing Research: Discovery, Analysis, and Interpretation. Wakefield, Mass.: Nursing Resources, pp. 123—130.

Wagner, T. (1985): Smoking behavior of nurses in western New York. Nursing Research, *34*, 58–60. *Use of random sampling.*

15

Observation as a Research Method

Research method refers to the way in which the researcher collects data, whether by observation, questioning, or measuring. The method of data collection is related both to the problem being studied and to the research design. The researcher uses methods of observation and measurement to collect data in the experimental design; questioning and measurement in the survey design; and all three methods in the historical design.

Observation, questioning, and measurement are basic (but not mutually exclusive) methods of data collecting. They are often used in various combinations. For the purpose of examination, however, the three methods will be separated. This chapter will concentrate on observation, while the following two chapters will analyze methods of asking questions and of measuring.

Upon completion of this chapter, the student should be able to: (1) state the factors that must be kept in mind to plan an observational study; (2) describe the observer's role in participant and nonparticipant observation; (3) explain what the observer watches; (4) describe classification as a means of observation; (5) define operational definition as a method of observation; (6) discuss instrumentation and its role in observation; (7) describe the role of scaling in observation; and (8) discuss the strengths and weaknesses of the observational method of data collecting.

OBSERVATION

Observation—the ability to see, examine, and record information—is the basis of all modern science. The role of the observer, and what the observer watches, require careful attention in research. Methods and means by which the researcher observes include sampling, classification, operational definition, instrumentation, scaling, and measuring. Sampling has been examined earlier (Chap. 14). Classification, operational definition, and instrumentation will be examined in this chapter, with some reference to scaling and measuring. Scaling and measuring will be examined in greater depth later (Chap. 17).

EXAMPLE FROM NURSING RESEARCH

Brown J., Tanner, C., and Padrick, K. (1984): Nursing's search for scientific knowledge. Nursing Research, 33, 26–32.

Brown et al. found that 11 percent of the research in 1980 reported the use of observational techniques. The use of unobtrusive observation lay fallow, despite the fact that Wooldridge et al. (1978, p. 2) wrote that "clinical patient care research is in the fortunate position of having the potential for many unobtrusive, nonreactive measures of patient welfare that can be used to evaluate the effectiveness of practice."

SCIENTIFIC OBSERVATION

While all human beings continuously observe throughout their lives, observation becomes scientific only when it fulfills certain conditions: (1) the observation is undertaken with specific objectives in mind; (2) it is systematically planned and recorded; (3) all observations are checked and controlled; and (4) the observations are related to scientific concepts and theories. Scientific observation is best exemplified by the true experimental design (see Chap. 12). However, the researcher may not always be able to fulfill all of the conditions for scientific observation. Aamodt (1972) points out that explanations for health and healing at the sociocultural level are neither well-understood nor well-described. In such cases, observation is (perforce) highly exploratory. Relying upon one observer, such research is at times as much an art as a science. Yet, such studies pave the way for studies that *can* meet the criteria for scientific observation. For example, the researcher who studies autistic children, catatonic schizophrenics, or people of different cultures may well rely solely on the observation of behavior over a considerable period of time to describe what is meant by *autism, schizophrenia*, or a particular *culture.*

In any observational study, a number of factors must be kept in mind. Kassenbaum (1970) suggests that the role of the observer involves considerable preparation. First, the researcher must be aware of the *selective attention* that he or she habitually displays as an observer; the researcher must also consider the selective attention that he or she wishes to display. For example, nurses may selectively observe patients on the basis of sex and age: men may be observed differently from women, and children differently from adults. The bias in the observations must be recognized and corrected. Second, the researcher must specify what he or she is reporting, whether overt behavior alone or inference from the behavior to the intentions of the subject. Third, the researcher must select, sharpen, and make explicit both what he or she plans to observe and what the researcher actually observes. Fourth, the researcher should think carefully about the experiences, reliving in his or her mind the observations made before, during, and after the researcher records them. Finally, the researcher should be sensitive to the impact of his or her presence upon those observed and should record these impressions often, in a systematic and careful manner.

A number of roles is available to the observer. The researcher may become an accepted member of the group being studied in order to participate in the processes being observed. Or, the researcher may stay aloof from participation and may observe only. Once the researcher selects the role, he or she must identify *what* to observe and measure and *how* the observations will be made; that is, the means of observing, measuring, and recording the data. Each of these processes is now examined.

The Role of the Observer: Participant and Nonparticipant Observation

The role of the observer may be one of full participation or of nonparticipation. In *participant observation*, the researcher finds a role that is acceptable to the subjects under study and assumes it full-time in order to interact with the subjects and observe behavior in its "natural" state. The objective of participant observation is to obtain a depth of experience that is not available by watching alone. In *nonparticipant observation*, the researcher remains aloof from interaction. In this case, the objective is to exchange depth of subjective experience for a more objective approach to data. Part-time participation may involve a combination of participant and nonparticipant observation.

Participant observation has been used by nurses such as Chapman, Horn, and Kendall to collect ethnographic data or clinical observations. For example, Chapman (1977, p. 17) conducted an experiment in the clinical area to study the effects of different nursing approaches upon the postoperative responses of male herniorrhaphy patients. She was able to use a number of previous studies reported in the literature to plan her study, check and control the experimental variables, and relate the observations to scientific concepts and theories. She assumed the role of participant observer by presenting herself to the patient as a member of the nursing staff. At the same time, she used a mechanical aid to enhance her observations—she wore a small tape recorder with a microphone to record nurse–patient interaction for later classification by independent judges. Chapman solved the ethical problem faced by researchers in such situations by obtaining the informed consent of all subjects prior to their admission to the study.

Horn (1978) spent 3 years as a participant observer in weekly well-child clinics on the Muckleshoot Indian reservation to observe and describe social and cultural factors influencing childrearing practices and health care. Similarly, Kendall (1978) conducted an ethnographic study in a small Muslim village in central Iran to study maternal and child nursing.

Instead of a participant observation study, Marshall (1972) used non-participant observation to study the reactions of patients to sounds in the intensive coronary care units. Marshall did not wish to become involved in patient care and, at the same time, she wished to protect the patients from additional stress. She used an instrument already in place (cardiac monitor) and added a tape recorder in an unobtrusive position to document the effect of sounds in the unit upon the patients' cardiac responses.

Both participant and nonparticipant observation may vary in terms of the degree of structure used. If it is not clear what data will be found or which measurements or scales are useful, then unstructured observation is necessary. However, unstructured observation is realistic only if the investigator has the time to spend observing and interacting with the study subjects, or devising and testing measures and scales. On the other hand, structured observations are used if the researcher knows what will be observed and has a system of classification, instrumentation, operational definitions, and scales with which to work. If more than one observer is at work, structure is essential. In such cases, the researcher must develop standardized methods of observation and must train observers to use each method, in order to ensure uniform observations.

Participant and nonparticipant observation are used to study all types of observable behavior. Observation is also used to examine records—or written observations of the past. In such cases, the observer's role is primarily judgmental and analytical. The researcher makes a judgment of whether the writer has made a valid observation and then uses techniques such as content analysis to analyze the material in terms of the concepts and theories being used. However, each research method must specify *what* will be observed and *how* it will be observed.

What the Observer Watches

What the observer watches depends upon the research design, the instruments available, and the theory that underlies the study. The experimental design is structured and controlled—it clearly specifies what will be observed and how. On the other hand, the survey depends upon indirect observation. The researcher questions the subjects about matters that the researcher cannot observe. The historical design depends upon the study of documented observations of the past. The methodological design, the ex-post-facto design, and the correlational design combine methods of observing, questioning, measuring, and evaluating.

What the observer watches is influenced by the instruments available. Electronic devices to monitor internal conditions enable the researcher to observe what he or she ordinarily could not. Audiotapes and videotapes capture processes that the researcher can examine later in detail. Such devices may be set to monitor observations at random times during the day and night—a feat not convenient or possible for the usual observer. Factors such as silence, duration of interaction, and fidelity of content may simultaneously be captured, a nearly impossible undertaking for one observer or even for several observers.

What the observer watches is structured by the theory or assumptions with which the observer begins. For example, observations of behavior modification may differ from observations of health practices in folk culture, and they may differ according to the unit of study and the site of the study. Observations of a family studied in its home will differ from observations of a family studied in the hospital setting. The observer may choose to watch individual behavior or processes, such as dying or sleeping.

What the observer watches is also related to the amount of control and manipulation that the observer can exert. Observations in a highly controlled experiment differ from observations in uncontrolled, opportunistic, "natural" environments. The observer who is manipulating an independent variable and watching closely the effect on the dependent variable is involved in a highly structured observation. On the other hand, the researcher who is collecting descriptive data has the advantage of watching a broader set of factors but must deal with a myriad of uncontrolled behaviors.

Uncontrolled observation, in which the researcher does not intervene, tends to fall into five categories of "simple observations" (Webb et al., 1966, p. 115). These simple observations include: (1) exterior physical signs, (2) expressive movement, (3) physical location, (4) language behavior, and (5) time duration. These categories were devised primarily for unobtrusive measures in the social sciences, but they are also helpful to the researcher in health science and may be adapted for use. Each of these categories will be examined, with examples from nursing studies where these are available.

1. Exterior physical signs *express current or past behavior and often may be observed unobtrusively*. These physical signs include voluntary changes of the body, such as beards, haircuts, tattoos, and clothing. Beards, length of hair, and haircuts are easily discernible signs related to lifestyle, affluence, state of mind, or occupation. For example, neglect of the hair may suggest certain emotional

factors at work. Webb et al. suggest that tattoos may be associated with delinquency, since more delinquents than nondelinquents are tattooed. On the other hand, tattoos may be a sign of military service and conformity to group pressure. Clothing is a particularly significant exterior sign that may reflect social status and image or the meaning of the situation to the patient. For example, Kane (1959) examined the meaning of clothing that outpatients wore to interviews. He followed this study with an examination of clothing worn by an outpatient (1959) and later examined the meaning of the form of clothing (1962). Klein et al. (1972) examined the use of clothing—uniforms or street clothes—worn by members of the psychiatric staff, while Petrovich et al. (1968) compared the use of uniforms and street clothes worn by psychiatric nurses. The white uniform of the nurse or physician may be associated with restraints or painful treatments, causing patients—especially children—to react with fear to anyone in a white uniform.

Exterior physical signs that have long been observed by nurses include: clinical signs of disease and physical disorder, such as the rash associated with measles; the color changes, edema, or dyspnea associated with heart disease; and vital signs, such as temperature, pulse, blood pressure, and respiration, which are used to infer or estimate internal physiology.

2. Expressive movements *communicate inner emotions that are ordinarily not observable. Kinesics*, the study of communication by observing body motion, is a fairly new field in nursing research, although kinesthetic needs have been examined by Hasselmeyer (1961), Barnard (1973), and others. Kinesics includes the unobtrusive study of facial expression, gestures, and body positions that express emotions. Wolff (1948) observed the gestures of mental patients at meals and at work and found evidence of a relationship between mental condition and the ways in which patients moved their hands. Other body movements that have been examined include touch, dance, and the expressive responses to music. McCorkle (1974) investigated the effects of touch on seriously ill patients, while Burnside (1973) examined the effects of touch on the care of the aged. Ammon (1969) studied the effects of music on children in respiratory distress, while Gunning and Holmes (1973) and Puttock (1972) investigated the use of dance therapy with psychotic children.

3. Physical position *or* physical location *refers to the clustering, dispersion, or position assumed by persons of different ages, sexes, and psychological states, such as fear or stress.* For example, certain persons assume the fetal position under stress. Webb et al. (1966, p. 124) report that fearful persons tend to cluster closely

to one another, while Leipold (1963) reports an increase in the spacing distance between individuals experiencing stress. The degree of space preferred at various times of the day, together with the degree of sociability manifested, was observed by Rodgers (1977), who reported that the amount of personal space preferred was greater in the morning than in the afternoon.

4. Language behavior, *or* conversation, *includes both the content and the persons who communicate with one another.* Baziak and Denton (1965) report that nurses and physicians often use medical words that are incomprehensible to their patients. Mahl's (1956) study of stuttering and slips of the tongue in the clinical setting reveals how the disturbances of speech and the silences are clues to inner meanings. Webb et al. suggest that conversation samples may be collected unobtrusively by noting who talks with whom, for how long, and about what. However, eavesdropping may raise ethical questions, although observations of public conversations may not. Communication with patients and families may be accompanied by silences, smiles, frowns, or humor that convey more to the patient than the content of the conversation. Robinson (1970, p. 117) noted the importance of such communication, but this has been little explored.

5. *The observation of time, duration, fluctuation, and time-movement studies, have received considerable attention in nursing.* For example, Alderson (1974) studied the effect that increases in body temperature have on the perception of time. Felton (1970, p. 1973) examined the effects of biological rhythms on nurses' efficiency, work shifts, and sleep patterns. Time-movement studies conducted to establish staffing standards in nursing are numerous.

MEANS AND METHODS OF OBSERVATION

The means and methods by which observations are made in research include: (1) classification, (2) operational definition, (3) instrumentation, (4) scaling, and (5) measurement. All of these processes are related (Fig. 15–1). *Classification,* the assignment of persons, places, or things to named categories, is an integral part of organizing observations. A scale may be an instrument that measures observations. Measurements that are incorporated into operational definitions, instruments, and scales may come before or after data are collected. In spite of the intimate interrelationships among the means and methods of observation, each of these processes may be separated from one another for analytical purposes. (See Appendix A, "Observational Aids.")

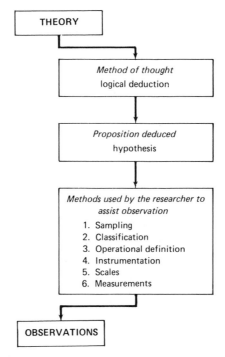

Figure 15–1. Relationships among theory, methods of observation, and observation.

Classification

Classification is the systematic assignment of subjects, objects, or ideas to named categories. The names suggest the basic units that will be observed. Basic units may be either specific motor behaviors, such as touching, or concepts such as anxiety, which must be defined by operational definition in order to be observable and measurable.

The names assigned to the categories should follow as closely as possible those defined in the literature. Once categories have been established according to theory, reclassifying or renaming them suggests a change in the theoretical approach. For example, changing the name of a mental illness from *dementia praecox* to *schizophrenia* suggests a change in the theory that explains such an illness.

Classification may be a goal in itself, or it may be a means to order what will be observed. For example, nursing research that seeks to establish categories such as "patient needs" or "nursing diagnosis" uses classification as a goal. Such classification identifies what needs to be observed and measured in nursing and, as such, is basic to the discipline. However, classification is more commonly used as a step in the research process that occurs before observation and helps the researcher organize what will be observed; or it is a step that occurs after observation and helps the researcher order similar observations that were made. Research that begins with theory, assumptions, or ideas from which hypotheses are deduced or objectives are developed uses classification before observation to specify exactly what the researcher predicts will be observed. Classification done after observation is inductive: the researcher develops categories from what was observed and assigns names or develops concepts that describe the similar data assigned to each category.

Classification begins with the formulation of the research proposal or working hypothesis that identifies what the observables will be. For example, the following hypothesis identifies four categories into which observations will fall: Infants born to mothers who smoke will have a lower birth weight than infants born to mothers who do not smoke.

The four categories of data to be observed are mothers who smoke; mothers who do not smoke; birth weights of infants born to mothers who smoke; and birth weights of infants born to mothers who do not smoke. Yet this fourfold classification is too broad for most research projects. For example, mothers who do and do not smoke include many different categories of mothers: those with the first child, those with many children, young mothers, older mothers, single mothers, married mothers, black mothers, and white mothers. Each of these categories contains variables that may influence birthweight as much as the independent variable, smoking. Therefore, the researcher must identify particular categories for study that control as many extraneous variables as possible. For example, selecting mothers with their first child will control the factor of multiparity. In order to be mutually exclusive and exhaustive, all categories must be carefully defined. In order to be observable and measurable, all variables must be defined by operational definition.

Mutually exclusive categories are those with data that unequivocally fall into one, and only one, category. In the example given above, mothers either smoke or do not smoke: mothers who fall into one category are excluded from the other. *Exhaustive categories* are those that include all possible cases of the variable to be observed. "Marital status" must include all possible types: never married; presently married and living together; presently married and separated; formerly married and widowed; formerly married and divorced. Such categories must be established before data are collected, not only to identify what will be observed, but to include such categories on interview schedules or check lists for observing, interviewing, or reviewing records.

After collecting data, the researcher may discover that an unexpected category of marital status exists: a mother whose marriage has been annulled. To assure that the categories are exhaustive, a new category must be established after data are collected to include this case.

To establish observable and measurable categories, precise definitions of the variables to be observed are mandatory before observation.

Two types of definitions are common: the verbal or normal definition, which defines concepts in words; and the operational definition, which defines variables in terms of observation and measurement. Formulating the operational definition prior to observing data is crucial.

The Operational Definition

The *operational definition* is a set of directions or procedures that designate precisely how to observe, measure, and record the phenomenon to be observed. In order for one researcher to be able to collect data in the same manner as another, the operational definition is essential. Few (if any) operational definitions are accepted by all scientists. No operational definition corresponds exactly to every researcher's view of what should be observed and measured. An operational definition is useful for a number of reasons: (1) it specifies exactly what a particular researcher plans to observe, (2) it communicates precisely how the variable to be observed will be measured and how the measurement will be recorded; and (3) it facilitates the possibility of detecting measurement errors and leads to a better interpretation of the observation. For example, Lindeman and Van Aernam (1977) developed a number of operational definitions, such as "subjects" and "stir-up routine," to study nursing intervention with the presurgical patient.

Subject was defined by six criteria: (1) 15 years and older; (2) admitted under nonemergency conditions; (3) scheduled for surgery other than eye, ear, nose, and throat; (4) scheduled for general anesthetic; (5) able to cooperate for tests of ventilatory function; and (6) not on intermittent positive pressure breathing therapy. *Stir-up routine* was defined as the conscientious application of three precepts at definite intervals during the postoperative period: (1) the patient must inflate his lungs adequately; (2) the patient must cough; and (3) the patient must move or be turned.

Touch was defined by McCorkle (1974, p. 115), using the following operational definition: "Gentle physical contact made by the investigator's hand at the patient's wrist during the entire interaction with an increase in pressure at the beginning of each one of the three specific questions asked by the investigator." McCorkle defined the seriously ill patient as: "A hospitalized patient admitted to a specified area for seriously ill patients, such as intensive-care and coronary-care units, or a patient designated seriously ill by his physician and diagnosis. The patient's condition had to be one in which there was a chance of recovery during the present hospitalization, but not necessarily a cure of his illness."

Using the operational definitions above, researchers may duplicate the "subject" studied by Lindeman and Van Aernam, and the "seriously ill patient" studied by McCorkle. The "stir-up routine" could be replicated, as could "touch."

Operational definitions are used to measure visible and invisible variables. For example, a rash may be visible to all observers, but no two may describe the rash in exactly the same way without an operational definition. On the other hand, anxiety may not be visible. To make anxiety observable and measureable, a set of directions that specify how to observe, measure, and record the phenomenon is necessary. The complexity of the concept and the lack of agreement in defining it are exemplified by the fact that at least 120 specific procedures to measure anxiety were extant in 1961 (Cattell and Scheier). Since that time, other procedures have been added.

The operational definition defines the phenomenon to be observed in a narrow manner in order to increase objectivity in observation and precision in measurement. However, as operational definitions become more and more specific, it is clear that data are lost, and the complexity of a concept such as *anxiety* is reduced to a simple level. This is a part of the price to pay in order that the study may be replicated and the phenomenon observed and measured.

For example, for two researchers to investigate the variable in the hypothesis just stated,* *smoking* and *mother* should be given an operational definition. Without an operational definition, questions immediately arise, such as what to do with the mother who was a heavy smoker but quit before she became pregnant. Such queries are answered by the operational definition, which removes ambiguity by giving the procedures for defining *mother*. For example, the following set of directions define what is meant by *mother* for the purpose of one study: (1) she is a primipara; (2) she is between the ages of 19 and 34; (3) she is currently married and living with her spouse; (4) she is not suffering from designated chronic diseases (diabetes, nephritis, etc.); (5) she was delivered of a living child in the public hospitals of Central City; (6) she was drawn by random sampling from the target population of primiparas in Central City during a designated time period; and (7) she gave informed consent to be interviewed.

Smoking mother may be more simply defined as: (1) a mother who meets the definition of *mother* above; (2) who reports that she smoked for five or more months during pregnancy; and (3) who reports that she smoked on the average of five cigarettes per day.

Although data are lost by the operational definition, precision in observation and measurement is gained. Once the researcher establishes the categories of observables, the researcher must next locate or devise the instruments for the observation.

---

*The hypothesis states: infants born to mothers who smoke will have a lower birth weight than infants born to mothers who do not smoke.

Instrumentation

In research, *instrumentation* refers to the construction and use of instruments in the observation, measurement, and analysis of data. Instruments are devices, tools, or implements; questionnaire items and response categories; and interview schedules, papers, or documents that facilitate observation and measurement. Instruments include both "hardware"—computers, thermometers, tape recorders, cameras, transducers to indicate various responses, timers, counters, and radio transmitters—and "software"—paper-and-pencil instruments, such as scoring charts; interview schedules; questionnaires; assessment guides; and scaling devices (Table 15–1).

TABLE 15–1. INSTRUMENTS TO ASSIST OBSERVATION

Instrument	Function
Accelerometer	A transducer; measures rate of change in a moving object.
Algesimeter	Measures pain threshold.
Audio analgesia	An audio signal for analgesia.
Biofeedback devices	Displays signals of a person to that person.
Calorimeter	Measures heat loss.
Cardiotachometer	Measures heart rate.
Dhronometer	Measures periods of time.
Decibel meter	Measures sound levels.
Dolometer	Measures subjective pain levels.
Dynamometer	Measures force.
Electrocardiograph	Measures electrical potentials of heart muscle.
Electrogoniometer	Measures angular positions of body limbs.
Electroencephalograph	Measures electrical activity of brain.
Electronystagmograph	Measures gastric motility.
Electromyograph	Measures electrical activity of muscles.
Electronystagmograph	Measures eye movements induced by electrical stimulation.
Ergodynamograph	Records work associated with muscular activity.
Esthesiometer	Measures touch sensibility.
Galvanic skin resistance device	Measures DC resistance of skin.
Kinesthesiometer	Measures ability to perceive own body position.
Mobat	Measures blood alcohol concentration viz. expired breath.
Opthalmograph	Measures movements of eye during reading.
Plethysmograph	Measures changes in blood volume.
Pneumograph	Records respiratory movements.
Stabilograph	Measures human motor response instability.
Transducer	Transfers energy between two or more systems.

Rugh and Schwitzgebel (1977).

The primary instruments of observation are the human sensory organs. However, these allow for the observation of only a small part of the phenomena in the environment. Instruments and the know-how to use these enable the researcher to extend the senses' accuracy and range. The most sophisticated instruments have been invented in the realm of time, motion, and weight, although the instruments used to observe human behavior, health, and sickness are becoming more highly developed. A number of these instruments may be used with little technical knowledge, while others require experts both to use the instruments and to interpret the data. For example, the use of an instrument to measure temperature or blood pressure may easily be learned, while the use of x-rays and computers is much more difficult. However, a review of the records that interpret data already collected by sophisticated instruments and analyzed by experts enables the researcher to gather such data second-hand.

Direct observation and assessment relies primarily on the well-trained observer, who watches, listens, palpates, smells, uses instruments that extend these senses, and records each observation precisely. The researcher may use one of the many instruments described in the literature or may devise his or her own instrument.

Hardware includes easy-to-use devices, such as the flashlight, tuning fork, tongue blade, thermometer, sphygmomanometer, stethoscope, and weight and height scales. Instruments that require more expertise are the tonometer (to show changes in intraocular pressure), Snellen chart and Rosenbaum pocket vision screener (to examine visual acuity), ophthalmoscope, otoscope (to examine the ear), nasal speculum, and vaginal speculum (see Table 15–2 for other instruments). If the client gives informed consent, hardware instruments, such as tape recorders, movie cameras, and videotapes, are invaluable to document observations. Such instruments collect data in the natural setting, hospital, clinic, or laboratory to be analyzed in detail at a later date. Other instruments include timing devices, such as wristwatches or stopwatches; infrared photography; two-way mirrors; electric eyes; and various instruments that measure moisture, pressure, or activity, or that count mechanical movement.

Software includes paper-and-pencil instruments, such as clinical assessment instruments that give a step-by-step procedure; instruments such as the Apgar score to determine need for resuscitation of the newborn; interview schedules; questionnaire forms; and numerous tests and schedules to assess or measure concepts such as *fear, depression,* and *anxiety.*

Instruments to observe and assess the physiological and psychological states include the devices noted and also those of considerable biomedical complexity. For example, instruments are available to convert a physiological event into an electric signal that may be recorded, transmitted, or displayed. The transducer, a device that transfers or converts

TABLE 15–2. SELECTED OBSERVATIONS AND INSTRUMENTS

Observation	Instruments
Achievement	Kahl's Achievement Orientation Scale (1968)
Activity	Activity Inventory, Brodie (1977)
Agression	Geen and Stonner (1971)
Angles of the limbs	Goniometer
Anal sphincter pressure	Kohlenberg (1973)
Anxiety	Anxiety Scale Questionnaire, Cattell and Scheier (1968); Timed Behavioral Checklist, Paul (1966)
Aptitude and ability	Eckland (1965)
Assertiveness	Rathus Assertiveness Schedule (1973)
Attitudes toward	Guttman Scales; Likert Scales; Semantic Differential Scales; see Miller (1970) for others
Physical fitness and exercise	Richardson (1960)
Mental illness	Cohen and Struening (1959)
Mentally retarded people	Bartlett, Quay, and Wrightsman (1960)
Blindness	Cowen, Underberg, and Verrillo (1958)
Disabled people	Yuker, Block, and Campbell (1960)
Menstruation	McHugh and Wasser (1959)
Mental hospitals	Souelem (1955)
Authoritarianism	F-Scale, Adomo et al. (1950)
Bacterial counts	Microscope
Blood alcohol concentration	MOBAT—commercial device to estimate via breath
Blood volume	Plethysmograph; commercial instrument
Blood pressure	Sphygmomanometer (mercury, anaeroid, electronic)
Community attitude	Community Attitude Scale (see Miller, 1970, pp. 272–277)
Community solidarity	Community Solidarity Index, Fessler (1952)
Development	Bayley Scale of Infant Development: Denver Developmental Screening Test. Frankenburg and Dodds (1967)
Depression	Depression Adjective Check List, Lubin (1965)
Distance	Social Distance, Boggardus Social Distance Scale
Electrical activity of organs	
Brain	Electroencephalograph
Heart	Electrocardiograph
Muscles	Electromyograph
Equilibrium	Movement of platform, Shipley and Harley (1971)
Eye-foot coordination	Mirror-visual instrument, Milkaelian (1972)
Fear	Fear Scale, Geer (1964)
Force	Dynamometer, commercial instrument
Galvanic skin response	Galvanic Skin Resistance Device, commercial instrument
Gross motor movement	Self-winding watch, Schulmann and Reisman (1979)
Gastric motility	Electrogastrograph, commercial instrument

TABLE 15–2. (*Continued*)

Observation	Instruments
Head movement of infant	Pressure change in air pillow. Vietze et al. (1974)
Hearing	Audiometer, commercial instrument
Heat loss	Calorimeter, commercial instrument
Heart rate	Cardiotachometer, commercial instrument
Length	Various measurement scales; Mecometer for infants
Life changes	Life Change Inventory, Costantini et al. (1974)
Locus of control	Rotter et al. (1972)
Micturition	Moisture Detection Device
Motion	Kinomometer, Kinesimeter
Morale	Minnesota Survey of Opinion (see Miller, 1970)
Occupational categories	NORC (1972)
Oral hygiene	Chemical agents, Evans et al. (1968)
Pain	Algesimeter, threshold; Dolometer, subjective pain
Respiration	Air flow, Pneumotachometer; volume, Spirometer; Pneumograph
Social desirability	Scale of Social Desirability, Crowe and Marlowe (1960)
Social participation	Chapin's Social Participation Scale (see Miller, 1970)
Salivation	Measurement method, Brown (1970)
Sleep	Rapid eye movements
Social interaction	Inventory, Methuen and Schlotfeldt (1962)
Social status	Hatt and North Occupational Ratings

energy from one form to another, is used with an amplifier, an instrument that amplifies or modifies the transducer's electric signal, and either an oscillograph, which writes down information, or an oscilloscope, which records information photographically. The electrocardiogram and the electroencephalogram require special training both to collect and to analyze data, but the researcher may use these instruments in a second-hand manner by examining experts' reports.

The sphygmomanometer and the stethoscope are familiar instruments used in physiological studies. Less familiar instruments are the pneumotachometer, which measures airflow; the spirometer, which measures pulmonary volume; the myograph, which measures muscular contraction; and the tromometer, which measures involuntary tremors of the muscles in the fingers. To measure the strength of muscles, a dynamometer is used. To measure reaction time, a chronoscope is used simultaneously with various watches and stopwatches that measure length of time, pressure, and movement.

Numerous other laboratory instruments, such as the microscope, enable the researcher to assess the health status of the subject. In addition, the patient's chart (or record) is an instrument itself for observing laboratory findings and physicians' examinations.

Scaling   ~Measure~

Scaling is a process of determining magnitude or quantity (see Chap. 17). Before observations, the researcher develops or locates a scale to help collect the data. A scale transforms an hypothesis into something that is observable.

Four general types of scales are: (1) the nominal, (2) the ordinal, (3) the interval, and (4) the ratio. The *nominal scale* names and measures whether subjects' characteristics are the same or different: sex (male *or* female); pregnant (yes *or* no); level of education (high school, college, graduate school). The researcher names the categories of observations to be made, and the nominal scale "measures" the frequency of the observation. The researcher can count the number of men and women, blacks and whites, and pregnant and nonpregnant females. However, the nominal scale is limited to such discrete and noncontinuous categories. Categories can be neither ranked nor measured in any other way.

Frequently used to plan for observations of attitudes, the *ordinal scale* allows the researcher to rank observations. For example, the quality of nursing care may be measured by an ordinal scale that asks the patient to rank the care received as good, better, or best.

The *interval scale* enables the researcher to measure quantitative observations that have no zero point: the temperature of a patient may be measured by a Fahrenheit or a Centigrade thermometer that is divided into equal units but without a zero point.

The *ratio scale* enables the researcher to plan to measure observations that do have a zero point, although this value may never be produced. For example, length, weight, and height may be measured by a ratio scale with equal intervals and a zero point.

Bias in Observation

Bias in observation—the tendency to observe subjects or processes in a manner that differs consistently from true observation—may be introduced in a number of ways. The *Hawthorne effect* refers to the change in subjects' responses because subjects know that they are participating in a study rather than because of factors the researcher wished to study. Another bias found in observation is the *halo effect*, the tendency of an observer to be influenced by one characteristic, such as a favorable impression of the person being observed, and to have this impression color other observations that are designed to be objective and unbiased.

Bias may also be introduced because observers may see the data differently: a short nurse may get a blood pressure reading different from that of a tall nurse. To reduce bias in observation, Simon (1978, p. 278) suggests that: (1) observers be carefully trained; (2) the area of discretion within which bias may operate be reduced by carefully specifying the observer's task; (3) detailed instructions be given; (4) immediate and detailed reporting be required; (5) mechanical devices, such as tape recorders and cameras, be used whenever possible for checking observations; and (6) several researchers observe, record, and compare observations.

SUMMARY

Research methods are the means by which data are collected. Common research methods used in nursing include observation, questioning, measurement, and a combination of these. Observation is the basis of all modern science and is used in experimental, descriptive, and historical research designs. The role of the researcher who uses observation as a primary means of collecting data may be one of participant or nonparticipant observer. Such roles may be used in various settings, including the clinic and the community. Both types of roles vary in terms of the degree of structure used and the selection of what will be observed. Highly structured observation is essential in experiments, while uncontrolled observation is used in cases of nonintervention, or simple observation. Five categories of simple observation useful in nursing research are: exterior physical signs (clothing, body markings, clinical signs), expressive movements (gestures, touching, expressions), physical positioning (clustering or dispersing), language behavior (conversation), and time observations (perception of time, time-movement).

The methods by which observations are made and summarized include classification, operational definition, instrumentation, and scaling. In addition, measurement may accompany or follow observation (see Chap. 17). Classification is the systematic assignment of subjects to named categories that are mutually exclusive and exhaustive. The operational definition is a set of directions or procedures that designate precisely how to observe, measure, and record observed phenomena. Instrumentation is the construction and use of tools to observe, measure, and analyze data. Numerous instruments have been devised to observe and assess people's health status. Scaling is a process of determining magnitude or quantity. Qualitative scales, such as the nominal and ordinal scales, determine the category of the variable to which study subjects belong. The ordinal scale not only determines the category but ranks the categories in terms of a graded order, such as poor, good, better, or best. An interval scale is a quantitative scale with equal intervals but no absolute zero point. Temperature measured in Centigrade is an example of the interval scale. The ratio scale is a quantitative scale that does possess an absolute zero point, although zero may not be produced. Examples of the ratio scale include length, weight, and height.

Bias in observation—the tendency to observe subjects in a manner that differs consistently from true observation—may be introduced by the study subject or by the observer. The Hawthorne effect refers to the change in subjects' responses because subjects know that they are participating in a study, rather than because of factors that the researcher wished to study. Bias may be introduced by the observer who sees data differently.

EXAMPLE FROM NURSING RESEARCH
Observation

Updike, P., Accurso, F., and Jones, R. (1985): Physiologic circadian rhythmicity in preterm infants. Nursing Research, 34, 160–163.

The authors report a study, utilizing observation, that investigated evidence of a circadian rhythm in six preterm infants. The study is reported to be one of the first of its kind to refute the belief that a preterm infant's physiologic activity is more or less a constant phenomenon. The observations included transcutaneous oxygen level, pulse rate, respiratory rate, sleep state, frequency of respiratory pauses, and skin temperature. The setting was in the Neonatal Intensive-Care Unit–Clinical Research Center of the university of Colorado Health Sciences Center. Environmental lighting conditions remained consistent throughout the 24-hour period. Feeding, repositioning, and other nursing-care measures occurred uniformly every 3 hours. Temperature in the isolettes was maintained constantly between 35 and 36 degrees Centigrade. The infants were monitored continuously for 24 hours for sleep state, respiratory rate, temperature, pulse rate, respiratory pauses, and $tcPO_2$ levels.

A value for each research variable was recorded every 30 minutes for 24 hours. Two hundred and ninety-four observations were made for each of the six subjects. Each observation for each variable was entered sequentially on a master data sheet in preparation for statistical analysis. The frequency of respiratory pauses was the number of episodes that occurred during each 30-minute interval. Sleep state was assessed by observation every 30 minutes throughout the study, using categories described by Anders et al. (1971) and others.

Interrater reliability of assessment for sleep state achieved a 95-percent agreement when assessments were simultaneously recorded. Data were summarized across the six subjects and were reported as means and standard deviations. Preterm infants exhibited evidence of a circadian rhythm in skin temperature, while both $tcPO_2$ and respiratory pause frequency exhibited a characteristic day/night pattern.

STUDY QUESTIONS

1. What is the connection between research methods and research designs?
2. Describe how you have used the three methods of research to

collect data in nursing. Is the same process used to collect data in nursing practice and nursing research?

3. What methods help the nurse observe in research?

4. If you are to observe scientifically, what conditions must you meet?

5. You are planning a research project that involves the observation of autistic children. What do you think your role as observer should be?

6. You have a grant to study the effects of visitors on patients in the intensive coronary care unit. What method could you use to protect the patients from stress and keep you from being involved in patient care?

7. In deciding what you can observe in a study of schizophrenic patients who come to a community clinic, what are some factors to consider?

8. What exterior physical signs can you observe in a prenatal clinic that may alert you to special problems of health care that need research?

9. You are the nurse in a home for the elderly who are able to care for themselves to a considerable extent. How would research on expressive movements enable you to encourage the patients to exercise more effectively?

10. Describe a research project on communication between student nurses and clinical supervisors that involves silences, smiles, frowns, or laughter.

11. Diagram the relationship among theory, methods, and observation.

12. In planning an observational research project, what are some methods that will help you observe?

13. You wish to study the effect of different methods of teaching diabetic patients to give insulin to themselves. What categories will help you observe the data and record it effectively?

14. Make an operational definition of *diabetic patient* that describes those you will teach in question 13 above.

15. Referring to Tables 15–1 and 15–2, identify any instruments with which you are familiar.

16. If you plan to use classification in research, what scale would be helpful?

17. What does the ordinal scale measure that the nominal scale cannot?

REFERENCES AND SUGGESTED READINGS

Aamodt, A. (1972): The child's view of health and healing. In Batey, M. (ed.), Communicating Nursing Research. Boulder: Western Interstate Commission for Higher Education, pp. 38–56. Response to critique. In Batey, M. (ed.), Communicating Nursing Research. Boulder: Western Interstate Commission for Higher Education, pp. 57–58. *A participant observation study: Aamodt lived for 13 months with a family and served as a volunteer teacher–aide in mission school, in order to observe children of the Papago in many settings.*

Alderson, M. (1974): Effect of increased body temperature on the perception of time. Nursing Research, *23*, 43–49. *The patient's perception of time associated with rise in temperature.*

Ammon, K. (1969): The effects of music on children in respiratory distress. In ANA Clinical Sessions. New York: Appleton-Century-Crofts. *A study of the effects of music on children with respiratory distress.*

Barnard, K. (1973): The effect of stimulation on the sleep behavior of the premature infant. In Batey, M. (ed.), Communicating Nursing Research. Boulder: Western Interstate Commission for Higher Education, pp. 12–33. *Behavioral observations of the sleep state of infants, during the 32nd to the 35th week of gestation, to collect data on sleep–wake patterns.*

Batey, M. (1973): Communicating Nursing Research. Boulder: Western Interstate Commission for Higher Education. *Fifteen studies in nursing research, many with critiques and responses to critiques. Includes participant-observation and nonparticipant-observation studies in the field and in the hospital.*

Baziak, A. and Denton, R. (1965): The language of the hospital and its effect on the patient. In Skipper, J. and Leonard, R. (eds.), Social Interaction and Patient Care. Philadelphia: J. B. Lippincott. *The medical jargon used by nurses and physicians is incomprehensible to laypersons.*

Brown, J., Tanner, C., and Padrick, K. (1984): Nursing's search for scientific knowledge. Nursing Research, *33*, 26–32.

Burnside, J. (1973): Caring for the aged: Touching is talking. American Journal of Nursing. *Therapeutic communication through touching is discussed.*

Carlson, C. (ed.) (1970): Behavioral Concepts and Nursing Intervention. Philadelphia: J. B. Lippincott. *Contains article by Robinson on humor.*

Cattell, R. and Scheier, I. (1961): Neuroticism and Anxiety. New York: Ronald. *Includes discussion of measures of anxiety.*

Chapman, J. (1977): Effects of different nursing approaches upon selected postoperative herniorrhaphy patients. In Downs, F. and Newman, M. (eds.), A Sourcebook of Nursing Research. Philadelphia: F. A. Davis, pp. 15–23. *Use of participant observation in clinical area experiment.*

Ciminero, A., Calhoun, K., and Adams, H. (eds.) (1977): Handbook of Behavioral Assessment. New York: Wiley. *Seventeen articles that review behavioral assessment comprehensively.*

Felton, G. (1970): Effect of time cycle changes on blood pressure and temperature in young women. Nursing Research, *19*, 48–58. *Biological rhythms, efficiency, and sleep patterns of nurses.* (1973): Rhythmic correlates of shift work. In Batey, M. (ed.), Communicating Nursing Research. Boulder: Western Interstate Commission for Higher Education. *Interval sampling of body temperature and urine every three hours to determine effect of biological rhythms.*

Grant, E. (1971): Facial expression and gesture. Journal of Psychosomatic Research, *15*, 391. *Contains a checklist of 100 units of muscle change associated with facial expression.*

Gunning, S. and Holmes, T. (1973): Dance therapy with psychotic children. Archives of General Psychiatry, *28*. *Communicating through dance.*

Habenstein, R. (ed.) Pathways to Data. Chicago: Aldine. *Thirteen articles report research in hospitals, home towns, etc.*

Hasselmeyer, E. (1961): Behavior Patterns of Premature Infants. Washington, D.C.: Government Printing Office. *Examines kinesthetic needs in the premature.*

Horn, B. (1978): Transcultural nursing and child rearing of the Muckleshoot people. In Leininger, M. (ed.), Transcultural Nursing. New York: Wiley, pp. 223–238. *Participant observations study of the culture of the Muckleshoot Indians of Washington State.*

Holsti, O., Loomba, J. and North, R. (1968): Content analysis. In Lindzey, G. and Aronson, E. (eds.), The Handbook of Social Psychology (2nd ed., Vol. 2). Reading, Mass.: Addison-Wesley. *An authoritative article on content analysis.*

Kassenbaum, G. (1970): Strategies for the sociological study of criminal correctional systems. In Habenstein., R. (ed.), Pathways to Data. Chicago: Aldine, pp. 122–138. *Outlines strategies for nonparticipant observer research, using participant observers as sources of data.*

Kane, F. (1958): Clothing worn by outpatients to interviews. Psychiatric Communications. *Nonparticipant observation of the clothing worn by outpatients.* (1959): Clothing worn by an outpatient: A case study. Psychiatric Communications. *Case-study method of unobtrusive observation.*

Kendall, K. (1978): Maternal and child nursing in an Iranian village. In Leininger, M. (ed.), Transcultural Nursing. New York: Wiley, pp. 399–416. *Participant observation in nursing research.*

Klein, R., et al. (1972): Psychiatric staff: Uniforms or street clothes? Archives of General Psychiatry, 26 (Jan.). *Street clothes worn by health personnel may be better than uniforms.*

Leininger, M. (1978): Transcultural Nursing. New York: Wiley. *Twenty-six articles, many of which report research that uses participant observation methods.*

Leipold, W. (1963): Psychological distance in a dyadic interview as a function of introversion–extroversion, anxiety, social desirability, and stress. Unpublished doctoral dissertation, Univ. of North Dakota. *Uses unobtrusive measures to note seats taken in interviews by introverted and anxious students.*

Lindeman, C. and Van Aernam, B. (1977). Nursing intervention with the presurgical patient—The effects of structured and unstructured preoperative teaching. In Downs, F. and Newman, M. (eds.), A sourcebook of Nursing Research (2nd ed.). Philadelphia: F. A. Davis. *Use of sound on slide instruments.*

Mahl, G. (1956): Disturbances and silences in the patient's speech in psychotherapy. Journal of Abnormal and Social Psychology, 53, 1–15. *Data collected in psychotherapy sessions by observation.*

Marshall, L. (1972): Patient reaction to sound in an intensive coronary care unit. In Batey, M. (ed.), Communicating Nursing Research. Boulder: WICHE, pp. 81–97. *Nonparticipant observation, using electrocardiographic oscilloscopes and tape recorders to study effects of ward sounds on heart rate.*

McCorkle, R. (1981): Effects of touch on seriously ill patients. Nursing Research, 23, 114–125. *Effect of touching observed.*

Petrovich, D. et al. (1968): Nursing apparel and psychiatric patients: A comparison of uniforms and street clothes. Journal of Psychiatric Nursing, 6. *Street clothes worn by health personnel compared with uniforms.*

Puttock, D. (1972): Dance therapy. Nursing Times, 68. *Nonverbal communication by means of dance.*

Robinson, V. (1970): Humor in nursing. In Carlson, C. (ed.), Behavioral Concepts and Nursing Intervention. Philadelphia: J. B. Lippincott. *Unobtrusive measure.*

Rodgers, J. (1977): Relationship between sociability and personal space preference at two different times of day. In Downs, F. and Newman, M. (eds.), A Sourcebook of Nursing Research (2nd ed.). Philadelphia: F. A. Davis, pp. 171–177. *Study of personal space, sociability, and time of day.*

Rugh, J. and Schwitzgebel, R. (1977): Instrumentation for behavioral assessment. In Ciminero, A. et al. (eds.), Handbook of Behavioral Assessment. New York: Wiley, pp. 79–113. *Good source of useful instruments for research.*

Simon, J. (1978): Basic Research Methods in Social Sciences. New York: Random House. *Chap. 19 deals with obstacles created by human observers.*

Skipper, J. and Leonard, R. (eds.) (1965): Social Interaction and Patient Care. Philadelphia: J. B. Lippincott. *Collection of articles dealing with patient care.*

Updike, P., Accurso, F., and Jones, R. (1985): Physiologic circadian rhythmicity in preterm infants. Nursing Research, *34*, 160–163.

Webb, E., et al. (1966): Unobtrusive Measures. Rand McNally. *Chapter Five deals with simple observation.*

Wolff, C. (1948): A Psychology of Gesture. London: Methuen. *Hand gestures studied to examine correlation between emotional make-up and gesture.*

REFERENCES FOR SELECTED INSTRUMENTS

Adorno, T., Frenkel-Brunswik, E., Levinson, D., and Sanford, N. (1950): The Authoritarian Personality. New York: Harper & Row. *Includes the F-Scale, which measures authoritarianism—a syndrome of organized beliefs and symptoms.*

Akutagawa, D. (1965): A study in construct validity of the psychoanalytic concept of latent anxiety and a test of projection distance hypothesis. Unpublished doctoral dissertation, Univ. of Pittsburgh. *Fear Survey Schedule—fifty items, self-rating schedule.*

Boggardus, E. (1959): Social Distance. Yellow Springs, Ohio: Antioch Press. *The social distance scale measures the grades and degrees of intimacy between social groups.*

Buros, O. (ed.) (1978): The Eighth Mental Measurement Yearbook. Hyland Park, N.J.: Gryphon Press. *Helps locate information on standardized tests.*

Cahell, J. and Warburton, F. (1967): Objective Personality and Motivation Tests. Chicago: University of Chicago Press. *Paper-and-pencil instruments.*

Chapin, F. (1970): Social participation scale. In Miller, D. (ed.), Handbook of Research Design and Social Measurement (2nd ed.). New York: David McKay. *General scale of participation in professional, civic, and social organizations.*

Chesney, M. and Tasto, D. (1975): The development of the menstrual symptom questionnaire. Behavior Research and Therapy, *13*, 237–244. *Fifty-one items distinguish between verbal symptoms of spasmodic and congestive dysmenorrhea.*

Chun, K., Cobb, S., and French, J. (1975): Measures of Psychological Assessment. Ann Arbor: Survey Research Center. *Psychological measure.*

Eckland, B. (1965): Academic ability, higher education and occupational mobility. American Council on Education. *Measures of intelligence and achievement.*

Fessler, D. (1952): The development of a scale for measuring community solidarity. Rural Sociology, *17*, 144–152. *Useful to determine relationships between community progress and solidarity.*

Geer, J. (1965): The development of a scale to measure fear. Behavior Research and Therapy, *3*, 45–53. *Fear scale.*

Gesell, A., et al. (1956): Youth: The Years from Ten to Sixteen. New York: Harper & Row. *Developmental approach.*

Hollingshead, A. and Redlich, F. (1958): Social Class and Mental Illness. New York: Wiley, pp. 390–391. *A two-factor index of social position is included.*

Kohlenberg, R. (1973): Operant conditioning of human anal sphincter pressure. Journal of Applied Behavior Analysis, *6*, 201–208. *Conditioning as an instrument.*

Lubin, B. (1965): Adjective checklists for measurement of depression. Archives of General Psychiatry, *12*, 57–62. *DACL—the Depression Adjective Checklist —one of the few scales considered sensitive to behavioral treatment programs. Subject rates self.*

Mikaelian, H. (1972): A technique for measuring eye-foot coordination without visual guidance. Behavior Research Methods and Instrumentation, *4*, 17–18. *A mirror-visual system to measure eye-foot coordination.*

Miller, D. (1970): Handbook of Research Design and Social Measurement. New York: David McKay. Part II: Guides to Methods and Techniques of Collecting Data in Library, Field, and Laboratory.

Moreno, J. (1972): Psychodrama. Beacon, N.Y.: Beacon House. *Sociometric technique.*

Osgood, C., et al. (1957): The Measurement of Meaning, Urbana, Ill.: University of Illinois Press. *The semantic differential technique to measure the affect feeling meaning of cognition.*

Rathus, S. (1973): A 30-item schedule for assessing assertive behavior. Behavior Therapy, *4*, 398–406. *The Rathus Assertiveness Schedule; subjects rate themselves.*

Reeder, L., et al. (1976): Handbook of Scales and Indices of Health Behavior. Pacific Palisades, Calif.: Goodyear. *Handbook useful to identify indices of health behavior.*

Richardson, F. and Tasto, D. (1976): Development and factor analysis of a social anxiety inventory. Behavior Therapy, *7*, 453–462. *Social Anxiety Inventory.*

Schulmann, J. and Reisman, J. (1959): An objective measurement for hyperactivity. American Journal of Mental Deficiency, *64*, 455–456. *Instrument to measure hyperactivity.*

Shipley, R. and Harley, R. (1971): A device for estimating stability of stance in human subjects. Psychophysiology, *7*, 287–292. *A linear-differential transformer senses movement of a platform to measure equilibrium and stability.*

Walk, R. (1956): Self-ratings of fear in a fear-invoking situation. Journal of Abnormal and Social Psychology, *52*, 171–178. *"Fear thermometer" assesses momentary anxiety level in response to a feared stimulus.*

Wallace, W. (1971): The Logic of Science in Sociology. Chicago: Aldine, Chap. 4. *Hypotheses, instrumentation, scaling.*

Zuckerman, M. (1960): The development of an affective adjective checklist for the measurement of anxiety. Journal of Consulting and Clinical Psychology, *24*, 457–462. *State of anxiety measured.*

16

Asking Questions as a Research Method:
The Questionnaire and Interview

When it is not possible or desirable to observe directly, questionnaires and interviews are the primary means of collecting data. Both methods are effective for obtaining information about attitudes, opinions, perceptions, beliefs, feelings, motivations, private behavior, past behavior, and anticipated behavior. In addition, both are useful for collecting demographic data that characterize a population, such as age, sex, occupation, marital status, and health status. Both rely heavily on verbal reports, either oral or written. However, they differ, in that the questionnaire obtains information from a respondent who answers a list of fixed questions with little or no assistance from the researcher, while the interview always involves interaction, either face-to-face or by telephone.

Brown et al. (1984), assessing the methods of data collection reported in research publications since 1952, found that nurses have relied mainly on questionnaires and interview schedules to collect data, with little change occurring over the three decades. In 1980, 41 percent of data collection was by questionnaire and 13 percent by interview.

Upon completion of this chapter, the student should be able to: (1) state how to construct a questionnaire and an interview schedule; (2) describe elements of the questionnaire, including the covering letter, instructions, questions, response categories and precoding, inducements to respond, and the informed-consent form; (3) differentiate among the structured, semistructured, and unstructured interview; (4) describe the focused interview and the clinical interview; (5) identify and define several projective techniques; (6) discuss other data-collection methods, such as the critical incident, content analysis, and Q methodology; and (7) contrast and compare the interview and questionnaire methods, listing advantages and disadvantages.

THE QUESTIONNAIRE

The construction of a questionnaire requires thought, planning, and testing. The researcher must convince and motivate an unseen respondent and must give the respondent clear, written instructions so that the respondent may understand, and respond properly to, the questions. The researcher must formulate clear, unambiguous questions, must arrange them in the proper order, and must organize the questionnaire so as to make taking data from it as easy and as accurate as possible. We shall examine how to construct a questionnaire, with attention to each of these factors.

Construction of the Questionnaire

The questionnaire is comprised of the following elements: (1) covering letter, (2) instructions to respondents, (3) questions, (4) response categories and precoding, (5) demographic data, and (6) inducements to respond. Each of these elements will be examined.

The Covering Letter. The covering letter begins with the identification of the sponsoring institution and the researcher. The sponsorship of the project refers to the person or agency who endorses or supports the study. The name of a highly respected person or agency is a guarantee to the respondents that the project is worthwhile, that the data will not be misused, and that confidentiality will be maintained. Colleges and universities consistently rate high, their sponsorship usually producing excellent cooperation. The name of a person who is important to the study subjects is likewise helpful. Thus, a covering letter on which the name of the sponsoring institution appears, or which is signed by a well-known person, is valuable in gaining cooperation, introducing the questionnaire, and introducing the researcher to the respondents. In general terms, the letter must explain why the research is being done, how the respondents were selected for the study, and why their answers are important. The letter should clearly state whether or not the respondents will be expected to participate further in the study, and it should guarantee anonymity and confidentiality to the respondents. A statement that information collected will be used for statistical purposes only, and that all data will remain completely confidential, will reassure the respondent that privacy will be guarded. An informed-consent form may follow the letter and precede the questionnaire, or it may follow the questionnaire. In either case, arrangements must be made to protect the respondent so that the respondent may return the signed consent form to the researcher with confidence.

Instructions to the Respondents. Instructions should appear throughout the questionnaire so as to enable the respondent to make appropriate responses. If only one response is proper, the instructions should clearly state this. Where more than one response is possible, this should likewise be indicated. It is particularly important to give directions each time the response pattern changes in any way. Since no explanation or interpretation beyond the written word is possible, clear and simple directions are mandatory. Instructions should be carefully tested by having persons who are not in the sample answer the questionnaire and indicate where the instructions are unclear or ambiguous. Where understanding is doubtful, sample questions and responses may be included in the instructions.

The Questions. The questions are the heart of the questionnaire. The researcher depends upon the questions to collect information about the research problem. Therefore, the questions should be carefully examined and tested for the following: (a) appropriateness, (b) content, (c) wording, and (d) order. (See Appendix B for sample questionnaire.)

1. *Two kinds of questions are appropriate in a questionnaire: the* standardized, *or* structured, *question, and the* open-ended *question.* The *standardized* question, also called the *fixed-alternative, closed-ended,* or *highly structured* question, consists of several alternative responses from which the respondent must choose the one most appropriate and accurate:

	Yes	**No**
There are plenty of opportunities on my job to use my nursing education.	☐	☐
I like the type of patients I work with in the community.	☐	☐
The doctors and nurses in the agency work as a team.	☐	☐

The fixed-alternative, closed-ended questions above may be answered quickly and are easy to analyze. However, there are disadvantages, such as the omission of possible alternatives to a simple *yes* or *no* answer, superficial examination of complex problems, and forced responses. In cases where the range of alternative responses is unknown or where the issues are sensitive or need exploration, an open-ended question may be more informative:

How much opportunity do you have on your present job to use your nursing education? _____

While the analysis of open-ended questions takes time and skill, the researcher gains a wealth of information on sensitive topics that cannot be explored with simple yes or no answers. In addition, material heretofore not investigated can be explored. In fact, both kinds of questions may be used.

2. *The content of the questions arises from the research problem and proposal.* Each facet of the problem must have questions in order to collect data. The researcher must decide the following: What data must be collected? How many questions is it practical to ask? How many questions should be devoted to collect data from each area? Given a specific number of questions, what must the content of each question be?

It is helpful to develop a question guide that includes the content that must be covered, content that may be helpful but is not essential, the estimated number of questions needed to cover the content, and the total number of questions that it is practical to ask. A choice may then be made either to increase the length of the questionnaire in order to ask all necessary questions or to reduce the number of questions.

Determining what should be the content of questions is not easy. A review of the literature to identify key concepts is often helpful. To study job satisfaction among nursing-service personnel, begin with a review of the literature in order to determine the concepts and definitions used in previous studies. Then define *satisfaction* and devise a questionnaire to measure job satisfaction.

3. *The wording of both the questions and the alternative responses is a crucial and difficult process.* The researcher should develop a checklist that includes all positive and negative characteristics of questions and should examine each question in the light of these attributes. Positive characteristics include clarity, brevity, simplicity, and applicability to the study sample. Negative characteristics include "double-barreled" questions, double-negative questions, embarrassing or sensitive questions, jargon-filled questions, complex questions, leading questions, questions that bias, and questions that are inappropriate to the study sample (Table 16–1 for a checklist).

"Double-barreled" questions ask two questions in one. They often contain words such as *either, therefore, or, and,* or *both.* Examples of such questions include the following: "Are nurses overworked, or do you think they are just inefficient?" "Nursing supervisors have more information about patients than student nurses do; therefore, do you think students should question procedures established by nursing supervisors?" "When did you stop keeping up with nursing research?"

"Double-negative" questions use two negatives to indicate a positive statement. For example, the respondents may be asked

TABLE 16-1. CHECKLIST FOR POSITIVE AND NEGATIVE CHARACTERISTICS OF QUESTIONNAIRE QUESTIONS

Positive Characteristics

1. Clarity: Can the question be interpreted in more than one way?
2. Brevity: Can the question be shortened and still retain its meaning?
3. Simplicity: Is the vocabulary at a simple level (such as that of a newspaper) that is appropriate to the study sample?
4. Applicability: Can the respondents in the study sample be reasonably expected to answer accurately?

Negative Characteristics

1. Double-barreled questions: Does the question ask two questions in one? Does it first make a statement with which the respondent may not agree, and then ask a question on the basis of that statement? Does the question have a hidden premise?
2. Double-negative questions: Does the question include words such as *don't* or *not*?
3. Leading questions: Is the question asked in such a way that the respondent knows that a particular response is desired?
4. Sensitive questions: Is the question asked in such a way that the respondent may become embarrassed, angry, or emotionally upset?
5. Jargon-filled questions: Does the question use professional, technical, or slang terms with which the respondents are not familiar?
6. Complex questions: Does the question use long phrases and complex sentences?
7. Questions that bias: Does the question contain information that would encourage the respondent to view one answer as more likely "right"? Does the question contain emotionally loaded words, such as *motherly, patriotic,* or *Communist*?
8. Inappropriate questions: Does the question assume prior knowledge inappropriate to the sample?

to state if they agree or disagree with the following double-negative question: "I don't think it is not a wise policy to have nursing students in the operating room." It is not immediately clear if a *yes* response means that the respondents feel that students should or should not be in the operating room.

"Embarrassing" or "sensitive" questions are any that are so blunt that they offend the respondent. Asking "Did you have premarital intercourse?" or "Did you ever have venereal disease?" may be important to the research proposal, but may be so embarrassing that the respondent will not answer.

"Jargon-filled" questions use language, either technical or slang, that is unfamiliar to the respondent. Questions about *urination* are preferable to those about *micturition*, while asking "How many marijuana cigarettes do you estimate you smoke per week?" is preferable to asking "How many times do you get stoned in one week?"

"Complex questions" must be read more than one time to understand their meaning. For example, the following question asks, "When nursing data are sought on matters such as wages in different specialties, such as maternal–child health, do you think a tabular form drawn up on the questionnaire itself, with all required items clearly stated, leaving blank spaces for proper entries, is preferable to a series of questions utilized to elicit the data?" Such questions must be simplified or discarded.

"Questions that bias" are phrased so that the respondent is encouraged to answer in one way rather than another. For example, using popular or unpopular persons or groups influences answers: "Do you agree with the A.N.A. president that . . ."; or "Do you think your country is wrong to . . ."; or "The Communists believe that . . . do you agree?"

"Inappropriate questions" use language that respondents are not able to understand, require information that study subjects will not likely have, request attitudes that few respondents have thought about, or call for a feat of memory that is unlikely for the average person. "How many patients have you cared for since you became a nurse?" is an inappropriate question, because an accurate response is improbable.

The way in which a question is asked may influence the respondent to answer in a more honest manner. The following suggestions may be helpful:

a. Substitute euphemisms for value-loaded language. Ask, "How do you discipline your child?" rather than "How do you punish your child?"

b. Indicate that other people have what might ordinarily be considered socially undesirable attitudes. For example, ask a question about suicide in the following manner: "Many people have thought about suicide at one time or another. Have you ever thought about suicide?" rather than bluntly asking, "Have you ever thought about suicide?"

c. If it is desired that the respondent express criticism, give the respondent an opportunity to voice praise where praise is due. For example, you may ask, "What was the most helpful nursing care you received?" before you ask, "What would you suggest to improve nursing care on Ward X?"

d. Rather than ask about a person or event with which the respondent may not be familiar, structure the question so that the respondent will be able to admit lack of knowledge gracefully. Ask first, "Have you ever had the opportunity to read about Madame Curie?"; then ask, "Do you think that Madame Curie is representative of women's capacity to be scientists?"

e. Achieve some balance of social desirability. Don't ask, "How often do you have intercourse a day?"; rather, ask, "Some couples engage in intercourse as many as several times a day, while others have intercourse as few as several times a year. How often do you have intercourse?"

f. Structure a question in such a way that any undesirable characteristic is assumed: "How many sexual partners did you have before marriage?" is more apt to get a response than "Did you engage in intercourse before marriage?"

4. *In general, the* ordering of questions *should precede from general to specific, regardless of whether the question is open or closed.* This procedure, beginning with broader questions and narrowing down to precise, specific ones, is sometimes called the *funnel technique.* The entire sequence of questions should follow some logical order, with no abrupt transitions. For example, the time sequence should move from questions about the past to the present and then to the future. The order in which questions are asked can influence what answers are given to subsequent questions. Ordering can also affect whether or not the respondent will answer the questionnaire: sensitive questions that are placed first may cut off response, while interesting but neutral questions that appear first may stimulate cooperation. Demographic data are sometimes placed in the beginning of the questionnaire but should generally be placed at the end, to avoid a dull beginning.

"Contingency questions" should be answered only by some respondents; therefore, they must be accompanied by clear instructions to avoid frustrating and confusing the respondent. Two methods for ordering contingency questions are:

Method 1. Have you ever nursed a dying child?
☐ Yes
☐ No
If yes, how many times have you nursed a dying child?
☐ Once
☐ 2 to 5 times
☐ More than 5 times
Method 2. Have you ever nursed a dying child?
☐ Yes. Please answer questions 6–10.
☐ No. Please skip questions 6–10. Go directly to question 11 on page 3.

The Response Categories and Precoding. Once the questions have been formulated, the researcher must provide the respondent with a good set of answers. Since the respondent must be able to communicate answers without error, the range and wording of answers must be considered with the same careful attention with which the questions were devised, or the questionnaire is in vain.

The response categories must be mutually exclusive and exhaustive:

the respondent must be able to choose one and only one alternative, but the alternative must be appropriate for each respondent. For example, the question that asks for religious affiliation should include the following categories:

☐ Protestant
☐ Catholic
☐ Jewish
☐ Other (please specify: _____)

Several different types of responses to fixed-alternative questions are: Likert-scale responses, rank-order responses, checklist responses, and other scale responses.

1. *Likert-Scale Responses*
   Instructions: Beside each of the statements listed below, please indicate whether you strongly agree (SA), agree (A), disagree (D), strongly disagree (SD), or do not know (DK).

	SA 1	**A** 2	**D** 3	**SD** 4	**DK** 5
Supervisors should have a master's degree.	☐	☐	☐	☐	☐

2. *Rank-Order Responses*
   Instructions: Please rank-order the following activities, in terms of what you prefer to do in nursing. Write *1* before the activity you prefer most; *2* before the activity you next prefer, and so on. Please rank-order all listed activities.

   _____ Bedside care
   _____ Administration of a ward
   _____ Giving medications
   _____ Teaching patients
   _____ Supervising students
   _____ Writing reports

3. *Checklist Responses*
   Instructions: Please check the data that you use to orient the disoriented patient.

	Always	**Frequently**	**Seldom**	**Never**
Nicknames	☐	☐	☐	☐
Have patients sign name	☐	☐	☐	☐

	Always	**Frequently**	**Seldom**	**Never**
Have calendar available	☐	☐	☐	☐
Radio	☐	☐	☐	☐
Holiday decorations	☐	☐	☐	☐
Identifying meal times	☐	☐	☐	☐

Precoding is the use of numerical codes on the questionnaire responses, so that responses may either be read by machine or be counted easily by hand. For example, the codes *1* for female and *2* for male may appear beside the response category:

Please indicate your sex:
_____ 1. Female
_____ 2. Male

Precoding may also be used to specify the positions of each response item on the machine-readable form (computer cards):

Please write the year and month of your birth:
_____ year   Columns 17–18
_____ month

Precoding at the response category saves time and effort when processing the responses for data analysis.

Demographic Data. Sometimes questionnaires begin with demographic questions, although many researchers prefer to end the questionnaire with these questions because they tend to be routine and somewhat dull. Demographic data include facts about age, marital status, occupation, educational level, sex, race, number of persons in the household, or other helpful information. For many such questions, standardized wording, such as that used in the United States Census, is helpful. Demographic data are often useful as a criterion measure (dependent variable) to identify the effect of independent variables, such as treatment or behavior, on different races, ages, or sexes of the respondents.

Inducements to Respond. Researchers have tried a number of approaches to encourage participation in a study. These include enclosing a small pencil with which to write, a coin, or the promise that results will be sent to respondents who request them. However, the most effective seems to be an appeal to the respondents' altruistic nature, by indicating the good that the study may accomplish. For example, letting the respondent know that he or she can help scientists better understand the phenomenon under study may be a considerable inducement to reply. The questionnaire's physical appearance is also important in eliciting a good return. The questionnaire should be attractive, with reasonable length, appropriate size, and inviting color and line-spacing.

Colors should be pretested for effectiveness but, in general, lighter colors (especially yellow and pink) have been found to elicit the highest percentages of returns. A questionnaire of several pages or a planned sequence of questionnaires may benefit by alternating light colors. However, regardless of color, it is important to show more paper than printing. A page of closely typed lines and questions may immediately discourage the respondent.

The size of the questionnaire may vary. A double postcard, with the questionnaire portion to be torn off and returned, has been successful in market surveys. Standard letter-size questionnaires ($8\frac{1}{2} \times 11$ inches) are widely used, since one-page forms encourage the respondent to answer immediately. However, it is important to provide adequate space for comments. A few well-answered questions are preferable to many undecipherable answers. In cases where the questionnaire must be long, successfully motivating the respondent may be more important than either the type or length of the form.

Hand delivery of questionnaires may be an important way to stimulate response. The researcher can deliver the form, explain the project, and elicit cooperation. The researcher may then collect the completed form or have the form mailed back in a self-addressed and stamped envelope. A variation of this technique is to first mail the questionnaire and covering letter and then visit the respondent to pick up the completed form, checking for completeness.

If the questionnaire is mailed, a follow-up mailing may be an effective method of stimulating returns that are not forthcoming. The follow-up mailing should occur 2 to 3 weeks after the initial mailing. Usually, the original mailing and two follow-up mailings result in a return from most people who care to respond at all. The overall response is one guide to assess how representative the sample return is. Statistics used to analyze research data often assume that all members of the sample return their forms; this is seldom true. Some social scientists regard a 50 percent return as adequate, 60 percent as good, and 70 percent as very good (Babbie, 1975). Others expect lower returns, from 10 to 20 percent (Parten, 1950).

Various Questionnaire Techniques

1. *The* Delphi technique *is a method of data collection that uses questionnaires that are mailed to a panel of experts in successive waves,*

with feedback from previous questionnaires included with successive questionnaires. Lindeman's (1975) use of this technique is probably the best-known example in nursing. Lindeman selected her panel of experts from persons identified by professional nursing organizations and funding agencies. To determine the five areas in which nursing research was needed, four rounds of questionnaires were mailed to 433 panel experts. Of the 433 experts, 341 responded to all four rounds of questionnaires. The first round asked the experts to identify five areas in which nursing research was needed. Of the 2,000 responses, 150 were selected as the most frequently mentioned. These were used in the second round, and respondents were asked to indicate three factors: whether nursing should lead research in this area; the value of the item for nursing as a profession; and the impact of the item on patient welfare. The third round of questionnaires included both the range of response and the average response from the previous questionnaire, and experts were asked to comment on these. The fourth round of questionnaires contained both summaries of the third round and comments obtained.

The findings of the study indicated that the highest priorities in the area of patient care were patient education, the alleviation of pain, and the development of indicators to measure the quality of nursing care. The highest priorities in the area of the nursing profession were research into the nursing process, the research process itself, and the development of instruments to measure the quality of nursing care.

EXAMPLE FROM NURSING RESEARCH

One study reports the results of a Delphi survey of 347 nursing administrators, clinical nursing staff, and nursing researchers in Veterans Administration hospitals nationwide designed to identify priorities for nursing research related to the care of veterans. The rounds included the following: In Round I, each participant submitted three questions related to issues in nursing believed to merit research. A group of three nurses then classified these questions and developed 73 statements related to the care of the veteran. In Rounds II and III, participants reviewed and rated each of the 73 statements on a scale of 1 to 7 to judge the following question: "What would be the magnitude of the impact on the care of the veteran patient if increased knowledge were available in this area?" In Round III, participants reviewed feedback from their own rating and from the group median for each of the 73 questions.

2. Sociometric data *are concerned with interpersonal and inter-organizational relationships and may be collected with questionnaires.* In this case, the questions asked may be "Who are your best friends?"; "Who are the persons that you respect most in the

group?"; "Who are the persons you would prefer to work with among your colleagues?" The respondents return a list of names indicating their social choices. The researcher then analyzes these data to find the chosen linkages among persons of the group. Analysis of sociometric data includes constructing graphs, such as the sociogram. A *sociogram* consists of dots that represent the persons, statuses, or offices involved. The lines connecting the dots represent the nominating and the nominated persons. The depicted relationships may be either *symmetric* (reciprocal, or mutual, choices), or *asymmetric* (nonreciprocal choices). The graphic approach is limited to the number of dots and lines that can be visually depicted.

Sociometric techniques have not been widely used in nursing. The Beard and Scott (1975) study of the efficacy of group therapy by nurses for hospitalized patients is one of the few studies that used this method.

3. *Use vignettes to measure broad concepts. Vignettes* are short, compact descriptions that exemplify a concept. Anthropologists were among the first to use "the hypothetical situation" as a technique of field research. According to Flaskerud (1979), Murray (1978) used eight vignettes to measure perceptions of problematic behavior by Appalachians, mental-health professionals, and lay non-Appalachians in the doctoral dissertation. The vignettes were part of a questionnaire to survey the response of two cultural groups to problematic behavior. The author was eliciting behavior that represented a norm in specific minority cultures. To establish the validity of the vignettes, three methods were used. First, 20 vignettes were developed based on actual case histories of members of the minority culture who had been hospitalized for mental illness. Second, the author used a panel of experts who had published research on the minority culture being studied. Third, the questionnaire was pretested. Flaskerud concluded that the use of vignettes as a measuring instrument is desirable, but efforts to establish validity are not conclusive.

Taylor, Skelton, and Butcher (1984) used vignettes in an experiment to examine features that distinguished chronic from acute pain syndromes and their influence on nurses' estimates of patient suffering, pain relief actions, and attitudes toward patients. Two hundred and sixty-eight nurses received a questionnaire that included a random assignment of one of the 24 variants of the instrument, one-paragraph descriptions of patients complaining of severe pain. Subjects estimated the intensity of the hypothetical patient's suffering, rated the patient on a series of trait dimensions, and indicated priorities for actions to relieve pain. The authors report that the vignette was constructed on the following model:

> Patient A, 40 years old, is admitted for evaluation of a history of low back (headache, joint) pain. The patient notes feeling sad and losing interest in most activities, including eating. (Sentence omitted in half the questionnaires.) Physical examination and lab data reveal (no) significant objective signs of pathology. As you enter the room, the patient says, "I am in severe pain."

Descriptions in the vignettes varied in terms of duration of pain (acute versus chronic), signs of physical pathology (positive versus negative), signs of depression (positive versus negative), and diagnostic category (low back versus headache versus joint pain). In addition to other assessments, the nurse respondents attributed less-intense pain when the patient had no signs of pathology and when duration was long-term and chronic. Data indicated that the chronic pain sufferer is negatively stereotyped by the nursing staff.

EXAMPLES FROM NURSING RESEARCH

The questionnaire is widely used in nursing research. For example, Moore-Nunnally and Aguiar (1974) developed two questionnaires—one to determine patients' attitudes toward the prenatal care that they were receiving, the other to determine patients' knowledge levels and attitudes toward their labor and delivery experiences. The prenatal questionnaire consisted of 52 items: eight questions on demographic data, 38 questions on attitudes and on care that patients did or did not receive, five open-ended questions, and one question that rated overall opinion on a 1-to-11 scale. The labor and delivery room questionnaire consisted of four parts: part A collected data not available on the patient's chart; part B elicited attitudes toward prenatal classes, labor, and delivery, in five open-ended questions; part C elicited further attitudes, in a series of 25 attitude statements; and part D collected data about pregnancy, labor, and delivery in nine multiple-choice questions.

In a study of the psychological preparation of surgical patients, Schmitt and Wooldridge (1981) used a questionnaire to measure attitudinal variables at the time of patients' discharge. Both the experimental group and the control group were asked to recall how well they had slept and the level of anxiety that they felt the evening before, and the morning of, surgery. Questions were designed to determine what the patients remembered about the surgery, including the operating room and the recovery room. In part, the questionnaire was expected to elicit whether or not the experimental group, which had extra preparation for surgery, would report less anxiety, better sleeping patterns, and would be better able to recall experiences about the surgery.

THE INTERVIEW

The *interview* is a method of data collection in which an interviewer asks questions of the respondent, either face-to-face or by telephone. The interview is comprised of three components: the interviewer, the interview schedule or guide, and the respondent. Each of these represents a wide range of variables. For example, the interview schedule may be highly structured, requiring the most formal type of interaction between interviewer and respondent. On the other hand, the schedule may be only a guide that the interviewer either has memorized or holds in hand, while encouraging the respondent to talk freely. In both cases, however, the interview schedule must be carefully formulated and the interviewer must be vigorously trained. First, we shall examine the interview schedule and the training of the interviewer. Following this, we shall investigate interviews that use various approaches.

The *interview schedule* or *guide* is a written form constructed with the same attention to instructions and questions that is used for the questionnaire. However, three differences are immediately apparent in the case of the interview: (1) the questions and responses are both spoken; (2) the face-to-face interaction commonly used may decrease the feeling of anonymity; and (3) the interviewer is able to observe as well as question. Each of these has important consequences in the interview.

Instructions on the interview schedule are of two kinds: instructions to the interviewer, which are not to be read, and instructions to the respondent, which must be read. In certain cases, instructions to the interviewer may contain instructions about how to proceed. An interview could be destroyed if the interviewer read his or her instructions aloud (Babbie, 1975, p. 120): "If the respondent is nearly illiterate, then . . . ." On the other hand, when a formal interview is used, instructions to the respondent must be delivered from a verbatim script from the beginning of the interview to the end. The questions must be clearly understood when spoken, and the interviewer must be able to record the responses quickly and accurately. To increase feelings of confidentiality and anonymity in cases of sensitive questions, a separate brief questionnaire may be filled out by the respondent to indicate responses such as income or sexual behavior. These may be placed in an envelope and attached to the interview schedule. A second technique is to hand the respondent a small card containing several categories and to have the respondent answer the question by indicating the appropriate category. For example, a question about income may include the following categories from which the respondent selects one:

- Category (A) income under $5,000
- Category (B) income between $5,000 and $9,999
- Category (C) income between $10,000 and $14,999

- Category (D) income between $15,000 and $19,999
- Category (E) income between $20,000 and $24,999
- Category (F) income over $25,000

The interviewer's observations increase the depth of the data collected. For example, the interviewer can note the quality of the dwelling, the condition of the yard and furnishings, the appearance of the respondent, the reaction of the respondent to various questions, and demographic data (such as sex and race).

The training of interviewers includes how to word questions, how to record responses, how to probe for responses when this is appropriate, and how to present one's self in the interview situation. As noted earlier, the interviewer must follow the exact wording and phrasing in a formal interview, without a single change. In the case of open-ended questions, the responses should be written precisely as they are spoken—bad grammar and all. Where gestures and tones are significant to reveal meaning, these may be added in the margin of the interview schedule. Probes may be required to elicit responses to open-ended questions, but these may take the form of silence or of simply asking, "Anything else?" (Babbie, 1975, p. 272) Probes should be neutral: all interviewers should use the same probes when these are necessary in a formal interview. Where more than one interviewer is used, interview training to deal with these and other questions should be conducted in a group. The researcher should begin with a description of the study, include general procedures, and then examine the interview schedule in detail, question by question. Demonstration interviews and return demonstrations by the interviewers who are being trained are also helpful. The pilot study helps test the efficiency of the training, and a discussion following pilot interviews can deal with troublesome issues. While actually collecting data, the researcher must work closely with the interviewers, supervising the process from beginning to end. In cases where student groups are working together on an interview project, meetings should be held frequently to compare notes and discuss problems.

In contrast with the standardized and structured questionnaire, the interview schedule may take a variety of forms. The interview may use a highly structured schedule, such as those in the formal interview described. Or, the interview may be partially structured or totally unstructured. Each of these will be examined.

Standardized and Structured Interview Schedules

This form of interview includes a schedule of questions that are asked in the same order, with the same wording, and according to identical procedures used by every interviewer. The goal of the interviewer is to be a neutral medium through which questions are asked and responses recorded. If the researcher affects the responses in any way, a bias is interjected that could be mistakenly interpreted as a characteristic of the respondent rather than an influence of the interviewer. Therefore, questions must be asked in a standard way, with as little interaction with the respondent as possible.

Partially Structured Interviews

In situations where the researcher wishes to conduct a more intensive and general study on a smaller sample, partially structured interviews are useful. In these cases, the interview is more fluid and allows the interviewer latitude to move in interesting and productive directions. Two partially structured interview techniques are the "focused interview" and the "clinical interview."

Focused Interview. This kind of interview is partially structured by a schedule of questions and topics that the interviewer wishes to cover. However, the interviewer is free to deviate from the schedule, so long as the material is covered by the conclusion of the interview. Focused interviews are useful to ascertain how the respondent defines certain situations, such as being in the hospital, in terms of variables such as age, sex, culture, social class, or diagnosis. The responses may be used for many purposes: to test hypotheses previously defined, to formulate new hypotheses from unanticipated responses, or to gather data on specified research problems.

Clinical Interview. A clinical interview combines observations with questioning. Nurses use the clinical interview to gather data on the status of patients or clients, to identify nursing needs, to diagnose, and to plan nursing care and intervention. The clinical interview is widely used in individual casework, in psychiatric clinics, and in field work with participant or nonparticipant observation.

The clinical interview may focus upon a specific situation, such as the development of an illness, the place of an individual within the family, or the relationship of an individual within the family and the community at large. The clinical interview combines observation and questioning with inductive reasoning to establish concepts and categories and to generate theory.

The clinical method begins with the observation of data, and then uses the inductive approach to summarize and categorize the data. The relationship between the concepts or categories may be established by an empirical generalization. Hypotheses may then be generated from the empirical generalization for testing. The clinical method may also include experiments, although the usual approach is to wait for processes to unfold rather than to make processes occur, as the experiment usually does.

The clinical method has its disadvantages. The case history of an entire life is complex and is beyond the researcher's ability to comprehend in its entirety. In addition, the researcher may introduce a bias in observation or questioning, or the client may fail to recall what happened in the past with complete accuracy. As a whole, clinical research may be more effective for formulating hypotheses than for extensive testing.

The Unstructured Interview

The unstructured interview may include elements of both the focused and the clinical interview, but these are integrated into a general approach that encourages the respondent to broach topics and to explore them as long as the respondent wishes. An unstructured interview may begin by simply asking the respondent to talk about whatever he or she has in mind or to "tell what things were like" when he or she was younger. While time-consuming, lengthy, and difficult, this approach helps the interviewer get inside the respondent's private world to discover factors that influence daily life, to investigate ways in which the external world is integrated with the respondent's internal world, or to uncover evidence of abnormal processes at work in the respondent's mind or personality. To assist in this process, the interviewer often uses projective techniques.

Projective techniques are designed to collect data in response to nonstructured or ambiguous stimuli that elicit behavior (often unconscious) on the part of the respondent. Projective techniques are often used in totally unstructured interviews, in which the respondent is encouraged to control the interview by expressing feelings, fantasies, fears, and doubts freely, without disapproval or even advice from the interviewer. In such cases, the function of the interviewer is simply to create an atmosphere of trust and to encourage the respondent to talk by using simple phrases, such as "tell me more" or "that is interesting." The researcher who plans to use projective techniques that require trained persons to analyze the data should recruit these people early in the research project.

The four major types of projective techniques are: (1) association, (2) construction, (3) completion, and (4) expressive tests. *Association* tests include the Rorschach Inkblot Test, the Holtzman Inkblot Test, and the word-association test. In each case, the researcher presents the subject with ambiguous pictures or words and asks for the first idea or word that comes to mind. The Rorschach is time-consuming to administer; special training is necessary to interpret it; reliability is low; and validity is questionable. The Holtzman Test is scored by reference to published norms; interrater reliability is satisfactory, and split-half and alternate-form reliability are acceptable. Validity data are promising. Word-Association tests can be interpreted using published norms; the test is easy to administer, and reliability is highest for tests with standard scoring procedures.

Construction tests include Murray's Thematic Apperception Test, Machover's Draw-a-Person Test, and Rosenzweig's Picture-Frustration Test. In these tests, the researcher presents a standard stimulus, and the subject is asked to construct a product in response. Reliability and validity are low for the Thematic Apperception Test and for the Draw-a-Person test. The Rosenzweig Picture-Frustration Test is relatively structured, with scoring procedures and established norms. Reliability is acceptable.

Completion tests include the Sentence Completion. Reliability varies with the type of stimulus used and with the specificity of coding. Some standardized measures have been published.

Expressive tests include play techniques and role playing. Reliability varies with the degree of structuring, standardization of instruction, and specificity of coding.

Projective tests commonly used in unstructured interviews include, among others, the following: (1) the Rorschach Test, (2) the Thematic Apperception Test, (3) word association, (4) sentence completion, (5) doll play, (6) figure drawing, and (7) psychodrama and sociodrama. Each of these will be briefly examined.

1. *The* Rorschach Test *consists of ten cards, each of which contains an inkblot—an unstructured, ambiguous stimulus.* The subject is asked, "What might this be?" and then tells what he or she sees in the inkblot, thereby giving it structure and revealing what is in his or her own unconscious. In order to interpret findings, the test requires training; therefore, it is useful only in extensive research. It has been used effectively in cross-cultural studies, such as that in which DuBois collected Rorschach material on the people of Alor. This material was independently analyzed by the psychiatrist Kardiner, who reached the same conclusion as DuBois and others about the Alorese basic personality structure (DuBois, 1944).

2. *The* Thematic Apperception Test *consists of a series of pictures of various situations, persons, or processes.* The subject is asked to tell a story about what he or she sees in the picture, thus revealing what is in the subject's own mind. Nineteen of the 20 cards contain black-and-white pictures; the last card is blank, allowing the subject to imagine a picture and describe it. The responses are scored according to the variable that the researcher is exploring. Some variables measured are achievement motivation, attitudes toward minority groups, attitudes toward authority, and the need for affiliation.

3. Word-association tests, *a variation of free association, attempt to draw from the respondent's mind all of the data that the respondent has stored in the process of daily life.* The subject is verbally pre-

sented with a list of words, one by one, to which he or she responds with the first word that comes to mind. The interviewer notes both the rate of response and the content, to analyze these for areas of emotional disturbance. In order to elicit internal conflicts or attitudes, the word list combines both neutral words and words with emotional implications, such as love or hate.

4. *The* sentence-completion *test is similar to the word-association test, in that the respondent is supplied with a stimulus—a set of incomplete sentences—and is asked to respond by completing the sentences in any manner desired.* The researcher later puts the responses into categories or rates them according to a previously set design.

5. Doll play *is a technique often used with children.* The child is given a doll or dolls, and the researcher observes what the child does with the dolls. At times, the researcher may tell the child the name of each doll, whether father, mother, or sibling; at other times, the research observes how the child names the doll and plays with it and what the child has the dolls say to one another.

6. Figure-drawing techniques *include those in which the subject is given paper and pencil with instructions to "draw a man" or "draw a tree."* Each technique has standardized methods of administration, scoring, and interpretation, although (like all of the projective techniques) questions are raised about the validity of the evidence.

7. Psychodramas *and* sociodramas *are as much observation techniques as they are interview situations.* However, the researcher does suggest to the subject that he or she act the part in a play —either playing the subject's own part (as if it were a life situation in the psychodrama) or the part of a designated other (such as wife, father, or brother) in the sociodrama. The researcher may then encourage the subject to tell why he or she played the part in a particular way.

The Telephone Interview

The telephone interview relies totally upon oral questions and responses, with little other interaction between the interviewer and the respondent. The major advantages are its low cost, the rapid completion of the interview, and the high response rates. In addition, large-scale telephone surveys may be conducted within a few hours of an occurrence that the researcher wishes to study; for example, an epidemic or a massive influenza inoculation. The interviewer is not required to travel to unfamiliar or dangerous neighborhoods in order to conduct a telephone survey.

However, there are several disadvantages to the telephone interview.

The chief of these is the problem of representativeness. Not everyone has a telephone; moreover, only those with listed telephones may be reached. But, the telephone interview may be used in conjunction with other techniques so as to be representative. In such cases, the telephone survey is useful when speed is important or when data are otherwise unobtainable.

OTHER METHODS OF DATA COLLECTION

Less frequently used methods of data collection include: (1) the critical incident, (2) content analysis, (3) the Q methodology, and (4) vignettes. These combine various methods of obtaining information.

1. *The* critical incident *requires a respondent to write an account of a particular situation.* For example, the researcher may ask the respondent to record a stressful incident that occurred in the past several months. The researcher then analyzes the content of the report. A large number of reports is necessary; 2,000 is the recommended number. This limits the method to those with sufficient time both to collect the data and to analyze it by content analysis.

2. Content analysis *uses communications as units of analysis.* Verbal or behavioral data are classified, summarized, and tabulated in order to understand: (a) the communication process itself, (b) the intentions behind the communication, and (c) the effect of the communication upon the audience.

    The steps used in content analysis include: (a) selecting the unit of content to be analyzed; (b) selecting theory to guide the formulation of categories and coding rules; (c) developing the categories; (d) collecting the observations; and (e) analyzing and interpreting the findings.

    Content analysis may consist only of counting words; for example, the number of times that a particular word is used to describe a depressed patient. Or the analysis may consist of inferring the intentions of the sender or the effect on the audience. The sampling process may include random sampling to select words, phrases, sentences, paragraphs, sections, chapters, books, writers, or contexts to be studied.

    The system of classification, or coding, used must be carefully established and tested before data collection begins, and the system must anticipate a quantitative analysis, especially if data will be processed by computer. Content analysis is useful for measuring attitudes, such as those of politicians toward health care, as well as to identify patterns of communication between health personnel and clients.

3. *The* Q methodology *is a method of collecting data in which the subject sorts a deck of cards on which words, phrases, or messages are written.* The Q *sort*, as the procedure is called, requires the subject to sort the cards according to a particular characteristic that the researcher has identified—approve-disapprove, high priority-low priority. The characteristics are usually placed on a continuum with several categories: category one indicates greatest approval; category five indicates disapproval; categories between one and five indicate less approval and more disapproval, respectively. The number of cards to be sorted ranges from over 50 to 100. Q sorts can be applied to a wide variety of problems and are helpful for studying individual attitudes objectively. However, to use large samples is time-consuming. But, without a fairly large sample, it is not possible to generalize.

EXAMPLES FROM NURSING RESEARCH

Interviews are often used in nursing research. For example, White and Maguire (1973) studied job satisfaction among hospital nursing supervisors, using 34 interviews ranging in time from 15 to 90 minutes. Each respondent was asked to describe a time when she or he felt satisfied with the job and a time when she or he felt dissatisfied. The total number of stories related was 62—31 satisfying and 31 dissatisfying. The interview was focused by the two questions but was otherwise unstructured, allowing the nurses to comment as long as they wished.

Davis and Underwood (1976) used a semistructured, focused interview to study the role of, function of, and decision-making process in a community mental-health center. Four areas of focus included role, function, decision making, and demographic data.

Downs (1964) used a semistructured interview to study maternal stress in primigravidas. She memorized the interview guide to preserve a more natural atmosphere. The average time per interview was 15 to 20 minutes.

In addition to their use in the interview, projective techniques are used in other ways. Christensen et al. (1979) used a version of the Thematic Apperception Test to devise a form to assess the need for achievement, affiliation, and power in nurse practitioners' professional development. Valadez and Anderson (1972) used ten captioned line-drawn pictures with a nurse and patient to ascertain the effect of a rehabilitation workshop on the attitudes of 60 nurses, before and after completion of the workshop. Porter (1974) used projective techniques to determine how grade-school children perceived their internal body parts, while LaFleur and Novotny (1981) studied human figure drawing by amputee children and verbalization of their general adjustment.

Hurwitz and Eadie (1977) used three methods of research in their study of the psychological impact on nursing students of participation in abortion: a series of questionnaires that were administered weekly; reports of dreams written by the student, either at the time of completing the questionnaires or not long afterward; and content analysis of the dream reports. The researchers were able to develop classification systems for dream subjects that included emotional states represented in the classifiable dreams, characters other than the dreamer mentioned in the reports, settings of the dreams, and primary themes of the dreams.

Freihofer and Felton (1976) used the Q method of data collection to study the nursing behaviors that family members or significant others desired most or least in the care of dying patients. Eighty-eight typed cards were given to a sample of 25 relatives or friends, who sorted the statements on the cards into nine piles that indicated most- to least-desired nursing behaviors.

COMPARISON OF THE INTERVIEW AND THE QUESTIONNAIRE: ADVANTAGES AND DISADVANTAGES

In comparison with the interview, the questionnaire is likely to cover a wider geographical area; to reach a larger number of people; to ensure respondents' anonymity, thereby eliciting more frank answers; and to require fewer skills and funds to administer. With careful pretesting, the questionnaire may provide more uniform responses than the interview, especially if it is necessary to have several interviewers, each of whom may affect the measurement situation differently. Questionnaires are especially useful for describing the characteristics of a large population, such as a student body, a hospital, or a community. Using a carefully selected probability sample, the questionnaires offer the possibility of making refined descriptive statements about existing behavior or conditions. No other method of observation can reach as large a population as rapidly with comparable accuracy. Many questions may be asked respondents on a given topic in the natural (and, presumably, less stressful) environment.

Yet, questionnaires (and surveys in general) are subject to serious weaknesses. Questionnaires can collect only self-reports of recalled past action or of prospective hypothetical action. What people do and what they say may differ, especially in cases where recall is selective. People likewise may not understand themselves; that is, they may not be able or willing to express unconscious attitudes and beliefs. Also, the requirement for standardization means that the least common denominator is represented. And response may be low—under 50 percent of the queries. Finally, the researcher cannot deal with context or social life, the "feel" of the situation, as one can in the interview, where observation plays a part.

Interviews may be the only way to reach a large proportion of the American population, especially if a long and complex set of questions is necessary. A mailed questionnaire may be risky, because the respondents may not be able to read or understand the questions. Not only can the skilled interviewer maintain interest, she or he can ask and, if permissible, can explain the questions of a complex schedule. Since the interviewer is also an observer, a much better picture of the respondents is obtained during the interview. Many people are willing to cooperate if all they have to do is talk. In addition, interviews may be granted by persons who would not be reached by questionnaire—the rich and secluded, the executive whose mail is screened by secretaries, or the very poor. Nevertheless, disadvantages of the interview technique are considerable: the method requires the time and money to train interviewers, transportation to move them to the point of the interview, and the ability to interpret the copious notes that may be taken in an unstructured interview.

Bias in the Questionnaire and Interview

Bias, the tendency to obtain data that differ from "true" data, may creep into both questionnaires and interviews. For example, the content of a question may be loaded in one direction; that is, it may be more likely to obtain answers in one direction than another. In addition, timing may introduce a bias; for example, publicity on abortion may affect attitudes reported on questions about abortion.

Bias may also be introduced by interviewers. Systematic differences may exist from one interviewer to another. Training and careful selection of interviewers helps minimize bias, but the interviewer's perception of the subject being interviewed may unwittingly influence responses. Such biasing factors may never be completely overcome, but they may be reduced by the use of highly structured interviews and carefully trained interviewers.

The *halo effect* is a type of bias that may enter into the use of rating scales. Generalized impressions may carry over from one rating to the next, or the rater may attempt to make ratings consistent. Halo effects may be reduced by having different raters rate the subject or process, or by having the same raters do the rating at different times, without being aware that they are rating the same subject or process as before.

SUMMARY

When it is not possible to observe directly, questionnaires and interviews are useful means for collecting data. The questionnaire obtains information from respondents who answer a list of fixed questions with little or no assistance from the researcher, while the interview always involves interaction. The construction of a questionnaire includes writing a covering letter; formulating the questionnaire proper, beginning with instructions to respondents, then the questions and response categories; precoding; and inducements to respond.

Questions are the heart of the data-collecting procedure. Questions must be appropriate; the content must be related to the research proposal; and the wording must be clear, brief, simple, and applicable. Negative characteristics, such as double-barreled questions or leading questions, must be avoided. The ordering of questions must be logical, proceeding from the general to the specific. The response categories must be mutually exclusive and exhaustive, and the instructions must be clearly written. Usually placed at the conclusion of the questionnaire, demographic data should include questions that may be used as a criterion measure. Many inducements to respond are available, the most effective being an appeal to the respondent's altruistic nature. The physical appearance of the questionnaire is also important, as is any factor that helps to motivate the respondent. The number of questionnaire returns considered sufficient has not been agreed upon, but 50 percent may be regarded as adequate.

Various data-collecting techniques use questionnaires in special ways. The Delphi technique uses successive, but different, waves (or rounds) of questionnaires to elicit particular responses from a panel of experts. Questionnaires are also used by persons seeking sociometric data, although the questions presumably could be asked in an interview.

The interview is a method of data collection in which the interviewer asks the respondent questions, either face-to-face or by telephone. The interview may be highly structured, semistructured, or totally unstructured. Highly structured and formal interviews require carefully trained interviewers, who must transmit questions and answers in a neutral manner. The partially structured interview includes the focused interview, which covers specific topics but which also leaves the interviewer free to pursue the data as he or she thinks best. The clinical interview is also partially structured and deals with patients or clients, nursing needs, or nursing diagnoses. It combines observation and questioning. The unstructured interview allows both the interviewer and the respondent to pursue topics freely. The interviewer often attempts to get inside the private world of the respondent to discover influences in the respondent's daily life. Projective techniques, such as the Rorschach test or the Thematic Apperception test, are at times used in conjunction with unstructured interviews.

The telephone interview relies totally upon oral questions and responses, with little other interaction between interviewer and respondent. The major advantage of the telephone interview is speed; also, costs are low and response rates high. Yet the telephone interview may not be representative because of factors such as unlisted telephones or persons without access to telephones.

The critical incident is a technique that gathers data either by interview or by questionnaire. Respondents recall an incident that has occurred in the past 3 months; then they write an account that the researcher analyzes. The large number of incidents necessary—some

2,000—limits this technique to those with enough time and expertise to collect and analyze the data.

Questionnaires and interviews both have their place in the data-collecting process. Generally, questionnaires reach a larger population at a lower cost, while interviews reach those who can neither read nor write and combine both questioning methods and observations. However, disadvantages accrue to each method, including questions of validity and reliability.

Content analysis is a method of data collection and analysis that uses communications as units of analysis. The researcher may count words in a communication process or may use a sampling process to select words, phrases, or chapters of a book to be studied. The researcher uses this method to classify, summarize, and tabulate who the sender was, what the message was, how the message was transmitted, the audience to whom the message was sent, why the message was sent, and the effect of the message upon the receiver. The *Q methodology* uses subjects to sort piles of cards with specific statements into categories that indicate attitude. Subjects place characteristics on a continuum, with various categories representing from greatest approval (first category) to disapproval (last category). The number of cards to be sorted ranges from over 50 to 100. Q sorts are especially helpful for studying attitudes objectively.

Bias in questionnaires and interviews may arise from the way in which a question is asked, the time when a question is asked, or by a systematic difference in interviewers. Bias may also be introduced by the respondent. The halo effect arises when raters carry over the rating from one item to the next. Halo effects may be reduced by having different raters rate the same subject, or by having the same raters do the rating at different times.

EXAMPLE FROM NURSING RESEARCH

The Questionnaire

Mary Jordan-Marsh (1985): Development of a tool for diagnosing changes in concern about exercise: A means of enhancing compliance. Nursing Research, 34, 103–107.

The author utilized a questionnaire comprised of two parts: The Stages of Concern for Exercise (SOCE) scale, which she adapted from an education tool in order to examine exercise behavior; and self-reports of minutes of exercise, history of exercise, enrollment in an exercise program, and ratings of expertise at exercise. The author handed out questionnaires to employees of a Southern California industry during a blood-pressure-screening program. The subjects were asked to fill out the questionnaire as they waited in line to have their blood pressure taken. The subjects were told that: (1) they did not have to fill out the questionnaire; (2) their names would not be included in the finished report; and (3) the questionnaires would not be available to the employer or health-care staff. Consent to participate was implied by the author when the subject filled out the questionnaire. The subjects returned either a blank or a completed questionnaire to a box for that purpose. Of the 232 questionnaires returned, 214 were completed.

The entire questionnaire consisted of a cover letter and one page asking for demographic information and details about the subject's exercise habits and sense of expertise in exercising. The last two pages consisted of the three-item original SOC, which was revised to the SOCE, which focused on changing exercise habits. The new format included minor wording changes to specify exercise as the behavior change of interest, or to change abstract terms to those more directly related to exercise. The finished product was a three-item, Likert-scale questionnaire with eight response categories ranging from 0 ("irrelevant") to 7 ("extremely true of me now"). The author notes that the large number of response categories was retained from the original scale.

Interpretation of the findings in the original SOC emphasized the importance of construing the interpretations as hypotheses to be confirmed with the client. The author suggests that interested persons refer to Hall's 1979 manual for the use of the SOC questionnaire. The simplest approach to interpretation was to focus on the highest stage score. High score peaks could serve as hallmarks for clinical intervention. The peaks indicate the client's area of greatest concern or interest, while stages with low scores indicate minimal or absent concern. The stage "Indifference" had to be interpreted in conjunction with other information.

STUDY QUESTIONS

1. You wish to study teenage obesity. Construct a ten-question questionnaire to examine what the teenager eats between meals. Include instructions to respondents, questions, response categories, and demographic data that you wish to collect. How would you encourage the teenager to respond?
2. Examine the following questions, and identify what (if anything) is wrong:

   - Do you prefer to lose weight by diet, or would you rather use medication?
   - Have you ever thought of killing yourself?
   - How often do you have intercourse in one week?
   - Don't you think it is not right for a nurse to wear street clothes on the job?

3. Construct a five-question questionnaire, using a Likert-type scale, to obtain information on the attitudes of student nurses toward dying patients.
4. Construct a five-question interview schedule for a telephone interview to examine knowledge of sickle-cell anemia.

5. You would like to study how children perceive nurses and doctors. Write a brief sentence-completion test that would collect such data.
6. Select a page from your nursing or research text. Use content analysis to identify words on the page associated with health care. What message is the writer attempting to transmit?

REFERENCES AND SUGGESTED READINGS

Aamodt, A. (1972): The child's view of health and healing. In Batey, M. (ed.), Communicating Nursing Research (Vol. 5). Boulder: WICHE, pp. 38–54. *Draw a picture and tell a story about it. Projective techniques to get at the meaning of health and sickness cross-culturally.*

Babbie, E. (1975): The Practice of Social Research. Belmont, Calif.: Wadsworth. *Chapter 5, "Questionnaire Construction," and Chapter 11, "Surveys."*

Beard, M. and Scott, P. (1975): The efficacy of group therapy by nurses for hospitalized patients. Nursing Research, *24*, 120–124. *Sociometric techniques.*

Brown, J., Tanner, C., and Padrick, K. (1984): Nursing's search for scientific knowledge. Nursing Research, *33*, 26–32. *Reports structure of research articles published in four major journals.*

Christensen, M., et al. (1979): Professional development of nurse practitioners. Nursing Research, *28*, 51–56. *Version of the Thematic Apperception Test used to assess needs for achievement, affiliation, and power.*

Davis, A. and Underwood, P. (1976): Role, function, and decision making in community mental health. Nursing Research, *25*, 256–259. *Semistructured focused interview.*

Downs, F. (1964): Maternal stress in primigravidas as a factor in the production of neonatal pathology. Nursing Science, *2*, 348–367. *Semistructured interview.*

DuBois, C. (1944): The People of Alor. Minneapolis: University of Minnesota Press. *An anthropologist cooperates with a psychiatrist. Projective testing.*

Flaskerud, J. (1979): Use of vignettes to elicit responses toward broad concepts. Nursing Research, *29*, 210–212.

Fox, D. (1976): Fundamentals of Research in Nursing (3rd ed.). New York: Appleton-Century-Crofts, Chap. 10.

Freihofer, P. and Felton, G. (1976): Nursing behaviors in bereavement. Nursing Research, *25*, 332–337. *Use of the Q-sort.*

Habenstein, R. (ed.) (1970): Pathways to Data. Chicago: Aldine. *Thirteen articles by various scholars report methods of data collecting.*

Holsti, O. (1969): Content Analysis for the Social Sciences and Humanities. Reading, Mass.: Addison-Wesley. *Content analysis.*

Hurwitz, A. and Eadie, R. (1977): Psychologic impact on nursing students of participation in abortion. Nursing Research, *26*, 112–120. *Content analysis of dreams; questionnaire.*

Jordan-Marsh, M. (1985): Development of a tool for diagnosing changes in concern about exercise: A means of enhancing compliance. Nursing Research, *34*, 103–107.

LaFleur, J. and Novotny, M. (1981): Study of human figure drawing by amputee children and verbalization of their general adjustment. In Krampitz, S. and Pavlovich, N. (eds.), Readings for Nursing Research. St. Louis: C. V. Mosby.

Lin, N. (1976): Foundations of Social Research. New York: McGraw-Hill. *Chapter 13: questionnaire and survey.*

Lindeman, C. (1975): Delphi survey of priorities in clinical nursing research. Nursing Research, *24*, 434–441. *Special type of survey.*

Moore, Nunnally, D., Aguiar, M. (1974): Patients' evaluation of their prenatal and delivery care. Nursing Research, *27*, *Questionnaire development.*

Parten, M. (1950): Surveys, Polls and Samples. New York: Harper & Row. *Surveys.*

Porter, C. (1974): Grade school children's perception of their internal body parts. Nursing Research, *23*, 384–391. *Projective techniques.*

Rose, M. (1972): The effects of hospitalization on the coping behaviors of children. In Batey, M. (ed.)., Communicating Nursing Research (Vol. 5). Boulder: WICHE. *Naturalistic observations at home; interviews.*

Schmitt, F. and Wooldridge, P. (1981): Psychological preparation of surgical patients. In Fox, D. and Leeser, I. (eds.), Readings on the Research Process in Nursing. New York: Appleton-Century-Crofts, pp. 126–137. *Questionnaires.*

Taylor, A., Skelton, J., and Butcher, J. (1984): Duration of pain condition and physical pathology as determinants of nurses' assessments of patients in pain. Nursing Research, *33*, 4 ff.

Valadez, A. and Anderson, E. (1972): Rehabilitation workshops: Change in attitude of nurses. Nursing Research, *21*, 132–137. *Projective techniques: captioned line-drawn pictures.*

Walizer, M. and Wiener, P. (1978): Research Methods and Analysis. New York: Harper & Row. *Chap. 10 describes question constructions, responses, questionnaires, interviews.*

White, C. and Maguire, M. (1973): Job satisfaction and dissatisfaction among hospital nursing supervisors. Nursing Research, *22*, 25–31. *Pilot study; interviews, thought-unit category analysis.*

Williams, M. (1972): A comparative study of postsurgical convalescence among women of two ethnic groups: Anglo and Mexican-American. In Batey, M. (ed.), Communicating Nursing Research (Vol. 5). Boulder: WICHE, pp. 58–73. *Interviews of 50 minutes each with 64 persons, using interpreter in two cases.*

17

Measurements and Scales:
Methods of Data Collection

All research aspires to produce accurate answers to scientific questions. However, accuracy must be demonstrated objectively. Therefore, to prove the accuracy of research, the scientist must specify how observations were made and measured, and which scales and instruments were used. Measurement is not only a unique process in itself; it is also interwoven with the processes of observation and questioning. The researcher must observe and question in order to measure. This chapter examines the measurement and the various scales used to measure. (The next chapters examine the validity and reliability of measurements and instruments.)

Upon completion of this chapter, the student should be able to: (1) define measurement; (2) discuss the relationship between measurement and reality; (3) name and define three ways of measuring; (4) identify levels of measurements and scales at different levels of measurement; (5) describe how to create an ordinal scale, such as the Likert scale, the graphic rating scale, the Guttman scale, and the semantic differential scale; (6) describe and give examples of the interval scale; (7) define and give examples of the ratio measurement and scale; and (8) discuss bias in measurement and other factors that may cause measurements to vary.

MEASUREMENT

Measurement is the assignment of numerals to objects or events according to rules (Stevens, 1959, p. 25). Measurements determine relationships, such as quantities, degrees, or extent of observations. Measurement assumes counting, comparing, or ranking. The symbols of the observations (such as numbers) can be summarized and represented economically in tables, graphs, and diagrams. Measurement is a central process in scientific research. Without measurement, observations cannot be summarized, and hypotheses cannot be tested. Thus, measurement is crucial to theory. Without measurement, theory would remain mere speculation.

Measurement and Levels of Reality

Measurement begins with the identification and definition of the concept or variable to be studied. The researcher attempts to link the abstract concept or variable to the "real" world. This is accomplished by using an operational definition to define the concept or variable in order to make it observable and measurable. Levels of reality involving human subjects include behavioral reality and verbal reality (Fox, 1982, p. 238). *Behavioral reality* is the subject's actual behavior in real-life situations, measured by observing, using instruments that aid observation, recording, counting, comparing, or ranking what was observed. *Verbal reality* is the subject's written or spoken responses to the researcher's verbal approximation of real-life situations. Creating instruments that bring together the reality of behavior and the reality of verbal responses is a difficult task for all researchers.

Researchers who measure physical attributes and observe behavior use instruments that correspond more closely to reality than do researchers who use instruments to measure attitudes, beliefs, and feelings. For example, measuring weight to study the effects of an experimental weight-loss diet, or making a documentary movie of a fearful child having a cast removed is closer to a type of reality than is measuring attitudes toward dieting, beliefs about nutrition, and feelings of fear. However, most measures are fallible. A "true score" is more a goal to be sought than a reality.

Nevertheless, measurement has a number of advantages that are essential to the researcher. For example, measurements communicate objective, precise, quantitative information with parsimony. Stating that a group of patients on a diet measures an average of five feet, five inches in height and an average of 200 pounds in weight conveys considerable information about reality in a few terms. In addition, an attitude test that uses an instrument revealing that the same group had experienced a loss of some kind in the past year and seeks comfort in food imparts succinct information about another kind of reality. Such measurements take away guesses and subjective evaluations and allow objective, precise, and independent verification by other researchers who use the same tools and who study the same, or an identical, group of patients.

Measurements in Nursing Research: 1952–1980

Brown et al. (1984) report that, in the 1950s, researchers tended to create their own instruments rather than use previously developed tests and measures. However, since the 1970s, about equal numbers of researchers have created their own tools or have used previously published tools. In fact, some researchers regard the use of instruments borrowed from other disciplines as a mixed blessing, since the reliability and validity of these instruments may not have relevance when used with nursing concepts.

Methods of Measuring

Methods and ways of measuring include counting, comparing, and ranking. _Counting_ is the oldest way of measuring. Fingers and toes were counted; knots placed on a length of string were counted; and rocks were used to stand for individuals or events, and were counted. The symbols, even the fingers and toes, could be manipulated more easily than the observations themselves. Such direct enumeration is measurement at the simplest level.

Comparison requires either a standard unit of measure with which to make a comparison or the units that have been measured with the same instrument, such as a test with which comparisons can be made. For example, official standards for comparing length and weight are preserved in national capitals, and standard tests exist (such as nursing state board examinations, which measure the level of knowledge of individual nurses who seek to obtain a nursing license). Comparative units or groups are those whose attributes or performances can be compared with those of a similar group. In addition, comparisons may be made through time. For example, comparison may be made of the measurements of similar units at one point in time (cross-sectional measurement studies), or comparisons may be made of the measurements of the same group at several points in time (longitudinal measurement studies). Experiments are structured to compare measurements at two points in time—before and after the independent variable is introduced into the experimental group.

Ranking involves measuring observations and then arranging the measurements in a series such as more or less, longer or shorter, larger or smaller, higher or lower, heavier or lighter. Quantitative scales measure variables with equal intervals (such as height, weight, length, time, and temperature) in these terms. Qualitative scales measure and rank qualities of an attribute (such as nursing care) in terms of poor, fair, good, better, or best.

Measurement Instruments

Measurement instruments, such as yardsticks, carpenter's rulers, thermometers, and scales to measure weight and height, are familiar to every researcher. All are quantitative measures that have rules to govern the measurement, and equal intervals that are marked on the measuring instrument. The relationship of these tools to reality is evident, and the amount of information that the measure affords is considerable. On the other hand, scales to measure coping, pain, and bereavement are not familiar to every researcher, nor does every scientist agree with the rules for measurement. For example, a number of instruments exist that measure the same concept (such as anxiety), including behavioral, cognitive, and physiological measures, yet none of these measures correlate highly with one another, according to Borkovec et al. (1976). On the other hand, a concept such as "burnout" is relatively new, with few measures, competing or otherwise, in existence.

LEVELS OF MEASUREMENT AND SCALES

A number of scholars identify four levels of measurement: nominal, ordinal, interval, and ratio. Others, like Fox (1982, p. 240), believe that only three levels should be considered as measurement: ordinal, interval, and ratio. In keeping with this view, he classifies variables into two categories: the discrete and the continuous. *Discrete variables* are those for which classification or measurement is possible only in whole units. For example, a group of persons having surgery on one day cannot be fractions of persons but are whole persons who can be classified into separate, mutually exclusive categories by operation (such as abdominal surgery, brain surgery, or bone surgery) or measured quantitatively to calculate average age, height, weight, or length of time in surgery. The researcher can both measure quantitative discrete variables and classify the qualitative discrete variable. In contrast, *continuous variables* are those in which measurement is possible in both whole and fractional units: 3½ hours; 5 feet, 11½ inches tall; and 160 ½ pounds in weight. Continuous variables can always be conceptualized as progressing from the smallest possible amount to the largest possible amount. However, continuous variables can only be measured, not classified into mutually exclusive categories, since "continuous" cannot produce mutually exclusive categories, only continuous fractional measurements.

With this reservation in mind, the levels of measurement common in the literature include the nominal level along with the ordinal, interval, and ratio. The ratio level is the strongest level of measurement, and the nominal (or ordinal, if only three levels are used) is the weakest level of measurement. Each of these levels has an associated type of scale: the nominal scale, the ordinal scale, the interval scale, and the ratio scale. A *scale* is a device for measuring the magnitude or quantity of a variable. The scale may be a series of steps or degrees, a scheme of graded amounts from highest to lowest, or an indicator of relative size. Levels of measurement, and the scales that accompany these, will be examined in turn.

Nominal Measurement and Scale

The *nominal scale* consists of a number of discrete, mutually exclusive, and exhaustively named categories. Numbers can be assigned to each category, but only for classification purposes. That is, Category 1 could stand for females and Category 2 for males, but this has nothing to do with quantification. There are not "quantities of being female" or "quantities of being male." The numbers are only for the identification of the category in case the data are to be entered into a computer. Qualitative attributes, such as sex (male or female), marital status (married or not married), pregnant (yes or no), and blood type (O or not O), refer to the names of attributes that are the same or that are different. There is no continuum between the two categories. No one is a little pregnant, or a little female, or a little married. The data derived from a nominal scale can only be counted to determine frequency: how many men, how many women, how many pregnant, and so on.

Examples of the use of nominal scales in research include that of Dixon (1984), who used a nominal scale on an evaluation form mailed to cancer patients at home. She wanted the respondents to record their perceptions of the helpfulness of the nursing interventions that she had used in a research project. Subjects were asked to check the scale indicating whether the intervention was "helpful" or "not helpful." An additional question was asked: "How do you feel about being involved in a research project?" Possible responses were "positive," "neutral," or "negative." Rottkamp (1976) used a nominal scale to categorize body position as "supine," or "prone," or "right-side lying," or "sitting," all mutually exclusive categories.

Nominal scales may be developed before data are collected to be included in questionnaires, interview schedules, or observation guides. After data collection, nominal scales may be developed to sort observations into categories that represent differences in the kinds of observation. For example, responses to questions may classify respondents as "assertive," "aggressive," or "submissive." The researcher then analyzes the data by counting or tallying frequencies—the number of observations that fall into various categories. Once the tallying is complete, statistical procedures that apply to frequency counts can be used. These include the mode, percentages, proportions, pi correlation coefficient, contingency coefficient, sign test, A and t tests for proportions, and the chi-square test, a statistical test to assess whether or not a relationship exists between two nominal-level variables.

The Ordinal Measurement and Scales

Ordinal scales permit an ordering of observations according to magnitude. Ordinal scales include information provided by nominal scales (distinctions in kind), as well as information on the ranking of individual observations in the total set of observations. Ordinal scales provide information on the relative positions of observations and on a measured dimension, but they do not include information on the distance between observations. Observations (such as the cheerfulness of nurses) may be divided into equal-appearing intervals, such as "cheerful," "more cheerful," and "most cheerful." But the intervals are not equal in the same way that the intervals of a thermometer or yardstick are equal. In order to be observed and measured, each of the ranks must be operationally defined, but the distance between the units cannot be calculated as equal. Nevertheless, there is a continuity between categories of cheerfulness as measured by the ordinal scale, whereas there is no continuity between categories of the nominal scale.

The grading or ranking of the ordinal scale may be according to some underlying continuum of intensity (most to least), distance (nearest to farthest), or preference (love to hate). The ordinal scale is capable of rank-ordering subjects or objects on a particular characteristic, although it cannot distinguish the exact degree to which one differs from the others. Ordinal scales commonly have only three to five categories, since it is difficult to make fine distinctions beyond this point. Applicable statistical procedures include all of those for the nominal scale. In addition, simple ranks, percentile ranks, median, interquartile range, rank-order correlation, median test, Mann-Whitney U test, and Druskal-Wallis K test may be used.

EXAMPLES FROM NURSING RESEARCH

Ordinal Scales

A number of ordinal scales used to measure attitudes or behavior are found in the nursing research literature, including (1) the Likert scale; (2) the graphic rating scale; (3) the Guttman scale; and (4) the sematic differential scale. Each of these will be examined.

1. *The Likert Scale* is one of the most commonly used scales in nursing research. The researcher creates a Likert scale by formulating a number of statements that are clearly favorable or clearly unfavorable to the attitude being studied. Respondents are asked to read the statements and then to select one of four or five (or more) categories, such as Strongly Agree, Agree, No Opinion, Disagree, and Strongly Disagree, that most clearly expresses their view.

    Cox (1985) reports a study of the Health Self-Determinism Index, a psychometric evaluation of a new measure of motivation in health behavior. The Index is comprised of 20 Likert format items divided evenly over the following four subscales: self-determined health judgments, self-determined health behavior, perceived sense of competence in health matters, and responsiveness in internal–external cues. The subscales correspond to the characteristics of an "intrinsically motivated person" who uses self-determinism in judgment and behavior and who has feelings of competence and responsiveness to internal cues. Half of the 20 items are worded in such a way that a "strongly agree" response indicates a strong sense of self-determinism and competence regarding health behavior. The other half are worded so that a "strongly agree" response indicates little or no self-determinism in health judgments and behavior, a lowered feeling of competence about health, and a greater response by the individual to external cues. Each item is scored on a scale of 1 to 5. A score of 5 indicates a maximum intrinsic response, while a score of 1 indicates the maximum extrinsic response.

Hubbard et al. (1984) report an investigation of the relationship between social support and self-care practices, using two instruments. The first instrument (Personal Resources Questionnaire) is structured to elicit responses to five dimensions of social support: intimacy, social integration, nurturance, worth, and assistance. Twenty-five statements were formulated to which the subjects responded on a seven-point Likert scale from "strongly agree" to "strongly disagree." The second instrument, the Lifestyle Questionnaire, contains 24 statements relating to six health-practice categories (nutrition, exercise, relaxation, safety, substance use, and prevention practices). Items are scored on a four-point Likert scale, with responses ranging from "regularly" to "never." Higher scores indicate more positive health practices.

2. *The graphic rating scale* is an evaluation scale in which the researcher develops a bipolar continuum, such as from "highest" to "lowest" or "most" to "least," and the respondent ranks the variables by placing a check at the appropriate point. The scale is a simple one to use and shows the relationship of one category to others. The disadvantage of the scale is that the respondent tends to avoid marking either extreme, causing a pile-up of scores in the central categories (Fig. 17–1).

McGuire (1984), reporting a study of the measurement of clinical pain, identified and classified available instruments, including the Verbal Descriptor Scale and the Visual Analogue Scale. The Verbal Descriptor Scale uses word descriptors for pain including: "None," "Slight," "Moderate," "Severe," and "Agonizing." The researcher asks the patient to select the single word on a checklist that most accurately reflects the patient's sensation. The scale is short and is easy for the patient to complete and for the nurse to score and analyze, but it may force the choice of a word that does not accurately reflect the patient's true sensation. For example, the patient may have more than moderate, but less than severe, pain. The Visual Analogue Scale uses a straight line that represents a continuum of pain intensity. On one end of the line is written "No pain" and on the other end

☐	☐	☐	☐	☐
Highest quality care	Very good care	Average care	Below average care	Very poor care

Figure 17–1. Nursing care assessment by a graphic rating scale.

"Pain as bad as it could possibly be." The length of the line is often about 10 cm. It may sometimes have word descriptors beneath the line, like a graphic rating scale. It tends to avoid the artificial categories of the Verbal Descriptor Scale and may produce more sensitive measurements, since respondents mark at any point on the continuum.

3. *The Guttman scale* measures attitudes by using a set of cumulative statements with which respondents are asked to agree or disagree. The researcher formulates a small number of statements (four or five) that comprise a homogeneous set with regard to one concept, such as "health care." The researcher constructs the scale so that the respondent who agrees with one item, such as Item #3, will also agree with all previous items; i.e., with Items #2 and #1, although not necessarily with Item #4. The statements increase in intensity with regard to the respondent's attitude toward health care. For example, Item 1 could state: "Health care should be available to all citizens"; Item #2: "Rich and poor will benefit from greater availability of health care"; Item #3: "Free health care for all would be in the interest of the country as a whole"; and Item #4: "Congress should make free health care available to all who need it."

The Guttman technique does not provide guidelines by which to determine how to form a cumulative scale, nor does the scale permit fine discriminations to be made. For these (and other) reasons, it is not found as often in the nursing research literature.

4. *Semantic-differential scale* is defined as a method for measuring the meaning of concepts, but has also proven effective for measuring the emotional-evaluative component of attitudes. The researcher asks the respondent to rate a concept on a series of seven-point bipolar rating scales. For example, the subject will be asked to check at the point that best represents what the concept "motherhood" means to the subject:

Motherhood is:

Bad	Good
Passive	Active
Weak	Strong
Irresponsible	Responsible

The semantic differential provides a wide variety of fixed-alternative formats from which to choose. It is easy to score and is versatile. It allows the ratings of two or more different concepts and groups of respondents to be compared. The disadvantage of the measure is that it, too, restricts the subject's response options.

The Interval Measurement and Scale

The *interval scale* measures the distance between points on a quantitative measuring instrument. The intervals can be added and subtracted, and the summaries can be subjected to all statistical tests appropriate with the type of sampling used. The interval scale does not have an absolute zero point. For example, Centigrade thermometers use an interval scale with an arbitrary zero point; the point at which water freezes. To deal with lower temperatures, the scale must go below zero.

Cassidy (1976) utilized a thermometer to study the relationship between daily life changes, physical symptoms, and the changes in the body temperature related to adjustment to life events. The thermometer used was the B-D Oral Basal Temperature Thermometer. This is a mercury glass thermometer with an extended scale of 96 to 100°F, which allows a much wider span between each tenth of a degree, making it easier to read and record slight temperature variations. During the study period, each subject was required to take and record measurements of oral temperature every 2 hours while awake. The data did not reveal that temperature ranges were greater on "days of greater-than-average life adjustment" or less on "days of average or less-than-average life adjustment."

The Ratio Measurement and Scales

The *ratio scale* is the highest level of measurement among the scales. In addition to having equal intervals quantitatively measured, the ratio scale has an absolute zero point. Examples include time, length, weight, and the Kelvin temperature scale. Many physical measures use scales at the ratio level, but few attitude or perception scales do. Winslow et al. (1985) used several ratio scales to study oxygen uptake and cardiovascular responses during bathing in both a control group of adults and in adults with acute myocardial infarction. Oxygen consumption was measured by a chain-compensated gasometer and was analyzed by a mass spectrometer from expired air collected via a Daniels one-way respiratory valve and 64-inch plastic tubing into a Doublas bag. A continuous electrocardiogram was recorded by a Holter monitor during both rest and bathing. Indirect blood pressure was measured by cuff sphygmomanometer during rest and immediately before and after each bath. The subject rated perceived exertion after each bath and completed a questionnaire after all three baths in which ease, enjoyment, and feeling of cleanliness were ranked. Data analysis included a three-way analysis of variance (ANOVA) and others. All statistical procedures used with this particular kind of sampling are appropriate for use with the interval scale data.

Bias in Measurement and Other Errors

A major factor that influences measurement is constant error, or *biasing*, that systematically affects the characteristic being measured. Bias may be caused by social desirability influence or by the acquiescent response set (Selltiz, 1976, p. 153). The *social desirability influence* is the tendency of respondents to give a favorable picture of themselves—to agree or disagree with a question to the extent that they think responses are

TABLE 17–1. SUMMARY OF MEASUREMENT SCALES

Scales and Statistics to Measure	Basic Definition	Examples
Nominal The mode, percentages, chi-square proportions, pi correlation coefficient	A noninterval scale that indicates "same" or "different" to permit the naming of the person, place, thing	Male–female category Blood-type category Diagnosis Questionnaire data
Ordinal chi-square median percentile, interquartile range, rank-order correlation, Mann-Whitney U test	A scale of "equal-appearing intervals"; however, size of intervals is not known; measures more or less	Course grades of A, B, C, D Status of patient, such as critical, serious, satisfactory Graphic rating scales Thurstone-type scales Likert-type scales and numerous others
Interval All statistical tests	A scale of equal intervals, with an arbitrary zero point	Temperature measured by Centigrade or Fahrenheit scale
Ratio All statistical tests	A scale of equal intervals, with an absolute zero point	Kelvin temperature scale; time; length; weight; certain types of test scores

socially desirable rather than to respond according to how they truly feel. The *acquiescent response set* is the tendency of respondents to agree or disagree with statements regardless of their content, especially when presented with a series of statements.

In addition to systematic or biasing errors of measurement, other factors may cause measurements to vary from one act of measurement to the next. These include the following: (1) transient personal factors (such as fatigue, health, attention); (2) a situational factor (someone is listening to the interview); (3) variations in administering the measure (bored researchers, tired observers); (4) differences in sampling of the items (questions or observations include only a few items from the total number possible); (5) lack of clarity of the measuring instrument (instrument may be too complex or instructions may be ambiguous); (6) mechanical failures (pencils break in answering questionnaires or machines break down); and (7) errors in processing and analysis (coding errors or errors in arithmetic).

SUMMARY

Measurement is a procedure whereby rules assign symbols and numerals to objects or events in order to determine relationships, such as quantities, degrees, or extent of observation. Ways of measuring include counting frequencies, comparing measurements against a known standard, and ranking observations (as larger or smaller, or better or worse) using quantitative or qualitative scales.

A scale is a device for measuring the magnitude or quantity of a variable. Four types of scales commonly used as levels of measurement include the nominal, the ordinal, the interval, and the ratio. The nominal scale, the lowest level of measurement, consists of a number of discrete, mutually exclusive, and exhaustively named, categories. The data derived from a nominal scale can only be counted to determine frequency. The ordinal scale is a qualitative scale comprised of equal-appearing intervals. Ordinal numbers indicate rank order only, not that the intervals between the ranks are equal. Some ordinal scales are the graphic rating scale, the differential scale, and the summated scale. The graphic scale is a simple scale in which the researcher develops a continuum from highest to lowest and the respondent ranks the variables by placing a check at the appropriate point. The Likert scale is a summated scale in which the respondents indicate their agreement or disagreement with statements. The graphic rating scale is an evaluation scale in which the researcher develops a bipolar continuum and the respondent ranks the variables by placing a check at the appropriate point. The Guttman scale measures attitudes by using a set of cumulative statements with which respondents are asked to agree or disagree, while the semantic-differential scale is a method for measuring the meaning of concepts and is used as well for measuring the emotional or evaluative component of attitudes, using a series of seven-point, bipolar rating scales. The interval scale measures the distance between equal intervals on a quantitative measuring instrument. However, the instrument does not have an absolute zero point. The ratio scale, the highest level of measurement, has both an absolute zero point and equal intervals. To be useful, all scales must be valid and reliable.

EXAMPLE FROM NURSING RESEARCH

Deborah McGuire (1984): The measurement of clinical pain. Nursing Research, 33, 152–156.

The author begins by identifying three problems experienced when measuring clinical pain: (1) the subjective nature of pain; (2) the limited number of reliable and valid instruments available to measure pain; and (3) issues such as type of pain, cause, and patient sample characteristics.

The subjective nature of the pain experience is the major problem. Subjective measures are considered unsatisfactory, because they cannot be readily verified, yet many researchers point out that only the individual who is experiencing the pain can accurately define the sensation.

Lack of qualifiable measures is the second major problem. Scales that have been used include Likert-type scales designed to measure the subjective experience of pain. McGuire considers this scale capable of providing quantifiable data, although some researchers question this. However, McGuire points out that even this scale does not measure the full experience of pain.

Lack of reliable instruments is the third difficulty. To ascertain that an instrument is capable of producing reliable data, McGuire writes, the instrument must be tested on individuals in different groups, settings, and times, and these responses must be similar. Another difficulty arises from the fact that published reports on the reliability of a particular instrument are not always available, although such data are critical, since reliability is necessary to determine whether an instrument is valid.

Validity is a particular problem in the measurement of pain. A clear operational definition is necessary in order to know what is being measured; otherwise, construct validity is not assured. In addition, due to the subjectivity of the experience, it is difficult to determine whether the construct pain or some other entity (such as anxiety) is being measured.

After noting the problems of measurement, McGuire gives a classification scheme for instruments to measure clinical pain, including the following: (1) scales such as verbal descriptor scales and visual analogue scales, both of which measure the intensity of pain; (2) physiological and behavioral measures, such as rating scales for pain (Hanken and McDowell, 1964) and pain-rating scales such as that of Chambers and Price (1967), which measures intensity, anxiety, attention paid to pain, and physiological parameters of pain; (3) multidimensional measures, including the two-component scale (Johnson, 1972, 1973), which measures physical intensity and emotional distress; (4) the McGill Pain Questionnaire (Melzack, 1975), which measures location, sensation, affective aspects, evaluation, intensity, and pattern of pain; and (5) the Card-Sort Method (Reading and Newton, 1978), which measures sensation, affective aspects, evaluation, and intensity. Of these, only the McGill Pain Questionnaire is reported to have both good reliability and good validity. The Verbal Descriptor Scale and the Visual Analog Scale have good reliability but only probable validity. All of the scales are easy to understand except the McGill Pain Questionnaire and the Card-Sort Method, which are described as being moderately easy to difficult to understand, with the McGill Questionnaire being easy to very difficult.

The nurse who selects a measuring instrument to measure pain must consider: (1) various definitions of pain; (2) the goals of the measurement problem; (3) the type of pain being measured; (4) characteristics of the sample; (5) ease of administration and scoring; and (5) the reliability and validity of the data. McGuire concludes that the advantages and disadvantages of any tool must be weighed, and that researchers and clinicians must steadily accumulate knowledge to assist in the difficult task of measuring clinical pain.

STUDY QUESTIONS _____

1. Define "measurement." Give examples of measurements that you have used in nursing, including counting, comparing, and ranking.
2. Name a nominal scale used in nursing practice or research.
3. Develop a Likert-type scale of ten questions to measure an attitude important in nursing care.
4. Identify ratio scales used in nursing when a patient is first admitted to the hospital.
5. What do "reality" and "measurement" have to do with each other?
6. Compare discrete and continuous variables. What do these types have to do with measurement?
7. Why don't some scholars (such as Fox) consider the nominal level to be measurement?
8. Compare the nominal and ordinal scales. What is the difference, and how are they similar in terms of measurement?
9. What is the semantic-differential scale? What are its advantages?
10. Contrast the interval and ratio scales.
11. What is bias in measurement?

REFERENCES AND SUGGESTED READING

Borkovec, T., et al. (1976): Assessment of anxiety. In Ciminero, A., Calhoun, K., Adams, H. (eds.), Handbook of Behavioral Assessment. New York: Wiley.

Brown, J., et al. (1984): Nursing's search for scientific knowledge. Nursing Research, *33*, 26–32.

Campbell, D. and Stanley, J. (1963): Experimental and Quasi-Experimental Designs for Research. Chicago: Rand McNally. *Includes factors jeopardizing internal and external validity.*

Cassidy, C. (1976): The relationship between daily life changes, physical symptoms and body temperature range: Temperature changes related to adjustments to life events. Image, *8*, 30–35.

Cox, C. (1985): The health self-determination index. Nursing Research, *34*, 177–183. *Likert scale used.*

Dixon, J. (1984): Effect of nursing interventions on nutritional and performance status in cancer patients. Nursing Research, *33*, 330–333. *Includes construct validity, discriminant and convergent validity.*

Fox, D. (1982): Fundamentals of Research in Nursing (4th ed.). Norwalk, Conn.: Appleton-Century-Crofts. *Chapter 17 includes reliability, validity, sensitivity, appropriateness, and objectivity of research instruments.*

Hubbard, P., et al. (1984): The relationship between social support and self-care practices. Nursing Research, *33*, 266–270.

Lin, N. (1976): Foundations of Social Research. New York: McGraw-Hill. *Chapter 10 includes validity, reliability.*

McGuire, D. (1984): The measurement of clinical pain. Nursing Research *33*, 152–156.

Nakagawa, H. (1972): An epidemiological study of psychiatric symptom pattern change. In Batey, M. (ed.). Communicating Nursing Research. Boulder: WICHE. *Measures of intercoder agreement.*

O'Neil, S. (1972): The application and methodological implications of behavior modification in nursing research. In Batey, M. (ed.), Communicating Nursing Research. Boulder: WICHE, pp. 179–191.

Rodgers, J. (1977): Relationship between sociability and personal space preference at two different times of day. In Downs, F. and Newman, M. (eds.), A Source Book of Nursing Research. Philadelphia: F. A. Davis.

Rottkamp, F. (1976): A behavior modification approach to nursing therapeutics in body positioning of spinal cord injured patients. Nursing Research, *2*, 181–185.

Selltiz, C., et al. (1976): Research Methods in Social Relations. New York: Holt, Rinehart, & Winston. *Chapter 5 discusses general problems of measurement.*

Simon, J. (1978): Basic Research Methods in Social Science (2nd ed.). New York: Random House. *Chapter 15 examines measuring.*

Stevens, S. (1959): Measurement, psychophysics, and utility. In Churchman, C. and Ratoosh, P. (eds.), Measurement: Definitions and Theories. New York: Wiley, pp. 18–63. *Defines measurement.*

Walizer, M. and Wienir, P. (1978): Research Methods and Analysis. New York: Harper & Row.

Winslow, E., Lane, L., and Gaffney, F. (1985): Oxygen uptake and cardiovascular responses in control adults and acute myocardial infarction patients during bathing. Nursing Research, *34*, 164–169.

18

Validity and Reliability of Measurements and Instruments

To be useful, all measures and scales must be valid and reliable. Both validity and reliability judge how good the various components and processes of research are. However, they differ, in that _validity_ refers to the extent to which various research elements measure what each purports to measure. Measurements, scales, instruments, and definitions must be valid in order to be good. _Reliability_ refers to the consistency, stability, accuracy, and dependability with which the scale or instrument measures. An instrument that is consistently reliable and dependable may not be valid unless it is also accurate. For example, a merchant's scale may weigh a steel ball exactly the same each time it is weighed, but the scale may be weighing ten pounds short each time. It is not accurate, so it is not valid. However, if the scale is accurate, reliable, dependable, and consistent, it is also valid. Validity and reliability are essential concepts in research.

Upon completion of this chapter, the student should be able to: (1) define validity; (2) define and compare content validity, face validity, predictive validity, concurrent validity, and construct validity; (3) define reliability; (4) define and discuss how to determine the stability of a measuring instrument; (5) define consistency (or internal homogeneity) and discuss how to determine consistency; (6) define equivalence and discuss how to determine inter-rater or interobserver reliability; (7) identify two tests that help the researcher to determine reliability; and (8) identify several additional criteria important in evaluating a measure or instrument.

VALIDITY

Validity is a judgment of the extent to which a component of research reflects the theory, concept, or variable that the researcher intends. A valid instrument measures what it purports to measure. Some methods of judging validity include: (1) content validity, (2) face validity, (3) predictive validity, (4) concurrent validity, and (5) construct validity. Each of these will be examined in turn.

1. Content validity *is concerned with the study's sampling adequacy.* It intends to judge whether all possible observations were sampled for use in a research study, whether by questionnaire, interview schedule, or checklist. It requires an examination of all possible questions, observations, or tests that potentially could have been used to measure the characteristics under study. This is seldom possible; nevertheless, the researcher can give careful consideration to exactly what is to be measured and how. Questions on a questionnaire should be as representative of as many appropriate questions as possible. Checklists should properly sample the items to be observed, and systems of classification should be exhaustive. It is helpful to have a panel of judges who are experts in the content area to review such items. Careful consideration and judgment act together to evaluate the validity of content. No objective method assures it.

EXAMPLE FROM NURSING RESEARCH

Newman and Gaudiano (1984) report a research project that studied depression as an explanation for decreased subjective time in the elderly. They defined depression as an affective state characterized by a negative self-concept associated with self-reproach and self-blame. To measure depression, the researchers used the Beck Depression Inventory. The inventory was validated by correlation with clinicians' rating of depression ($r = .65$), and is sensitive to changes in clinical rating.

2. Face validity *is the extent to which the instrument (checklist, scale, system of classification, etc.) appears to be logically appropriate.* However, judging the validity of a scale or instrument by merely looking at it entails subjective judgment and is therefore weak. Its primary virtue is that it requires little time. An experienced researcher can quickly spot gross errors by examining whether or not the scale seems to be actually measuring what the researcher intends it should, or whether or not the researcher has provided a relevant sample of the variable under study.

3. Predictive validity, *sometimes called* empirical validity, *is the ability of the instrument to measure and predict.* For example, an I.Q.

test is valid if it predicts accurately which students will do well in academic work. Predictive validity may also be judged by comparing the results of one test or instrument with results of a test or instrument of known validity. For example, the age and sex distribution found in a research sample may be validated by comparing it with the findings of the United States Bureau of the Census, which collects demographic variables from the total population and, therefore, measures what the researcher wants her or his instrument to measure. The predictive validity of an instrument designed to identify characteristics of neurotics or psychotics may be validated by comparing it with instruments that have examined these characteristics in known neurotics or psychotics. Projective tests, such as the Thematic Apperception Test or the Minnesota Multiphasic Personality Inventory, are validated in this way.

4. Concurrent validity *is derived from the ability of the instrument or design to measure present observable behavior.* It distinguishes those who differ in their present state. However, certain states may not be directly observable; instead, these may be examined by finding visible factors that are logically linked to the state. For example, the amount of support that a mental patient has from kin and friends may be determined by how many visitors, letters, cards, or phone calls the patient has. However, for many characteristics, such as attitudes, few such methods have been identified. In such cases, the researcher uses construct validity to judge the extent to which the research tool is valid.

5. Construct validity, *the validity of concepts (constructs), judges the extent to which the research tool measures the concept or variable that the researcher wants it to measure.* Construct validation is an indirect approach that estimates the extent to which a subject actually possesses the characteristic presumed to be reflected by a particular scale or test. In such cases, multiple measures of the same concept are often used. For example, attitudes toward euthanasia may be first measured by giving respondents a questionnaire; later, an interviewer may question the same respondents. Then, the researcher may examine the behavior of the respondent: how the respondent acts when asked to sign a petition for or against euthanasia. Thus, construct validity may be established by using multiple measures.

EXAMPLES FROM NURSING RESEARCH

McGuire (1984), assessing the validity of six instruments to measure pain, notes that the validity of three of the instruments—the Verbal Descriptor Scale, Visual Analogue Scale, and Card Sort Method—is only probable, while the validity of the Chambers-Price Pain Rating Scale is questionable and that of Johnsons' Two-Component Scales is unclear. Only the McGill Pain Questionnaire was considered to have good validity. This questionnaire measured the following dimensions of pain: location, sensation, affective aspects, evaluation, intensity, and pattern.

Burckhardt (1985) reports that the McGill Pain Questionnaire has discriminant validity, as indicated by its ability to differentiate various painful conditions.

Knapp (1985) defines measurement as the process of translating reality into numbers, noting that three concepts are involved in the translation: the construct, the true score on the variable, and the obtained score on that variable. Validity issues arise when the fit between the construct and the true score is studied. Knapp, critical of certain authors, writes that construct validity of a theory and the validity of a test cannot be tested simultaneously. In addition, he writes, confusion exists in differentiating between construct validity, where all variables are on equal footing, and criterion-related validity, where one or more of the variables has superior status.

Weiss and Davis (1985) studied the validity and reliability of two scales, the Collaborative Practice Scales, to measure features of collaboration within the specific relationship of nurse and physician. One scale measured practices of physicians, and the other measured practices of nurses, each utilizing specific relationships of the nurse and the physician. The nine-item nurse scale measured direct assertion of professional expertise-opinion and active clarification of mutual responsibilities. The ten-item physician scale measured acknowledgment of the nurse's contribution to patient care and consensus development with nurses. The objectives of the research were to determine construct, concurrent, and predictive validity of the scales, as well as their internal consistency and test–retest reliability. Sex of physician and the physician's behavior (as rated by peer evaluators) predicted scores on the physician scale; educational preparation and type of professional responsibility predicted nurses' collaborative practice. Six-week test–retest reliability was significant for both scales.

Factors Jeopardizing Internal and External Validity

Validity may be judged as internal or external. *Internal validity* refers to judgments of the measures or designs within the study sample; *external validity* refers to the researcher's ability to generalize from the study sample to the larger population from which the sample was drawn.

For example, the internal validity of an experimental design deals with the question of whether the independent variable (the experimental treatment, or stimulus) actually made a difference to the research findings. Internal validity is the basic minimum for every experiment—its reason for being. Without the assurance that the experimental treatment made a difference in the observed effect, there is no way to interpret the findings of the experiment. On the other hand, external validity deals with the extent to which the study subjects or objects were representative of the larger population from which they were drawn; that is, the extent to which the findings of the small sample may be generalized to the larger population.

The selection of a research design or tool that is internally and externally valid is every researcher's ideal. Yet, this goal is not always reached. As noted earlier, Campbell and Stanley (1966) identify a number of extraneous variables that jeopardize the internal validity of the experimental design: (1) history, (2) maturation, (3) testing, (4) instrumentation, (5) statistical regression, (6) differential selection bias, and (7) experimental mortality, as well as interaction among these factors.

History refers to specific events that occur between the first and second measurement of the experimental group. A lapse of time may allow events to occur that influence the second measurement. An exciting afternoon, emotional disturbances, or drinking lots of coffee could change the response from the first measurement to the second, thereby interfering with the action of the independent variable. A control group that undergoes all of the experiences (except the independent variable) helps control the effects of history.

Maturation is the process that occurs within the respondent as time passes. Biological and psychological processes may cause the respondent to become tired, hungry, or bored. Or, the problem under study may go into a stage of remission or may cure itself independently of the experimental treatment, thus confusing the effect of the independent variable. These effects are controlled by randomization and by the use of control groups.

Testing refers to the effect that taking the first test has upon subsequent tests: respondents may do better on the second test because they have practiced by taking the first test, rather than because of the effect of the independent variable. This effect may be controlled by avoiding the first test.

Instrumentation refers both to the measuring instrument and to the researcher who uses the instrument. *Instrument decay*—autonomous changes in the measuring instrument, such as the stretching or fatiguing of a spring scale—may interfere with valid measurements. The researcher, too, may experience fatigue or a decline in efficiency. Changing researchers may also interfere with the validity of the instruments. Instrument error is controlled by pretesting before research and by using the same instrument for all measurements. Observer error is controlled by using equivalent random samples of interviewers. Using double-blind studies (which keep the interviewers ignorant of which is the experimental and which is the control group) is also helpful.

Statistical regression is a process that occurs when groups have been selected for study on the basis of extreme scores. For example, students chosen because of their low scores tend to average higher on subsequent tests. The tendency to move closer to the average score is called *regression toward the mean*, a ubiquitous phenomenon. Random assignment from an extreme pool of scores to either the experimental or the control group controls regression.

Differential selection is the method by which subjects are chosen for research groups. If random sampling is not used, a bias may be introduced into the study. *Matching*—the process of equating the subjects in terms of certain variables—may be used, although it should be used as an adjunct to, and not instead of, random sampling.

External validity is the ability to generalize from the study sample to the population. External validity is jeopardized by any factor that interferes with the representativeness of the sample. The effects of testing, selection biases, reactions to the unnatural environment of the laboratory, and prior experiments may jeopardize external validity. Another threat is the *Hawthorne effect*—the unnatural behavior that results when subjects know that they are being observed.

RELIABILITY

Reliability is the extent to which a specified procedure, such as measurement, yields consistent observation of the same facts from one time to another and from one situation to the other. Reliability refers to the stability, consistency, accuracy, and dependability of an instrument or measurement. If a test is reliable, repeating it will yield the same result. However, reliability has accrued a variety of meanings over time, due in part to the context in which it was developed and used. Reliability was developed in the context of various tests of ability at a time when extraneous variables received little attention (Selltiz et al., 1976, p. 182). Inconsistence in the results of repeated use of the same instrument was thought to represent errors of measurement rather than the influence of unrecognized and unknown extraneous variables. But, it began to be recognized that inconsistencies of results did not necessarily mean measurement error. New concepts and theories of reliability began to appear. Terms formerly lumped together under the concept *reliability* began to be differentiated. Some are not yet in wide usage. Characteristics of reliability that are examined today include stability, equivalence, and homogeneity.

Stability of Reliability

Stability is the extent to which repeated administrations of an instrument or measure give the same results. A stable instrument of measurement remains consistent with repeated applications.

To determine the stability of the measuring instrument, the researcher may compare repeated measurements: the same test may be given to a sample of study subjects on two or more occasions and the scores then compared. Such assessments are called *test–retest* reliability.

Test scores are compared by computing a *reliability coefficient*, or *correlation coefficient*, between the two sets of scores. If the two scores are unrelated, the correlation is equal to zero; if the scores are perfectly correlated, the correlation coefficient would be +1.00; if negatively related, the score will lie between 0.0 and −1.00. The Pearson product-moment correlation (Pearson r) is the most commonly used correlation index.

EXAMPLE FROM NURSING RESEARCH

Miles, M. (1985): Emotional symptoms and physical health in bereaved parents. Nursing Research, 34, 76–81.

Miles (1985), studying emotional symptoms and physical health in bereaved parents, used five scales in the study: (1) the Hopkins Symptom Checklist; (2) the Bereavement Health Assessment Scale; (3) the Illness Problems Scale; (4) the Drug Usage Appetite Change and Sleep Problems Scale; and (5) the Review of Life Experiences Scale. The Hopkins Symptom Checklist is a 58-item self-report inventory that measures emotional symptoms. There are normative data for the inventory on 1,800 psychiatric outpatients and 700 normal controls. Test–retest reliability for the five subscales ranged from .75 to .82. Internal consistencies, as measured by coefficient alpha, were uniformly high, ranging from .84 to .87. Factorial invariance ranged from .65 to .96.

For the Illness Problems Scale (IPS), the reliability coefficient (Cronbach's alpha) for the scale was .77. Construct validity for this subscale was supported by its correlation with the Somatization scores (a subscale) on the Hopkins Symptom Checklist: $r = .29$ with a given probability.

For the Drug Usage Scale, construct validity was found in the inverse correlations between use of drugs and the grief level; that is, how far along the bereaved individuals perceived themselves to be in the grief process: $r = -.35$ with a given probability.

The content and construct validity of the Review of Life Experiences were based on its use of items from two other validated life-events scales, with the addition of items identified as important life stressors in the authors' pilot studies. The internal consistency of the scale was .53.

Internal Homogeneity

Internal homogeneity, or *consistency*, is the extent to which all of the subparts of an instrument or scale measure the same characteristic. To determine internal homogeneity, the items on a test are split into two parts, and each of the parts is scored independently. The scores on each of the two parts are then used to compute a correlation coefficient. If the instrument is internally homogeneous, the correlation should be high.

The test may be split in two ways: the first half of the test may be split from the second half. For example, a test of 50 questions may be split into one test comprised of questions 1–25 and a second test composed of questions 26–50. Another way in which the test may be split is by the number of the questions. For example, odd questions may comprise one test, and all even questions the second test. In the past, the split-half method was often used. It was soon noted that the first half of the test often contained items not found on the last half, and vice versa. In addition, the subjects could become fatigued toward the end of the test or could make guesses and perform less well. Therefore, the split-half method began to be replaced by splitting the test by odd- and even-numbered questions. If a test is internally homogeneous, every subject should get about the same score on both tests. The extent of internal homogeneity was measured by correlating the scores on the two tests.

The Spearman-Brown prophecy formula uses the reliability obtained by correlating scores on the two halves of the test to predict the maximum reliability of the entire instrument. The split-half, which uses a first-half/second-half split, may obtain a different reliability estimate from one that uses an odd–even split. However, other procedures may be used, including the Kuder and Richardson procedure (KR–20), available on programs for computers, which is based on reliability estimates on the relationship of the response pattern to each separate item and the data from performance on the total instrument.

Equivalence

Equivalence refers to two processes: inter-rater (or interobserver) reliability, and the extent of agreement between the measurement of two instruments. Inter-rater, or interobserver, reliability is estimated by having two or more researchers observe or measure the same study subjects at the same time. The coefficient of equivalence indicates the extent to which these measurements agree. Different instruments may attempt to measure the same thing. For example, a measure of anxiety may use a number of instruments: pulse rate, blood pressure, perspiration, etc. The extent to which these measures agree estimates the equivalence.

EXAMPLES FROM NURSING RESEARCH

O'Neil (1972) used simultaneous measurements of several behaviors to study the effect of behavior modification procedures on the motor problems of a child with cerebral palsy. Two observers recorded simultaneously, for a total of 18 sessions. Percentage of agreement between observers' data was calculated using the formula:

$$\frac{\text{Number of agreements}}{\text{Total number of agreements + disagreements}}$$

Nakagawa (1972) reports an historical epidemiological investigation, using records of first admission to a state mental hospital to study the pattern of psychiatric symptom change. A detailed system of coding was developed to classify presenting complaints. To determine the level of intercoder agreement, 10 percent of the records were double-coded. A reliability test (Scott's) was then applied to the double-coded cases. The reliability of the coders was calculated to be 0.85, indicating reasonably good reliability.

ADDITIONAL CRITERIA

Other criteria important in evaluating a measure or instrument include sensitivity, efficiency, generalizability, objectivity, and appropriateness.

Sensitivity is the ability of an instrument to make discriminations. A scale that measures tons of coal will not do for the measure of a dosage of medication. In addition to the ability to make discriminations, a sensitive instrument can detect change. More and more instruments are being invented to detect changes in the body associated with cancer. As other factors of interest to nursing acquire more sensitive instruments, the quality and the level of knowledge will increase.

An *efficient instrument* is one that requires a minimum of effort and expense and still measures with validity and reliability. A questionnaire or interview schedule should only be as long and as complex as is necessary to achieve credible reliability and validity. A perfect instrument that is too complex and expensive to use will not collect much data. The advantage of computer analysis is the efficiency and speed with which it is completed.

The *ability to generalize* refers to the expectation of the researcher that instruments that are reliable and valid in one study will be found so in another. However, previously used instruments found to be reliable and valid in the original study are often found to be less so when used on other kinds of groups. Therefore, current studies should indicate whether the instrument previously found valid and reliable is being used to study the same kind of group as did the original study or whether it has been retested for use with the present one.

Objectivity refers to the extent to which two or more independent researchers can apply the same instrument to measure the same phenomenon. This is particularly important in interviewing. The characteristics of the interviewer, such as age, sex, race, and apparent social class, can affect the way in which the subjects respond. Other factors that demand scrutiny include the role that the researcher plays in the determination of the nature of the data and the instrument used to collect the data. For example, a person with strong feelings one way or the other about abortion issues may not produce an objective instrument to measure attitudes toward abortion.

Appropriateness is defined by Fox (1982, p. 270) as the extent to which the respondent group can meet the demands imposed by the instrument. For example, the use of a questionnaire should be geared to the literacy and culture of the responding subjects. Middle-class English, for example, may not always be appropriate when studying members of other ethnic groups or classes.

SUMMARY

Validity is the extent to which a component of research, such as a scale, method, instrument, design, or measure, reflects and measures what the researcher intends it to measure. Methods of judging validity include content validity, face validity, predictive validity, concurrent validity, and construct validity. Content validity is concerned with the sampling adequacy of the study; that is, whether or not all possible observations were included. The researcher strives for content validity by using representative measures where possible. Face validity is the extent to which the element of research, such as the scale, questionnaire, etc., appears to be logically appropriate on examination. It is a weak judgment, due to the subjective element and limited time of study involved. Predictive validity is the ability of the instrument to measure and predict: accurate predictions tend to validate the measure. Concurrent validity is the ability of the instrument or scale to measure present observable behavior. When certain states are not directly observable, visible factors may be found to measure a factor logically. Construct validity judges the extent to which the research tool measures the concept, variable, or construct that the researcher wants it to measure. Multiple measures of the same concept are often used to establish validity.

A number of factors may jeopardize internal validity (validity within the sample) and external validity (the ability to generalize from the sample to the population from which the sample was drawn). Internal validity is jeopardized by history, maturation, testing, instrumentation, statistical regression, differential-selection bias, and experimental mortality. Using randomization, control groups, and double-blind experiments helps to control these factors.

Reliability is the extent to which a specified measurement yields consistent observations of the same facts from one time to another and from one situation to another. Characteristics of reliability include stability, equivalence, and homogeneity. A stable instrument or measure remains consistent with repeated applications. To determine stability, the researcher may use a test–retest, giving the same test to the same study subjects on two or more occasions. The scores are then compared by computing a reliability coefficient. Internal homogeneity is the extent to which all subparts of an instrument or scale measure the same characteristic. To determine internal homogeneity, the items on a test may be split, either by dividing the test into halves (first half and last half) or by using all odd questions for one test and all even questions for another. The extent of internal homogeneity is measured by correlating the scores on the two tests. Equivalence refers to inter-rater reliability and to the extent of reliability between two different instruments. Inter-rater reliability is estimated by having two or more researchers observe the same study subjects at the same time; the coefficient of equivalence indicates the extent of agreement. Instruments such as tests are examined by developing two different forms of the test that are given one after the other to the same subjects. If the correlation coefficient between the scores is high, the instrument is estimated to have good reliability.

EXAMPLE FROM NURSING RESEARCH

Jalowiec, Anne, Murphy, Suzanne, and Powers, Marjorie, (1984): Psychometric assessment of the Jalowiec coping scale. Nursing Research, 33, 157–161.

The authors report a study designed to provide more detailed analysis of the reliability and validity of the Jalowiec Coping Scale. (The report is summarized with parenthetical remarks by the author of this book.) Jalowiec developed the scale to examine the coping methods used by hypertensive and emergency room patients. She used 40 coping strategies on the scale, identified from a review of the literature on stress, coping, and adaptation. An ordinal scale was developed with the descriptive endpoints of "never" and "almost always" on one-to-five intervals.

Twenty judges classified each item of the scale as primarily "problem-oriented" or "affective-oriented." *Problem-oriented* was defined as coping strategies that tried to deal with the stressful situation itself; and *affective-oriented* was defined as strategies designed to handle the distressing emotions evoked by the situation.

Reliability: The instrument was tested for reliability, including the stability and homogeneity (or internal consistency) of the instrument. Stability was first evaluated by test–retest using 28 subjects from a general population, with retesting after two weeks. The authors report that the Spearman's rank-ordering of the test–retest data yielded significant reliability coefficients of .79 for total coping scores, .85 for problem-oriented scores, and .86 for affective scores. Later, a one-month retest interval with 30 subjects yielded similarly significant rhos: .78 for total scores, .84 for problem, and .83 for affective, supporting the stability of the scale.

Tests of homogeneity, looking for the internal consistency of sampling items, used the SPSS (Statistical Package for the Social Sciences) to analyze Cronbach's coefficient alpha. The authors note that Cronbach's coefficient alpha does not measure all sources of measurement error but, if test instructions are clear and uncomplicated, and if scoring is objective, other errors make little difference. A coefficient alpha of .86 was obtained, indicating overall homogeneity of the content on the scale.

Validity: Internal consistency, the authors write, is concerned with whether something in common (such as the subparts of an instrument) is being measured; knowing the internal consistency of an instrument is the first step that must be taken in assessing construct validity. Construct validity (the degree to which an instrument measures a complex concept, such as coping) is concerned with determining what the common element is that is being measured. The authors assessed the content validity by a judgment of: (a) the systematic manner of tool development, (b) the large number of items used to tap the domain, and (c) the inclusion of diverse coping behaviors. They assessed the construct validity by factor analysis, which identified clusters of related variables by showing which items share a common variance, and are thus able to measure the same attribute.

Factor analysis supported the earlier, problem-oriented classification of coping scale items; however, the affective-oriented classification did not demonstrate cohesiveness when statistically examined. The authors write that further testing is necessary in order to determine the soundness and replicability of this structure of coping behavior.

The authors conclude by quoting a statement from Goosen and Bush (1979, p. 51), who are interested in adaptation: "As the link between health and adaptation becomes more evident, nursing interventions directed toward assisting the client to adapt to an ever-changing environment may become a unique theoretical framework for nursing." Information gained from a sound coping scale, the authors note, can be a salient component of that theoretical framework.

STUDY QUESTIONS _____

1. What is validity?
2. What does judgment have to do with validity?
3. Define, discuss, and compare content validity, face validity, predictive validity, concurrent validity, and construct validity.
4. Define reliability.
5. Define and compare stability, equivalence, and homogeneity of reliability.
6. Name additional criteria important in evaluating an instrument.
7. Describe what the Spearman-Brown formula does.
8. What is the Kuder and Richardson procedure?

REFERENCES AND SUGGESTED READING

Borkovec, T., et al. (1976): Assessment of anxiety. In Ciminero, A., Calhoun, K., Adams, H. (eds.), Handbook of Behavioral Assessment. New York: Wiley.

Campbell, D. and Stanley, J. (1963): Experimental and Quasi-Experimental Designs for Research. Chicago: Rand McNally. *Includes factors jeopardizing internal and external validity.*

Cassidy, C. (1976): The relationship between daily life changes, physical symptoms, and body temperature range: Temperature changes related to adjustments to life events. Image, *8*, 30–33.

Cox, C. (1985): The health self-determination index. Nursing Research, *34*, 177–183. *Likert scale used.*

Dixon, J. (1984): Effect of nursing interventions on nutritional and performance status in cancer patients. Nursing Research, *33*, 330–333. *Includes construct validity, discriminant and convergent validity.*

Fox, D. (1982): Fundamentals of Research in Nursing (4th ed). Norwalk, Conn.: Appleton-Century-Crofts. *Chapter 17 includes reliability, validity, sensitivity, appropriateness, and objectivity of research instruments.*

Hubbard, P., et al. (1984): The relationship between social support and self-care practices. Nursing Research, *33*, 266–270.

Jalowiec, A., Murphy, S., and Powers, M. (1984): Psychometric assessment of the Jalowiec coping scale. Nursing Research, *33*, 157–161.

Lin, N. (1976): Foundations of Social Research. New York: McGraw-Hill. *Chapter 10 includes validity, reliability.*

McGuire, D. (1984): The measurement of clinical pain. Nursing Research, *33*, 152–156.

Miles, M. (1985): Emotional symptoms and physical health in bereaved parents. Nursing Research, *34*, 76–81.

Nakagawa, H. (1972): An epidemiological study of psychiatric symptom pattern change. In Batey, M. (ed.) Communicating Nursing Research. Boulder: WICHE. *Measures of inter-coder agreement.*

Newman, M. and Gaudiano, J. (1984): Depression as an explanation for decreased subjective time in the elderly. Nursing Research, *33*, 137–139.

O'Neil, S. (1972): The application and methodological implications of behavior modification in nursing research. In Batey, M. (ed.), Communicating Nursing Research. Boulder: WICHE, pp. 179–191.

Rodgers, J. (1977): Relationship between sociability and personal space preference at two different times of day. In Downs, F. and Newman, M. (eds.), A Source Book of Nursing Research. Philadelphia: F.A. Davis.

Rottkamp, F. (1976): A behavior modification approach to nursing therapeutics in body positioning of spinal cord injured patients. Nursing Research, *2*, 181–185.

Selltiz, C., et al. (1976): Research Methods in Social Relations. New York: Holt, Rinehart, & Winston, p. 182.

Walizer, M. and Wienir, P. (1978): Research methods and analysis. New York: Harper & Row. *Chapter 14 discusses reliability and validity.*

Weiss, S. and Davis, P. (1985): Validity and reliability of the collaborative practice scales. Nursing Research, *34*, 299–304.

PART VI

Data Analysis

19

Data Analysis

Data analysis is the process by which the researcher summarizes and analyzes the data that have been collected. The kind of analysis utilized depends on the research design, the method of sampling, and the method by which the data were collected and measured. Data collected by a descriptive or historical research design, or from unstructured questions in other designs, often produced extensive qualitative data of considerable depth. The researcher organizes such data into categories by content analysis and uses various processes to analyze and interpret the categories. These processes include a count of the frequencies, a calculation of percentages and proportions, and the construction of tables and graphs for a visual depiction of data. Statistical tests that use nominal data (such as the chi-square test) may be used to compare groups in terms of qualitative variables.

The researcher who has used a quantitative design to collect sets of data may use the techniques to analyze data that qualitative analysis uses and, in addition, may utilize both descriptive statistics (to calculate the central tendency and variance) and inferential statistics (to test statistical hypotheses and to judge whether relationships observed in the sample are likely to occur in the population from which the sample was drawn).

This chapter begins with the analysis of qualitative data, then examines the analysis of quantitative data by means of descriptive statistics. (Chapter 20 then examines the use of inferential statistics.)

Upon completion of this chapter, the student should be able to: (1) compare qualitative and quantitative data analysis; (2) describe procedures used to organize and analyze qualitative data; (3) identify, define, and compare measures of central tendency and variance; and (4) identify and define the tests designed to analyze correlations.

ANALYSIS OF DATA

Qualitative data are produced from research designs, such as the descriptive, documentary, or historical, and from unstructured questions utilized by other designs, such as the survey. Qualitative data are narrative in form and are often extensive, but may be counted (and thus, quantified) to show differences in kind or rank. In contrast, quantitative analysis shows differences in amounts.

The first task of the researcher in qualitative analysis is to distinguish general patterns, such as descriptions of mental patterns, verbal patterns, behavioral patterns, or institutional patterns. Since the data may have been collected from two perspectives—that of the subjects (the *emic* perspective) or that of the observer (the *etic* perspective)—these must also be identified and distinguished. Then the researcher organizes the data utilizing the following procedures: (1) content analysis; (2) counting and summarizing frequencies; (3) tabulating the data; (4) creating tables and graphs for visual depiction of data; and (5) using statistical procedures appropriate for the use of the nominal scale (such as calculation of the mode and the range). In quantitative analysis, the researcher begins with numerical data, using descriptive statistics to summarize data and inferential statistics to test estimations and statistical hypotheses. Each of these will be examined in turn.

Content Analysis

Content analysis is the systematic and objective procedure used to identify and analyze significant written, verbal, or visual data in order to tabulate, classify, summarize, and compare the contents. Analysis may begin with the establishment of categories of data or, if the contents to be analyzed are unknown, categories may be developed during the process of analysis. The categories should be homogeneous, inclusive, mutually exclusive, exhaustive, and useful. If more than one researcher is used to code the information, inter-rater reliability should be determined early.

The purpose of content analysis may be to analyze semantic content or to establish the meaning or intent of the content. *Semantic content analysis* is a process designed to develop a set of categories that represent the actual content of the material being analyzed. The researcher decides what should be coded and how it should be coded, and then may submit the code to experts to judge how to weigh the responses. The meaning and intent of the content is a judgment made by the researcher.

Six basic elements of content analysis, identified by Holsti (1968), include comparisons of: (1) the *source* (the sender of the message); (2) *encoding* (the process that resulted in the message); (3) the *message*; (4) the *transmitting channel* (how the message is sent); (5) the *detector* (the recipient of the message); and (6) the *decoding process* (the effects of the message).

Messages are compared in terms of each of the elements above. For example, the source can be compared in terms of whether it was a single source over time, a single source but in varying situations, a single source but to several audiences, or messages from two or more sources. Concepts used from a source with a single message can also be compared. Descriptions and comparisons may be made of the themes or trends apparent in the communication; the attributes of the senders, receivers, and situations vis-à-vis the message sent; and the responses to the message. Responses may be judged to be positive, negative, or mixed. The units in the message to be analyzed may include words, phrases, concepts, or themes.

EXAMPLES FROM NURSING RESEARCH

Content Analysis

An example of content analysis in the nursing literature is the research report of Caty, Ellerton, and Ritchie (1984). The authors used content analysis to study the contents of 39 published case studies of hospitalized children. The researchers established the categories to be used in the analysis from the Lazarus stress-and-coping paradigm. The articles to be analyzed were assigned at random to two of the researchers. Inter-rater reliability had been calculated prior to beginning the analysis. The researchers first analyzed the material for the type of behavior described by the author of the case study, then classified this material according to the category system previously established for their own purposes. The researchers met at frequent intervals throughout the coding process to discuss and agree on problem areas. Frequency counts were made where appropriate. Suggestions for further research included: (1) looking for answers to the question: "Coping with what?" and (2) identifying a mechanism to determine whether the category system used was sensitive to variations in coping behaviors across various stressful situations.

Kendall (1977), writing on her field work in an Iranian village, identified five themes, including dominance and submission, paternalism, familism, a male–female dichotomy, and fatalism. She described how these themes permeated the Iranian society, influencing patterns of childrearing.

Psychologists, such as Evans (1982), report content analysis of themes that are useful in nursing. Examples include themes found by Shneidman in a content analysis of suicide letters and notes: strong emotion; a pervasive quality of forlornness; an overwhelming need for love; a disappointing relationship; unusual thought processes (such as illogical chains of reasoning); and specific instructions to those who are to be left behind. Evans suggests that content analysis such as this should aid in understanding the dynamics of suicide and should assist mental-health professionals to identify people most likely to carry out a suicide threat.

Procedures for Counting and Summarizing Frequencies

Both qualitative and quantitative analysis of data include counts of the frequencies with which data appear. Quantitative analysis often begins with such a count. The researcher, confronted with a mass of returned questionnaires and filled interview schedules, must first count in order to summarize the data contained in these instruments. Analysis of qualitative data also includes counting the frequency of data, but only *after* considerable prior analysis of the descriptive material has been made.

Fox (1982, pp. 292 ff.) recommends the use of hand analysis and tally sheets to analyze quantitative data in projects of limited scope and sample. The same process is helpful in counting the frequency of qualitative data, once all the preparatory analysis is complete. The first step in hand analysis is to construct a tally sheet or a table for counting data in certain categories (Fig. 19–1), or both.

The purpose of the tally sheet is to help the researcher to organize the raw data into frequencies, in a visible form that enhances comparison. The information in the tally sheet depicted in Figure 19–1 is interpreted from a study by Flaskerud (1984), who compared data from nominal

Minority Group	Sex		Occupation				Marital	
	Male	Female	PT	H	UL	CS	M	NM
App. N = 18	卌 | |	卌 卌 |		卌 卌	卌 |	| |	卌 卌 卌	| | |
Bl N = 20	卌 卌 | |	卌 | | |		卌 | | |	卌 卌	| |	卌 卌 | | |	卌 | |
NA N = 28	卌 卌 | | |	卌 卌 卌		卌 | | |	卌 | |	卌 卌 | | |	卌 卌 | | |	卌 卌 卌
MA N = 30	卌 卌 | |	卌 卌 卌 卌 | | |		卌 卌 卌 | | |	卌 卌	| |	卌 卌 卌 卌 卌	卌

Figure 19–1. A tally sheet. Key: *App = Appalachians, Bl = blacks, CS = clerk/secretary, H = home, M = married, MA = Mexican Americans, NA = Native Americans, PT = professional title, UL = unskilled labor, and UM = unmarried.*

categories: the perceptions of problematic behavior by six minority groups and a group of mental-health professionals.*

Qualitative data may be summarized from the tally sheet as ratios, proportions, rates, and index numbers; and data may be tabulated and frequency counts made. Data from the nominal categories may be presented visually in tables and graphs.

Ratios, Proportions, Percentages, Rates, and Index Numbers

Data obtained from qualitative scales, such as the nominal and the ordinal, can be summarized as ratios, proportions, percentages, rates, and index numbers.

The *ratio* equals the frequency of A divided by the frequency of B, where A is one category of observations and B is another category:

$$\text{Ratio} = \frac{\text{Frequency of A}}{\text{Frequency of B}}$$

For example, to find the sex ratio of a category containing 150 males and 250 females, divide the number of males by the number of females (which gives .6 males per female); then multiply the answer by 100 to remove partials (such as .6, since .6 of a male does not exist, in reality). This gives a ratio of 60 males in the group for every 100 females:

$$\text{Ratio} = \frac{150}{250} = .6$$

or, to remove partials: .6 × 100 = 60 males per 100 females

A *proportion* is the relation in size of one thing compared to another, an equality of ratios. (It is also a method of finding the fourth term of such a proportion, when three are known). A *percent* is a convenient way to express many proportions; for example, ten percent of the children were absent because of illness. Percent is the parts in each hundred: ten percent is 10 parts in each 100, or 10/100 of the whole. In the example above,

---

*Flaskerud reported the number of persons falling into each minority category; and the mode, a summary of raw data used in qualitative analysis, for education, sex, religion, marital status, occupation, and family type. From the numbers in each category, and the report of the mode, a reconstruction of raw data was estimated.

where a category contained 150 males and 250 females, the portion and percent of males to the total population is:

$$\frac{\text{Males}}{\text{Total people}} = \frac{150}{400} = 0.375;$$

or, expressed as parts per 100: $0.375 \times 100 = 37.5$ percent of the total population is male.

$$\text{Proportion} = \frac{\text{Category frequency}}{\text{Total number}}$$

$$\text{Percent} = \frac{\text{Category frequency}}{\text{Total number}} \times 100$$

A *rate* is a quantity, amount, or degree that is measured in proportion to something else. For example, the standard population is a norm or standard of reference based on a particular, actual census of a living population, in proportion to which the distribution of age, sex, and race may be measured.

$$\text{Rate} = \frac{NA}{NA + NB} \times \text{Base}$$

In the formula above, NA equals the number of times that event A occurs; NB equals the number of times that the event might have occurred but did not; and the base is a standard, preselected number, such as 100 or 1000, all of which are related to a given period of time.

An *index number* is an average that indicates change between sets of data over time. A familiar index is the value of the dollar, with the value of the dollar during a particular year serving as the base. The index number equals the value in period A, divided by the value in the base period, times 100. The problem in making an index is selecting an appropriate based period, preferably one of relative stability, and one that was not unique. If the researcher wishes to establish an index number of the changes in the cost of health care over time, periods of depression, recession, or inflation should not be selected for the base. The formula is:

$$\text{Index number} = \frac{\text{Value in period A}}{\text{Value in base period}} \times 100$$

Tabulation of Data

Tabulation of data is the process of arranging the material in a concise and logical order. An *array* is a list of data ranked from lowest to highest. For example, if data have been collected on the ages of persons in the sample, the data may be ordered from youngest to oldest in a list: 18, 19,

20, 21, 22, 24, 29, 30, and so on. The array organizes the data in a form that is easily described and summarized.

The next step is to count the number of cases that belong to the various categories. The result of such a count is called a frequency, designated by the lower-case letter "f." The frequency tells how often a characteristic occurs, such as the number of persons that are aged 20 or are female. In qualitative studies and in studies using the nominal level of "measurement," the frequency count is the only kind of quantitative data that it is possible to obtain.

In quantitative analysis, however, constructing an array and counting frequencies are only the beginning steps. The researcher may next construct a *frequency distribution* to indicate how certain characteristics are spread across different locations or categories. Frequency distributions deal with continuous data, such as age or temperature, and cannot be made for discrete data. To make a frequency distribution, the researcher first establishes the set of categories into which the data will be grouped. The categories must be exhaustive, mutually exclusive, homogeneous, logical, and consistent. All categories must be the same size, spanning the same number of units of measurement. For example, to make a frequency distribution for adult males of various ages, the researcher must first put all of the ages into mutually exclusive and exhaustive categories: men from 20–29, 30–39, 40–49, and so on, until all ages are included. The categories are called *class intervals*, designated by the lower-case letter "i." *Class* is the category, while *interval* is the standard size of each category (ten years in the example). Frequency distributions using class intervals help to analyze interval data, which may then be depicted visually in a graph or table.

Tables

After the frequency of data in the category has been counted, the researcher may arrange the data in tables. Tables are useful in data analysis for the following reasons: (1) space is conserved—tables present data in such a way that the narrative may be reduced (although not omitted, since a table without an explanation is not helpful); (2) relationships among data may be visualized, a process that facilitates the process of data comparison; (3) data are summarized and put into individual cells —errors and omissions in the categories can be easily noted; (4) comprehension is enhanced—tabulated data are easier to understand and remember; and (5) statistical computations are possible—statistical tables (such as the 2 × 2 contingency table) are the basis for statistical computation (such as the chi-square).

A *table* may be either a general-purpose table or a special-purpose table. The *general-purpose tables* are the original, primary tables, designed to include large amounts of data that will supply information for

(1) TABLE. (2) A MODEL OF A TABLE AND ITS COMPONENTS* (3) A SUGGESTED • LAYOUT OF A SECONDARY TABLE, TO BE INCORPORATED INTO THE TEXT OR THE REPORT.

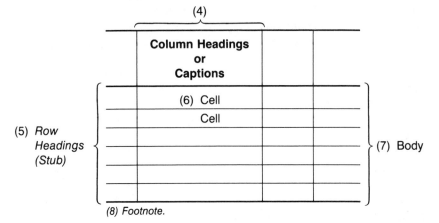

Key to the elements of the above table:
(1) Table number—center above title or place on line with title; may be Arabic or Roman.
(2) Table title—describes the data contained in the table.
(3) Headnote—infrequently used; this further describes the data referred to in the title.
(4) Column—shows data for one category, according to categories contained in the rows or stubs.
(5) Row—shows data for a category, according to data contained in column head.
(6) Cell—intersection of a row and a column.
(7) Body—all of the cells in a table.
(8) *—explanatory footnotes concerning the table itself, using asterisk or dagger to alleviate confusion with textual footnotes.

Figure 19–2. A model of a table.

other tables and graphs. *Special-purpose tables* are secondary tables drawn from the general-purpose tables and designed to analyze, summarize, or interpret selected material. Special-purpose tables also illustrate significant relationships found in primary data. For example, a 2 × 2 contingency table is a special purpose table that organizes data for statistical tests, such as the chi-square, which is designed to compare groups in terms of qualitative variables.

Every table has both a title (placed above the body of the table) and a number (Arabic or Roman), which is either centered above the title or is placed on the first line with the title (Fig. 19–2).

The parts of a table include the *columns* (vertical data), *rows* (horizontal data), and *cells* (small spaces defined by the intersection of a column and a row). The *line headings* of the rows comprise the *stub*, which is at the left margin of the table. The *column headings* are at the top of the table and are over the stub. A *box heading* may extend over more than one column; if so, the headings under the box heading are called *subheadings*.

In statistics, the size of a table depends upon the number of individual frequencies, or cells, contained in it. Size is determined by first noting the number of horizontal cells or rows and then the number of vertical cells or columns.

Graphs: Visual Depictions of Data

A *graph* is a diagram or line that shows how one quantity depends on, or changes with, another. Among commonly used graphs are the bar graph, the pie graph, the histogram, and the frequency polygon.

The *pie graph* is a circle (360 degrees) that represents 100 percent of the sample—the various parts of the sample being converted to degrees (i.e., angle values of the circle). It is used to represent frequencies for categories that are discontinuous, such as those formed by a nominal scale (Fig. 19–3).

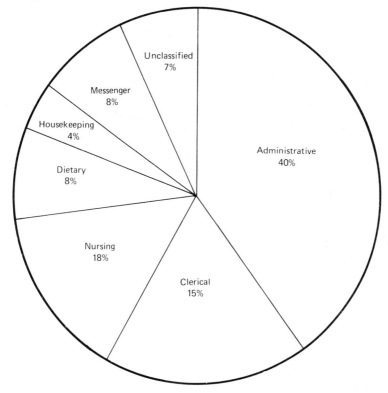

Figure 19–3. Pie graph showing percentage of activities performed by the staff nurse by skill level.

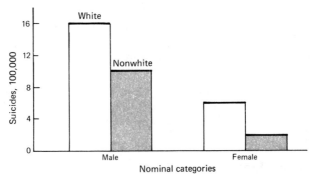

Figure 19–4. Bar graph depicting suicides by race and sex.

The bar graph, histogram, and frequency polygon utilize the vertical scale or axis of a graph (called the *Y-axis* or *ordinate*) to record frequency, and the horizontal scale or axis of a graph (called the *X-axis* or *abscissa*) to record categories.

The *bar graph*, like the pie graph, represents frequencies for discontinuous categories that arise from the nominal scale. The bar graph utilizes the X- or Y-axis of a graph to record its data, the frequencies being recorded on the ordinate and the categories on the abscissa. The bars are discrete and nontouching (Fig. 19–4), reflecting the nature of nominal data.

The *histogram* is a *frequency distribution graph* that records continuous data from ratio and interval scales. Assuming equal class intervals, the frequency of a class is represented by the height of the bars and the class interval by the width of the bar. Thus, to construct a histogram, bars of equal width should be made to stand for the size of the class interval. The height of the bars represents the frequency with which the occurrence in each category takes place. The frequency always goes on the vertical axis (or ordinate), while the categories or class intervals go on the horizontal axis (or abscissa).

The bars of a histogram touch one another, indicating continuous data. A space, however, should be left between the ordinate and the first bar. Frequencies should start at zero, and the proportions of the graph should be reasonable, having the frequency units and the class intervals properly divided (Fig. 19–5). A narrow abscissa with tall ordinates, or a wide abscissa with short ordinates, form misleading graphs.

A *frequency distribution polygon* may be made from a histogram by putting a dot in the center of the top of each column and connecting the dots with a line.

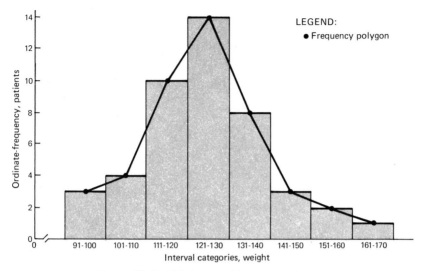

Figure 19–5. Histogram and frequency polygon.

ELEMENTARY DESCRIPTIVE STATISTICS: CENTRAL TENDENCY AND VARIANCE

Data from quantitative scales may be described by two descriptive summary measures: the measure of central tendency (the mean, median, and mode) and the measure of variance (range and standard deviation). A single value—a *univariate statistic*—represents a group of values. For example, the *mean* represents the average value in a set of scores; the *median* is the middle score in a set of scores, and the *mode* is the most frequent score in a set.

Central Tendency

The most typical, common, or average value for all of the subjects studied is called the *central tendency*. *Central* refers to a middle value, while *tendency* refers to the general trend of the numbers, in terms of their central or middle value. For example, if all of the ages in a sample were being studied, an observation of one age may be compared with all ages; i.e., with the distribution of the variable "age" in the population. Once all of the ages are listed, the array organized, and the data summarized, then the age that is most frequently found in the sample (the mode) may be determined, along with the average age of the sample (the mean), and the middle age in the sample (the median).

The Mean. A simple descriptive statistic, and the one most widely used, is the *mean*, or *average*. It is obtained by adding together all of the values or scores and dividing this number by the total number of scores. The mean is symbolized by $\overline{X}$; the formula for calculating the mean is:

$$\overline{X} = \frac{\Sigma X}{N}$$

where $\overline{X}$ stands for mean or average; Σ (the Greek letter *sigma*) stands for the sum of; X stands for the individual scores; and N stands for the total number of scores. The mean is affected by the value of every case; thus, the extreme and erratic items may be given undue weight. For example, if the researcher wished to calculate the average monthly salaries of ten persons who made $280, $300, $310, $320, $330, $340, $350, $370, and $10,000, respectively, to get the mean $\overline{X}$, the researcher would add up the sum (Σ) of all of the individual scores (X) and would divide by the total number of scores (N). The mean ($\overline{X}$) would be $12,920 divided by 10, or a monthly average of $1,292.

However, the mean should not be used if the distribution of scores is very skewed; i.e., asymmetrical or distorted. In the example used here, the one large income has pulled the mean income far above what it would have been if the scores were symmetrical. If the sample of scores has a reasonably symmetrical distribution, the mean is a good measure of central tendency.

The mean is often advantageous to use, merely because it is so well-known and so well-understood. If there are fewer observations than 30, the items may be treated individually. However, if a larger number exists, the data should be arranged in a frequency distribution first, then the mean of the distribution calculated.

The Median. The *median* is the middle score that divides a set of scores into two equal parts. The median is the measure of central tendency most commonly used with a skewed distribution of scores. It is also used with scores based on an ordinal measurement scale, which ranks scores from largest to smallest, with intervals not exactly determinable. For example, if a researcher wished to have the patients on a ward rank the efficiency of nursing care with the categories "excellent," "good," "fair," "poor," and "terrible," each of these categories could be assigned a code number from one (for "terrible") to five (for "excellent"). However, it is important to remember that these are not scores in the usual sense but simply numerical codes or guides to the categories. If 15 patients were to rank the nursing care, the scores might look something like this:

$$5,5,5, \quad 4,4,4,4,4, \quad 3,3,3,3, \quad 2,2, \quad 1$$

In these scores, the median score is a 4, which stands for the category "good." The median is the middle score. It lies between the two middle scores (if the total number of scores is even) or it is the middle score (if the total number of scores is odd).

Based on values lying immediately on either side of it, the median is not as influenced by the size of extreme items, as is the mean; thus, it may be used effectively where individual values are extreme and atypical.

The Mode. The mode is the simplest measure of central tendency to calculate, defined as the most frequent score. The mode may be used with any scale, but it is the only measure of central tendency usable with the nominal scale. Like the median, the mode is useful in cases where it is desirable to eliminate the effects of extreme variations. In a frequency distribution, the mode is that point on the scale of the variable where the frequency is the greatest. At times, there may be one mode (unimodal), two modes (bimodal), or three modes (trimodal), unless there is a distinct central tendency. In a large sample, the mode may have little significance.

Thus, if the nominal scale is used, the best measure of central tendency is the mode. If the measurement scale is ordinal, the best measure of central tendency is the median. With equal-interval scales, when scores have reasonable symmetry, the best measure is the mean. Where the measurement is equal intervals but the scores are skewed or asymmetrical, the best measure of central tendency is the median.

Variance

The purpose of describing the central tendencies of the data is to provide a single value to represent a group of unlike values. For example, averages accent the best single representative of a set of scores or numerical values. On the other hand, the variance examines dispersion, or how observations are spread out. The variability of the scores may be of as much interest as the central tendency, since the actual observations are not totally concentrated but, instead, are spread out or distributed among many values or categories. The extent to which these observations are dispersed around the central values, whether clustered close around the average or widely scattered, may be measured. The three principal measures of variance are the total range, the interquartile range, and the standard deviation.

The Range. The simplest measure of the dispersion of data is the *total range*, a relatively crude and unstable measure of dispersion that defines the difference between the largest and smallest observations in a set. Therefore, the total range is limited, taking into account only these two specific observations—the largest and the smallest. In spite of this, the range, like the mode, is useful for reading tables or for quickly scanning data for a rough picture of the scope of observations and their tendency to be dispersed. The formula for obtaining the total range is as follows:

$$\text{Total range} = (\text{the largest } X) - (\text{the smallest } X)$$

where X is an individual score.

Knowing the total range is sometimes a better indicator of the nature of the data than knowing the mean. For example, examine the grades below that two groups of eight students each made on a test:

Group A	Group B
100	60
80	55
60	50
50	50
50	50
40	50
15	45
5	40
400	400

where Group A $\overline{X}$ = 400/8 = 50 and Group B $\overline{X}$ = 400/8 = 50.

Adding the individual test scores X together and dividing by the total number of test scores, eight in each case, the mean $\overline{X}$ (50) for each group is found to be identical. Yet, the scores for each group vary considerably. If the total range for the two groups were known, more useful information would be in hand about the variation among the scores than could be gained by knowing the mean alone. The total range for Group A is 95 (100 − 5 = 95), while for Group B it is only 20 (60 − 40 = 20). This means that a greater variation exists within the scores of Group A than within Group B, although the mean of both is identical. Therefore, the range gives a better understanding of the variability of ten scores.

The range does have limitations. For example, a change in one individual score, the lowest or the highest, can alter the total range drastically. If Group B had one score of 100, the entire range would change. In addition, the range fails to give the overall variability within the group of scores. To correct this problem somewhat, another measure of range, the interquartile range, is often employed.

The Interquartile Range. The *interquartile range* is a positional value found by making an array of values; i.e., lining up the values in order of size and dividing the array into quarters. The range of categories or scores that includes the middle 50 percent of the scores is the interquartile range, the range between the scores comprising the lowest quartile (or quarter) and the highest quartile (or quarter). The formula for obtaining the interquartile range is:

$$\text{Interquartile range} = Q_3 - Q_1$$

where Q_3 is the category in and below which are ¾ of the scores, and Q_1 is the category in and below which are ¼ of the scores. Q is the symbol for quartile.

Using the test scores of Group A, the interquartile range may be identified:

Group A

100	
80	Q_4
60	Q_3
50	
50	Q_2
40	
15	
5	Q_1

where $Q_3 - Q_1$ = the interquartile range.

Normal Frequency Distribution and Standard Deviation. The *normal frequency-distribution curve*, also called the *bell-shaped curve*, the *normal curve*, or the *Gaussian curve* (after its inventor), has properties that are valuable in the statistical analysis of data. The curve indicates that most of the values of the measurements of a variable under study cluster together and possess about the same scale value, forming the mode, the median, and the mean. A much smaller number of the variables (or study subjects) possess more extreme (or deviant) values on either extreme of the curve (Fig. 19–6). In the normal curve, 68 percent of all values fall

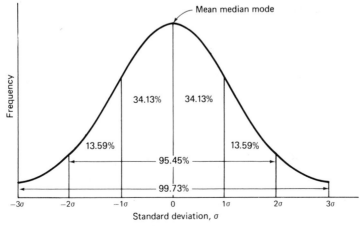

Figure 19–6. The normal frequency distribution curve and standard deviation.

TABLE 19–1. AN ARRAY OF WEIGHTS OF TEN CHILDREN

Individual Weights (X) (in pounds)	
20	70
50	70
60	80
60	100
70	120

Where ΣX = 700 pounds, N = 10 individual weights, $\underline{X} = \dfrac{\Sigma X}{N}$ = 70, $\underline{X}$ = 70 pounds.

within one standard deviation on either side of the mean ($\pm$ one SD), 95 percent of all values fall within two standard deviations from the mean (± 2 SD), and 99 percent fall within three standard deviations from the mean (± 3 SD).

To understand standard deviation and its relationship to dispersion, it is helpful to consider a simple example of how individual scores deviate from the mean, and how they are dispersed around the central tendency, represented by the average score of the group; i.e., the mean (Table 19–1).

With the calculation of the mean for the group, it is now possible to calculate how much each individual deviates from the mean score (Table 19–2).

Having averaged all of the scores, the deviations of each individual score from the mean fall one-half on the positive side and one-half on the negative, resulting in a summated score of zero. Therefore, this method cannot be used to find an average deviation, or variance.

TABLE 19–2. WEIGHTS OF CHILDREN EXPRESSED AS DEVIATION FROM THEIR MEAN

Original Weights (X)	Deviation Scores $(X - \bar{X})$
20	-50
50	-20
60	-10
60	-10
70	0
70	0
70	0
80	$+10$
100	$+30$
120	$+50$

Σ of all deviation scores = 0

TABLE 19–3. SQUARED DEVIATION SCORES OF WEIGHTS OF CHILDREN

Individual Scores (X)	Deviation Scores ($X - \overline{X}$)	Squared Deviation Scores ($X - \overline{X}$)²
20	− 50	2500
50	− 20	400
60	− 10	100
60	− 10	100
70	0	0
70	0	0
70	0	0
80	+ 10	100
100	+ 30	900
120	+ 50	2500
		6600

To solve this problem, each number may be squared to eliminate the negative signs. This procedure gives the following: the average variability of the squared deviation scores may be obtained by dividing 6,600 by N, or $6,600 \div 10 = 660$ (Table 19–3). This average squared deviation is in units of the pounds squared; therefore, to return the measure to the original units, the square root of the average squared deviation must be calculated: $660 = 25.69$ pounds—the standard deviation, or SD. To sum up:

$$SD = \sqrt{\frac{\Sigma(X - \overline{X})^2}{N}} = \sqrt{\frac{6600}{10}} = \sqrt{660} = 25.69 \text{ pounds (Fig. 19–7).}$$

Thus, to calculate the standard deviation, the following procedure is followed: (1) determine the mean $\overline{X}$ of all of the values; (2) find the difference between each individual value X and the mean $\overline{X}$; (3) square each deviation; (4) find the sum of the squared deviations and divide by the total number of values to get the mean or average squared deviation; (5) take the square root of the average squared deviations to obtain the standard deviation SD, or the average of the extent to which each score deviates from the mean.

Complementary to the arithmetic mean, the standard deviation is the most widely used measure of variability. It is used when the frequency distribution approximates a normal curve relatively well. *Standard* comes from the fact that the standard deviation indicates a group average spread of scores (or values) around their mean. *Deviation*, indicating the spread of scores around the mean, is measured by how much each score deviates, or is scattered, from the mean.

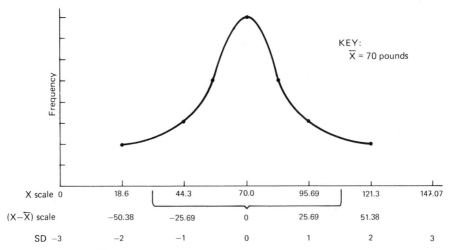

Figure 19–7. Standard deviation of weights of children.

Standard Scores. Symbolized by the lower-case letter "z," *standard scores* tell how many standard deviations away from the mean the particular raw score is. The formula for standard score is:

$$z = \frac{(X - \overline{X})}{SD}$$

where z = standard score, X = individual score, $\overline{X}$ = mean, and SD = standard deviation.

For example, standard scores with a mean set at 500 and a standard deviation set at 100 are used by Medical College Aptitude Tests. Many intelligence and achievement tests use standard scores with a pre-established mean and standard deviation.

BIVARIATE DESCRIPTIVE STATISTICS: CORRELATIONAL PROCEDURES

Bivariate descriptive statistics are those derived from the analysis of two variables simultaneously. This process contrasts with both *univariate statistical analysis*, which summarizes data from a single variable to describe the mode, median, mean, and variance, and *multivariate statistical analysis*, a complex statistical procedure that analyzes three or more variables and which is best undertaken with the use of the computer (to save time and effort). *Bivariate statistical analysis* is concerned with one independent variable and one dependent variable. The researcher wants to know how these two variables are associated, or correlated. Procedures to assess these associations, or relationships, include the use of contingency tables and correlational procedures.

The *contingency table* summarizes descriptive data and provides a cross-tabulation of data. Frequency relationships may be examined using nominal data from qualitative studies, depicted in a 2 × 2 contingency table and analyzed using the chi-square test, which assesses whether a relationship exists between two nominal-level variables (such as tuberculosis and sex). Contingency tables are also used with data from ordinal scales that contain few ranks. The tables are easy to construct, and they summarize considerable information at a glance.

Correlational studies examine how variables change in terms of one another—how a variation in one variable is associated with a variation in another variable; for example, how lung cancer is associated with cigarette smoking. The researcher does not intervene in the process of change but, rather, examines how the variations are interrelated with one another. Correlations form a scale from minus one (− 1) through zero (0) to plus one (+ 1). Minus one is a perfect negative relationship, 0 is no relationship at all, and + 1 is a perfect positive relationship. Correlations reflect a two-way association, a numerical estimate of the magnitude of the relationship between two sets of data.

A *correlation coefficient* is an index that summarizes the extent of the relationship from − 1 to 0 to + 1. If two variables are perfectly correlated, the relationship is 1.00; if the relationship is not perfect, the correlation is less than 1. The closer the correlation is to 1, the stronger it is; the closer it approaches 0, the weaker it is. If two variables are not related at all, the correlation coefficient is 0. If two variables are perfectly inversely related, the correlation coefficient is − 1. *Inverse relationship* means that an increase in one variable is associated with a decrease in the other variables. As the correlation coefficient moves from − 1 toward 0, the inverse association is weakened—i.e., an increase in one is barely associated with a decrease in the other.

The researcher commonly uses correlational procedures to describe the relationship between two measures from ordinal, interval, or ratio scales. For example, they are used to assess the stability, or the reliability, of an instrument. The reliability of an instrument is stable if the researcher can administer the same test to a sample of individuals on two occasions and can establish a high correlation coefficient (usually greater than .70) between the two. Correlations can be established graphically or by the calculation of the index to indicate the magnitude of the association.

The *scatter diagram*, or *scatter plot*, is a graphic representation of correlation between two variables (Figure 19–8). To create a scatter diagram on a rectangular coordinate graph, the range of values for one variable is scaled on the horizontal axis, and a dot or point is placed at the proper place on the scale. The range of values for the second variable is scaled on the vertical axis by placing a dot or point at the proper place on the scale. From either the scatter or the concentration of the points,

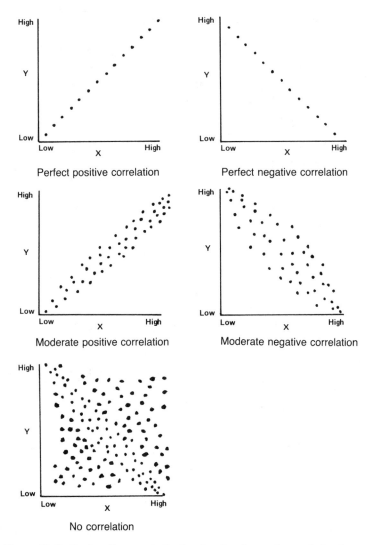

Figure 19–8. Scatter diagrams indicating the direction and magnitude of a correlation.

the direction and magnitude of a correlation are depicted. A positive correlation is evident if the slope of the points begins at the lower-left corner and extends in a line to the upper-right corner. The denser, or closer, the points are to one another, the stronger the relationship. A negative correlation is evident if the slope of the points begins at the upper-left corner and extends in a line to the lower-right corner. The more closely packed the points in a line, the stronger the negative correlation. A weak relationship is indicated by the width of the lines; the broader the width, the weaker the relationship. No relationship is indicated by a scatter of points all over the graph.

The *correlation coefficient index* is considered better than graphs to express the direction and magnitude of a relationship between two variables. Two such indices are *Spearman's rank-order correlation rho* and *Kendall's tau*. Both of these procedures are recommended by Fox (1982, p. 343) when both variables have been measured on the ordinal scale with more than six, but fewer than 20, gradations of response (such as the number of units in a hospital). Both of these procedures rank the two sets of data and compute a correlation by which to estimate the extent to which the ranks are associated. Ranking seldom has meaning when there are fewer than seven gradations by which to rank.

The *Pearson product-moment correlation*, symbolized by "r" and the correlation ratio are recommended if both variables have been measured at the interval level, thereby providing continuous data. Both are computationally similar, and both range from -1.0 through 0 to $+1.0$.

Perfect correlations are rare, and the determination of a strong or weak relationship varies. For physiological associations, the correlation should be greater than .07 to be considered strong.

Correlations at the level of multiple variables may use several techniques. A *correlational matrix* is used to compute the correlations between all possible pairs of variables. To estimate the minimum number of separate variables, or factors, necessary to provide the information contained in a correlational matrix, the researcher uses factor analysis as a procedure. *Factor analysis*, rather than addressing the nature of the interrelationships among several variables, analyzes the structure of the interrelationships in order to determine the number and kinds of variables needed to explain it.

MULTIVARIATE METHODS: CORRELATIONAL PROCEDURES FOR THREE OR MORE VARIABLES

Multivariate methods of data analysis refer to those statistical procedures that analyze the relationships among three or more variables. For example, Hasselmeyer (1961) used six measures of behavior in her study of the effect of the use of a diaper roll on the behavior of premature infants. These included eating ability, crying behavior, sleep behavior, bodily movements, and time required to regain initial birth weight.

Multivariate methods of data analysis are becoming more common in nursing as researchers have increasing access to computers for statistical procedures (such as the Statistical Package for the Social Sciences, or SPSS). However, there are not as many techniques for the analysis of correlations among multiple variables as there are for two variables. Those commonly used include the correlational matrix, factor analysis, and multiple regression.

The *correlational matrix* takes the multiple variables of a study and correlates each of the variables with every other variable, obtaining as many different correlations as there are variables to correlate. The matrix presents the interrelationship, allowing the researcher to make observations that are otherwise impossible to make.

Factor analysis is a technique for interpretation. It estimates the minimum number of variables (factors) needed to provide the information contained in a correlational matrix. It identifies which variables are interrelated as unified concepts; i.e., it interprets the correlations so as to find functionally unitary traits in two or more correlated variables. Rather than answering questions about the nature of interrelationships among variables, it looks for the underlying structure of the interrelationship in order to determine how many variables, and what kinds of variables, are needed to explain the interrelationship. For example, Jalowiec et al. (1984), assessing the Jalowiec Coping Scale, used the SPSS to perform a factor analysis on coping-scale data from 141 subjects. Principal factor extraction (the first step to reduce the variables) was used to determine the minimum number of independent factors that would satisfactorily produce the correlations between variables. Further analysis was then performed on the significant factors extracted in order to maximize the high correlations and minimize the low ones, thereby making the clustering of variables more obvious, so as to enhance factor interpretation. Factor analysis thus reduced a large set of variables to a smaller, more manageable set.

The *coefficient of concordance* is a procedure for ordinal data, used if ranks for several variables for a set of respondents are available. The coefficient of concordance computes the rank-order correlation for each separate pair of variables, as well as the arithmetic mean of the several rank-order correlations.

Multiple regression is a correlational procedure that analyzes the effects of two or more independent variables on a dependent variable, the criterion measure. It predicts future performances of the variables under study, utilizing knowledge of several predictor variables to predict one variable, the criterion variable. Multiple regression begins with the process of simple regression; i.e., with data for predictors and criteria needed for one group. A correlational matrix is then developed from these data that shows the relationship between the predictor variables and the relationship of each predictor to the criterion measure. For example, Miles (1985), in her study of emotional symptoms and physical health in bereaved parents, used All Possible Subsets Regression Analysis to evaluate the relative contribution of selected person–situation variables to the emotional symptomatology scores in the combined group of bereaved parents. Woods (1985), in her study of the relationship of socialization and stress to perimenstrual symptoms, disability, and menstrual attitudes, used the SPSS Multiple-Regression Procedure to test the proposed relationships among stressful milieus, socialization, menstrual attitudes, and disability for three groups of symptoms. Cowan and Murphy (1985), in their study of postdisaster bereavement risk predictors, used Multiple-Regression Analysis to determine the extent to which six risk variables combined (age, gender, life stress, social support, centrality of relationship, and belief of preventability) could predict high-risk health outcomes, such as depression, somatization, and risk to physical health.

Analysis of covariance (ANCOVA) is a procedure for controlling extraneous variables. It combines both multiple regression and analysis of variance. It is used in experimental and quasi-experimental designs to give added control. For example, Harris and Hyman (1984), in their record review of clean versus sterile tracheotomy care and level of pulmonary infection, sought to determine if clean tracheotomy care was more effective than sterile care, as measured by levels of postoperative pulmonary infection. The researchers used the analysis of covariance to analyze the data obtained. Laboratory data supported practicing clean procedures as those associated with the lowest levels of postoperative infection.

Discriminant analysis is the use of multiple-regression analysis with a dependent variable at the nominal level to predict group membership on the basis of two or more independent variables.

INTERPRETATION OF DATA SUMMARIES

Interpretation of the data summaries consists of extracting meaning and conclusions from the data. The method of interpretation is reasoning, from data summaries, tables, graphs, tests, and comparisons. The researcher summarizes what was found; draws conclusions about the significance and importance of the data findings for nursing; compares findings to other studies; and relates findings to the research problem, assumptions, hypotheses, or existing theory. The researcher states the extent to which it is possible to generalize from the findings of the study sample to a larger population. The researcher also identifies gaps in knowledge that need to be filled by future research; suggests specific areas for additional research; and criticizes his or her own work, pointing out strengths and weaknesses. When possible, the researcher makes recommendations for using the findings in practice or suggests the extent to which it is possible to prescribe, given the current level of knowledge.

SUMMARY

The summary, analysis, and interpretation of data begin when all of the data are collected, although the researcher plans for this step from the beginning of the project. Qualitative data are summarized as frequencies, rate, ratios, proportions, and percentages. Quantitative data are summarized by additional measures, including mean, median, mode (central tendency), and standard deviation (variation).

Analysis of qualitative data includes content analysis, counting, and constructing tables and graphs. Content analysis includes the development of a set of categories to represent the content being analyzed; comparisons of the source of the message; the process that resulted in the message; transmitting the message; the recipient of the message; and the effects of the message. A technique for counting and recording frequency includes the construction of tally sheets and all-purpose tables that record the counts and summarize the raw data. Bar graphs and special-purpose tables summarize data further and provide visual depictions of the data. Ratios, proportions, percentages, rates, and index numbers use frequencies to summarize data further.

A ratio between two quantities is the number of times that one number contains the other. A proportion is the relation in size of one thing compared to another—an equality of ratios. A percent is the parts in a hundred that a portion of the whole represents. A rate is the quantity, amount, or degree measured in proportion to something else.

An analysis of quantitative data includes the use of elementary descriptive statistics and correlational procedures. To begin analysis, raw data must be organized in a form suitable for descriptive summaries. If computer analysis is planned, data must be coded.

To begin a data summary, data may be tabulated—arranged in a concise and logical order—by using an array, a frequency, or a frequency distribution. An array ranks the observation from lowest to highest. A frequency counts the number of cases that belong to various categories. A frequency distribution indicates how certain characteristics are spread across different categories.

Tables and graphs are helpful ways by which to depict data summaries. Tables may take many forms, but all include basic information, including title, stub, box head, line, column, cell, body, and source of data.

A graph is a diagram or line that shows how one quantity either depends on or changes with another. Commonly used graphs are the pie graph, bar graph, histogram, and frequency polygon. The pie graph is a circle that represents 100 percent of the sample. It is used to represent discontinuous frequencies, such as those measured by the nominal scale. The bar graph is also used to depict data measured by the nominal scale, but it uses the X or Y axis of a graph to record its data. The histogram is a frequency-distribution graph that records continuous data from ratio and interval scales. The frequency of a class of data is represented by the height of the bars; the interval, by the width of the bars. A frequency-distribution polygon may be made from a histogram by putting a dot in the center of each column and connecting the dots with a line.

Measures of central tendency include the mean (or average score), the median (or middle score), and the mode (or most frequent score). The mode is the only measure of central tendency usable with the nominal scale; the median is useful if the distribution of the scores is skewed; and the mean is the most widely used measure and represents the average score.

The variance examines the dispersion of scores around the central values. The range is the simplest measure of dispersion; it defines the difference between the largest and the smallest observations. The inter-quartile range includes the scores between the lowest quarter of an array of scores and the highest quarter. The standard deviation is an index that measures the extent that individual scores, on the average, deviate from the mean.

Bivariate descriptive statistics are those derived from the analysis of two variables simultaneously, with one independent and one dependent variable. The contingency table summarizes descriptive data and provides a cross-tabulation of data. Nominal data from qualitative studies may be depicted in a 2 × 2 table for use in chi-square testing. Correlational studies examine the change in two variables in terms of one another. Correlations form a scale from − 1 through 0 to + 1. Minus one is a perfect negative relationship; when one variable increases, the other decreases. Plus one is a perfect positive relationship; when one variable increases, the other increases. Zero indicates no relationship. The closer to zero the correlation is, the weaker the correlation is. A correlation coefficient is an index that summarizes the extent of the relationship. The Spearman's rank-order correlation rho and Kendall's tau are two indices of correlation that are recommended for use when both variables have been measured on the ordinal scale with more than six, and fewer than 20, ranks of response. The Pearson product-moment correlation, symbolized by the lower-case letter "r," and the correlation ratio, are used if both variables have been measured at the interval level. The scatter plot is a graphic representation of a correlation between two variables.

Multiple variables require techniques such as the correlational matrix. Factor analysis is used to examine the nature of the interrelationships among several variables in order to determine the number or kinds of variables needed to study a particular relationship.

Interpretation of data summaries means extracting the meaning from the data. The researcher uses reasoning and comparison to draw conclusions or to relate findings to the research problem's hypothesis or theory. The researcher must determine the following: the extent to which it is possible to generalize, the gaps in knowledge that continue to exist, and the research needed to fill those gaps. In addition, the researcher criticizes the research, noting its strengths and weaknesses. When possible, the researcher makes recommendations for the use of the research findings in practice. The current level of knowledge must be noted in making such recommendations.

The function of data analysis is to provide a summarization of completed observations in order that research questions may be answered. The function of interpretations of data is to bring the intellectual focus of the researcher to bear upon the data in order to elucidate the meanings of the research findings.

EXAMPLE FROM NURSING RESEARCH
Data Analysis

S. Penckofer and K. Holm, (1984): Early appraisal of coronary revascularization on quality of life. Nursing Research, 33, 60–63.

To assess the impact of bypass surgery, the researchers compared two groups of bypass patients three to eight months postoperatively. Patients were asked to rate themselves in relation to past, present, and future life satisfaction. In addition, the patients were asked to report the level of angina before and after surgery; the level of physical activity before and after; and satisfaction with family life, social life, and sexual life.

The researchers utilized an analysis of variance (ANOVA) to indicate the association between the patients' view of future life satisfaction compared to their life satisfaction prior to open-heart surgery. To analyze demographic characteristics, the researchers used percentages, range, averages, and standard deviation. For example, 88 percent of the patients were white, 15 percent were professional, and 41 percent were skilled or unskilled. The age range was from 40 to 61 years, the average being 48.823 years, and the standard deviation equaled 6.90. A two-way ANOVA with repeated measures on pre-operative and postoperative angina ratings yielded a significant difference for time periods; patients in both groups reported less angina after surgery ($\bar{X}$ = 4.73 and SD = .89). A two-way ANOVA with repeated measures was also computed on ratings of activities before and after surgery, with a significantly higher level of activity found after surgery. Statistics for satisfaction of family life, social life, occupation, and sexual life utilized the mean and the standard deviation. A two-way ANOVA with repeated measures indicated that patients experienced greater satisfaction with social life and sexual life postoperatively.

STUDY QUESTIONS _____

1. You are studying all personnel in the hospitals of Central City who are involved with bedside nursing care. Make a list of the categories you would expect to find. How could the categories be transformed into numerical symbols?
2. You have a category (race) that contains 400 persons, 150 of whom are black. What proportion—what percent of the category—is not black?
3. Construct an array for the following set of blood pressure scores, with attention first to the systolic and then to the diastolic:

130/60 190/100 110/50 240/120 120/80 90/40 185/100

4. Below is a set of test scores. What is the median? the mean? the mode?

100, 100, 40, 60, 70, 70, 70, 65, 65, 65, 65, 80, 95, 85, 30, 70, 70, 80, 80

5. Below is a group of weights. Construct a frequency distribution.

105	120	138	155	161	170	178	181
110	123	150	157	165	173	179	185
118	130	151	160	169	175	179	189

6. With the same data, construct a histogram.
7. Drawing on the data in Question 5, construct a table indicating a relationship among weight, sex, and race. Columns one and two are white women, columns three and four are black women, columns five and six are black men, and columns seven and eight are white men.
8. Construct a bar graph showing the relationship between the weights of all of the men, compared with the weights of all of the women.
9. Compare measures of central tendency with those at variance.

REFERENCES AND SUGGESTED READINGS

Abdellah, F. and Levine, E. (1979): Better Patient Care Through Research. New York: Macmillan. *Chaps. 8 and 9 examine data processing and analysis.*

Armstrong, F. (1981): Parametric statistics and ordinal data: A pervasive misconception. Nursing Research, *30*, 60–62.

Byrne, T. and Edeani, D. (1984): Knowledge of medical terminology among hospital patients. Nursing Research, *33*, 178–181. *Use of percentages, mean, standard deviation, Pearson correlational analysis, correlation coefficient.*

Caty, S., Ellerton, M., and Ritchie, J. (1984): Coping in hospitalized children: An analysis of published case studies. Nursing Research, *33*, 277–282. *Content analysis.*

Cowan, M. and Murphy, S. (1985): Identification of postdisaster bereavement risk predictors. Nursing Research, *34*, 71–75.

Evans, J. (1982): Invitation to Psychological Research. New York: Holt, Rinehart, & Winston. *Content analysis.*

Flaskerud, J. (1984): A comparison of perceptions of problematic behavior by six minority groups and mental health professionals. Nursing Research, *33*, 190–197. *Use of chi-square test, percentages, mode, mean.*

Fox, D. (1982): Fundamentals of Research in Nursing (4th ed.). Norwalk, Conn.: Appleton-Century-Crofts. *Chap. 19, "Techniques for the analysis of quantitative* data"; Chap. 20, "Descriptive statistics"; Chap. 21, "Correlational procedures;" Chap. 23, "The analysis of qualitative data."

Fox, D. and Ventura, M. (1984): Internal psychometric characteristics of the quality patient care scale. Nursing Research *33*, 112–117. *Factor analysis.*

Gortner, S., Hudes, M., and Zyzanski, S. (1984): Appraisal of values in the choice of treatment. Nursing Research, *33*, 319–324. *Spearman rank order correlations; factor analysis.*

Harris, R. and Hyman, R. (1984): Clean vs. sterile tracheotomy care and level of pulmonary infection. Nursing Research, *33*, 80–85.

Hasselmeyer, E. (1961): Behavior Patterns of Premature Infants. Washington, D.C.: Government Printing Office.

Holsti, O. (1968): Content analysis. In Lindzey, G. and Aronson, E. (eds.), The Handbook of Social Psychology. Reading, Mass.: Addison-Wesley. *Content analysis.*

Hubbard, P., Muhlenkamp, A., and Brown, N. (1984): The relationship between social support and self-care practices. Nursing Research, *33*, 266–270. *Mean, standard deviation, and range.*

Jalowiec, A., Murphy, S., and Powers, M. (1984): Psychometric assessment of the Jalowiec coping scale. Nursing Research, *33*, 157–161.

Lin, N. (1976): Foundation of Social Research. New York: McGraw-Hill. *Includes a chapter describing one variable.*

Kendall, K. (1977): Maternal and child nursing in an Iranian village. In Leininger, M. (ed.), Transcultural Nursing. New York: Wiley. *Qualitative study, identifies themes; reliability assessment; factor analysis; use of SPSS.*

Maxwell, A. (1961): Analysing Qualitative Data. New York: Barnes & Noble. *Studies the chi-square.*

Miles, M. (1985): Emotional symptoms and physical health in bereaved parents. Nursing Research, *34*, 76–81. *Use of the chi-square.*

Penckofer, S. and Holm, K. (1984): Early appraisal of coronary revascularization on quality of life. Nursing Research, *33*, 60–63.

Van Ort, S., Gerber, R. (1976): Topical application of insulin in the treatment of decubitus ulcers. Nursing Research, *2*, 9–12. *Pearson's r.*

Volicer, B. and Bohannon, M. (1970): A hospital stress rating scale. Nursing Research, *24*, 32–39. *Spearman's rank-order correlation.*

Woods, N. (1985): Relationship of socialization and stress to perimenstrual symptoms, disability and menstrual attitudes. Nursing Research, *34*, 145–149. *Mean.*

20

Statistical Inference

Statistical inference is a combination of mathematical processes and logical principles that allows the researcher to test estimations and statistical hypotheses (null hypotheses) against actual data. The researcher uses statistical inference for two purposes: (1) to estimate the probability that data found in the randomly drawn sample accurately reflect the target population or universe from which they were drawn; and (2) to test the null hypotheses formulated from the research hypothesis.

Upon completion of this chapter, the student should be able to: (1) define concepts used in the study of inferential statistics; (2) compare descriptive and inferential statistics; (3) describe samples, populations, standard errors of the mean, and chance factors; (4) describe how to estimate population parameters; (5) compare the estimation of population parameters with the testing of statistical hypotheses; (6) describe the relationship between the research hypothesis and the null hypothesis; (7) explain how to formulate a null hypothesis; (8) describe Type I and Type II errors; and (9) define, describe, and contrast parametric and nonparametric statistical tests.

CONCEPTS USED IN THE STUDY OF INFERENTIAL STATISTICS

Like research in general, inferential statistics has a language of its own. Learning the concepts used in the study of inferential statistics enables the student, not only to read research reports with better understanding, but also to understand the general process associated with the ability to generalize from a sample to the target population from which the sample

TABLE 20–1. DEFINITIONS OF SELECTED CONCEPTS

Chance Factors—the residual, unknown factors that affect events after the factors that determine events have been isolated.

Hypothesis

 Null—likewise known as H_0, the *statistical hypothesis*, the *test hypothesis*, the *benchmark hypothesis*; refers to any hypothesis that is subject to nullification by a sample statistic; a hypothesis formulated to state no relationship between specified variables and populations.

 Statistical—same as null hypothesis.

 Research—likewise known as the *scientific*, *experimental*, or *theoretical hypothesis*, or as H_1, a statement of the predicted interrelationships among a number of variables that the researcher expects to find in the sample data.

Level of Significance—the probability that an observed relationship or value could be attributed to the tendency for the sample statistic to fluctuate from one sample to the other. The probability of rejecting the null hypothesis when it is true. Used in research involving human subjects; often set at .001, but no lower than .01.

Mean—the average value.

Population—any set of persons, things, or measurements having an observable characteristic in common. A universe.

 Parameter—a hypothetical *true* value for a population; any measurable characteristic of the population, such as the population mean.

 Target Population—the specified subjects or cases from which the study sample was drawn and about which the researcher intends to generalize. May be distinguished from the accessible population, which refers to that population actually available for a study.

Sample—any subset of a population.

 Sample Statistic—a value computed entirely from the sample, such as the mean or average, that the researcher computes from observations.

Sampling—the process of selecting a subset of a population for inclusion in a study.

 Random Sampling—affording each unit in the population an equal chance or probability of being chosen for the study sample.

 Sampling Distribution—data that represent characteristics of samples.

Statistic—both a summary value (such as the mean) that is calculated from a sample of observations, and an estimator of some population parameter (i.e., the *true value* of a population).

Statistics—Descriptive—summary measures such as means, medians, modes, percentages, ratios, and standard deviations, calculated from measurements of sample units.

 Inferential—the process by which the researcher is able to generalize from the sample data to the target population.

Tests of Statistical Significance—a technique of testing that allows the researcher to determine whether or not summary measures could be independent estimates of the same population parameter.

was drawn. Table 20–1 summarizes very briefly some of the concepts used in this chapter.

A COMPARISON OF DESCRIPTIVE AND INFERENTIAL STATISTICS

A *statistic* is both a summary value (such as the mean) that is calculated from a sample of observations and an estimator of some population parameter (i.e., *true value*). A statistic is both the factual data and the use of such data to infer or estimate population parameters from sample statistics.

Descriptive statistics (such as the mean) summarize research data from a sample, while *inferential statistics* use the data from randomly drawn samples, both to infer characteristics of the population from which the sample was drawn and to test statistical hypotheses. Descriptive statistics may be used whether or not random sampling has been used, but inferential statistics require the use of random sampling and other processes based on the principles of probability. Researchers in the clinical area often use random assignment alone, rather than in combination with random selection, but base their inferences to the larger population (that is, the external validity of their study, or the ability to generalize) on the findings of repeated study of samples. Descriptive statistics summarize the unwieldy mass of raw data, transforming it into frequencies, means, and other summaries that point out the characteristics of the sample. While of basic importance, such findings are usually limited to the sample under study, unless the process of random sampling has been used.

Inferential statistics allow the researcher to go beyond the description and summary of data. An inferential statistic is a tool that enables the researcher to use findings summarized from randomly collected samples in order to make judgments about a population and to test a statistical hypothesis about the characteristics of a population. The researcher can infer (or estimate) the extent to which relationships observed in the study sample would occur in the population from which the study sample was drawn by the use of random sampling.

Populations, Samples, and Chance Factors

Central to the study of statistical inference is the relationship among the concepts of population, sample, and chance.

Any set of persons, things, or measurements having an observable characteristic in common constitutes a *population* or, as it is sometimes called, a *universe*. A *population parameter* is a hypothetical *true value* for a population—any measurable characteristic of the population, such as the population mean or variance. A population may be finite; for example, all patients who come to City Clinic for the treatment of cancer. Or, the population may be infinite; for example, all persons who have had, or ever will have, cancer. Population parameters are usually designated in the literature by Greek letters such as *mu* (μ), which stands for the population mean, or small *sigma* (σ), which stands for the population standard deviation.

A *sample* is any subset of a population, symbolized (as a rule) by English letters, such as $\overline{X}$ (the mean), and X (a single score). A *sample statistic* is a value computed entirely from the sample—a numerical descriptive measure (such as the mean or average) that the researcher summarizes and computes from observations. Samples may be variously collected but, to be used to infer, a sample must have been selected by random sampling.

Chance factors are the residual, unknown factors that affect events after the factors that determine events have been isolated. The observable world is not a world of complete certainty; there is always some degree of uncertainty. But neither is the world one of chance alone. The researcher attempts to reduce the number of factors of which he or she is ignorant. Where uncertainty remains, the researcher tries to calculate the extent of such factors and the risk of error that they introduce. The laws of probability provide the basic ingredient in inferential statistics and enable the researcher to calculate the element of risk as inference is made from sample to population.

Estimation of Population Parameters

To estimate a population parameter, such as the population mean, the researcher begins after the data are collected. As the researcher knows, the data found in the sample may differ from those found for the "parent" population. For example, 100 different samples randomly drawn from the same population may differ somewhat in statistics (such as the mean), both from one another and from the population. Yet, sampling is the most economical way, in most instances, to study a population. The size of the population, the cost in time and money necessary to observe all of the elements, and the difficulty of being able to observe all of the subjects make the study of the total population prohibitive. Moreover, measuring the total population could destroy or change the units, or affect the subsequent state. To determine the characteristics of the total universe of a person's blood, it is not necessary to take all of the blood from the body. Therefore, the researcher takes a sample and, from this sample, estimates (or infers) the parameters of the population.

However, a number of problems are inherent in such an approach. First, the researcher, in all likelihood, has data from only one sample, which contains about 30 subjects. Due to the vagaries of chance sampling, there is the probability that a discrepancy may exist between the sample statistic and the population parameter. A *sampling error*—the deviations of all sample means drawn from a population from the true mean of the population—may have occurred as a result of random sampling. The sample statistic, such as the mean, may deviate from the true mean of the population. Second, the researcher determines how close the mean of the sample is to the mean of the population that may be unknown. How is the mean of an unknown population estimated?

It is possible to demonstrate that the mean of a sample, not only tends to gravitate toward and to cluster around the population means, but also that the pattern of distribution of a large number of sample means drawn from the same population tends to assume a shape approaching that of the normal (bell-shaped) curve.

To examine these assertions, it is necessary to understand the process of obtaining a sampling distribution, although few researchers will actually go through this time-consuming, tedious process.

Sampling distributions are data that represent characteristics of samples, not individual cases. For example, individual cases may be put into various categories whose mode, median, and mean may be calculated, revealing the characteristic of one sample. But a sampling distribution of the mean uses an infinite number of samples drawn from the same population. To construct a sampling distribution of the means of a large number of samples, the researcher would take the following steps:

1. Designate the target population.
2. From this population, draw (by random sampling) a very large number of samples (for example, thousands of samples); each of these samples must be of equal size and must contain no less than 30 subjects.
3. Compute the mean for each of the samples.
4. Put all of the sample means into a frequency-distribution graph.
5. Calculate the mean of the sample means.

According to the *central-limit theorem*, the mean of this distribution will probably approach the population mean, and the shape of the frequency distribution graph will probably fit the characteristics of the normal, bell-shaped (Gaussian) curve. Thus, the researcher can be assured that the statistic from the sample will always bear a relationship to the corresponding population parameter, which may be unknown. The sample statistic tends to cluster around the population parameter in a recognizable manner. The researcher with data from a single randomly drawn sample may feel assured that, while the data may vary from the population parameter, they usually will not vary far, especially if the number of observations in the sample is large. In addition, the variance of the sample can be calculated with techniques of inferential statistics. Should the researcher be able to increase the size of the sample, the average sampling errors will decrease, although the researcher must quadruple the sample size to cut errors in half. The fact that the sampling distribution of means approaches a normal curve allows the researcher to treat the distribution in much the same way that he or she treats any normal distribution.

The *standard error of the mean* is the standard deviation of a sampling distribution—i.e., the standard deviation of a theoretical distribution of sample means. The smaller the standard error (that is, the less the sample means vary), the more accurate the means are as estimates of the population's "true value." The standard error of the mean is used to construct the normal curve as a model for inferences about the difference between two means. The standard error of the mean is computed by dividing the standard deviation of the sample by the square root of the sample size.

$$\begin{array}{c}\text{Standard error} \\ \text{of the mean}\end{array} = \frac{\text{The standard deviation of the sample (SD)}}{\text{The square root of the sample size}(\sqrt{n})}$$

The number of points computed is used to construct a normal curve of the sampling distribution of means. The probability, then, is that 68 percent of the cases will lie within one standard deviation above and below the mean, 95 percent within two standard deviations, and nearly 100 percent within three standard deviations above and below the mean.

Testing Statistical Hypotheses

The two general types of statistical inference include the estimation of population parameters, which has just been examined, and the testing of statistical hypotheses, which will be examined now. The estimation of a population parameter begins *after* the data are collected. The testing of statistical hypotheses begins *before* the data are collected: the researcher formulates the statistical (null) hypothesis from the research hypothesis,* specifies the "level of significance" at which the null hypothesis is to be rejected, and then collects the data that she or he will analyze to test the hypothesis.

Both procedures, estimating population and testing statistical hypotheses, are based upon probability theory and the use of random sampling. Both are concerned with population parameters (as these are related to sample statistics), both must deal with sampling error, and both must rely upon the sampling distribution of a statistic. However, the estimation of a population parameter begins with the sample data and ends with a range of values (the confidence interval and its accompanying confidence level), within which the population parameter probably lies. On the other hand, testing the statistical hypothesis begins with the null hypothesis, which predicts that the relationship between variables stated in the research hypothesis is probably only due to chance. It ends with a decision to accept or reject the null hypothesis on the basis of sample data. The use of inferential statistics in testing the null hypothesis, in order to arrive at a decision to accept or reject it, will now be examined.

The Null Hypothesis and Related Concepts

A null hypothesis is formulated in order to be rejected. The researcher uses principles of probability to test the statement that observed effects are only chance occurrences. Data that fail to support the null hypothesis indicate to the researcher that the findings probably are *not* due to chance alone, a crucial point in the interpretation of the data. However, the researcher can make two types of errors in deciding to accept or reject

---

*The *research hypothesis* is a statement of the *expected relationships* among phenomena being studied; the *null hypothesis* states that the differences obtained in the values between the groups being compared could have occurred by chance alone.

TABLE 20–2. ERRORS IN HYPOTHESIS TESTING

The Decision of the Researcher is to:	The Null Hypothesis is Actually:	
	True	False
1. Reject the null hypothesis	Type I error, with a given probability of alpha*	Correct decision
2. Accept the null hypothesis	Correct decision	Type II error with a given probability of beta†

*Alpha: the level of significance or the degree of risk involved in rejecting the null hypothesis.
†Beta: the degree of risk involved in failing to reject the null hypothesis.

the null hypothesis, Type I or Type II (Table 20–2). A *Type I error* arises when the researcher decides to reject the null hypothesis when it is actually true. A *Type II error* is made when the researcher decides to accept the null hypothesis when it is actually false. The researcher controls the risk of making a Type I error (rejecting a true null hypothesis) by selecting a level of significance. The *level of significance* is simply a phrase used to designate the probability of rejecting a null hypothesis when it is true. It does *not* indicate the findings' importance or meaning.

Steps to follow in the formulation and testing of a null hypothesis include the following, each of which will be discussed:

1. Formulate the research hypothesis.
2. Formulate the null hypothesis, which states that the results observed are due to chance alone.
3. Specify the level of significance at which the null hypothesis is to be rejected. The level of significance is usually set at .05 or at .01. A level of significance of .05 means that a true null hypothesis would be rejected in only five samples out of 100. A level of significance of .01 means that a true null hypothesis would be rejected in only one sample out of 100.
4. Complete all of the steps in the planning phase of the research project.
5. Obtain the study sample by using random sampling.
6. Collect and summarize the numerical data.
7. Complete analysis of data, using appropriate statistical tests to calculate the probability that the null hypothesis is true.
8. Make a decision to accept or reject the null hypothesis at the given level of significance.

Step One: Formulate the Research Hypothesis. The *research hypothesis*, likewise known as the *scientific hypothesis*, the *experimental hypothesis*, H_1, or the *theoretical hypothesis*, is a statement of the predicted interrelationships among a number of variables (at least two) that the researcher expects to find in the sample data. The research hypothesis is formulated during the planning period, with reference to the theory or empirical generalization from which it is deduced. The purpose of hypothesis testing is to ascertain the extent to which the relationships observed in the sample statistics may be generalized to the population from which the sample was drawn. Ultimately, the researcher hopes that the data will support or clarify theories designed to explain what is present in the empirical world, how phenomena change, how things remain the same, or how events or variables are interrelated.

For example, the experimental hypothesis is tested by observing the specified variables both before and after an independent variable has been introduced; by comparing the changes in the experimental group with any changes in the control group; and by inferring whether the hypothesis should be rejected or accepted on the basis of the findings. However, the researcher does not know whether the findings are the result of his or her manipulation of the independent variable or of sampling error. Therefore, the researcher formulates a statistical (null) hypothesis in order to test statistically the probability that the findings are due to chance alone. Rejection of the null hypothesis tends to strengthen the research hypothesis.

Step Two: Formulate the Null Hypothesis. The *null hypothesis*, likewise known as H_0, the *statistical hypothesis*, the *test hypothesis*, and the *benchmark hypothesis*, was conceived to refer originally to any hypothesis that is subject to nullification by a sample statistic. However, it is often used, in a more restricted sense, to refer to a hypothesis formulated to state no relationship—no correlation or causality—between specified variables or specified populations.* The formulation of a null hypothesis from an experimental hypothesis is illustrated with the following example modified from Simon (1978, p. 406).

Simon formulates a null hypothesis (which he calls a *benchmark hypothesis*) to examine whether an independent variable "removes" a

---

*The formulation of the null hypothesis is complex, involving not only the hypothesis but a number of related statements included in the following steps:

1. The null hypothesis is formulated from the research hypothesis before data are collected.
2. The null hypothesis states that the statistics observed are due to chance alone.
3. A statement that accompanies the null hypothesis specifies *alpha*—the "level of significance" (Type I error).
4. If possible, the statement specifies the number of observations (N) that will minimize *beta* (Type II error).
5. The statement identifies statistical tests to be used to analyze the data.

All of these steps are taken in Phase 1—the planning phase of the research.

sample under study from the original population. In this case, the original population consists of patients who have cancer. The researcher proposes to test the experimental hypothesis that a drug (drug A) cures cancer, using a sample of 12 patients who are selected from the population of cancer victims. The researcher, first, randomly divides the sample of 12 into two groups: the experimental group, who will receive drug A, and the control group, who will not. He then introduces the drug, the independent variable, into the experimental group. After the drug is given, 5 of the 6 patients in the experimental group are said to be well, while 2 of the 6 in the control group who did not receive the drug are likewise pronounced well. Did the drug affect the rate of recovery from cancer? Will patients who take the drug in the future have a higher rate of recovery than they would have had if they had not taken the drug? Specifically, did drug A remove the patients in the experimental group from the original population of cancer victims with its original chances to get well?

In this case, the null hypothesis states, "Patients who take drug A still belong to the original population of cancer victims, with its original chances to get well." That is, the patients have the same chance to get well as if they had never taken the drug. According to the null hypothesis, the drug will make no difference; any differences observed are due to chance alone. If the researcher can test this null hypothesis and find evidence that leads him *not* to accept it, the researcher thereby strengthens the hypothesis that drug A is related to the rate of recovery—that drug A removed the experimental group from the original population, with its original probability of recovery, and provided the patients with a different (and better) probability of recovery.

To formulate the null hypothesis, the researcher first states the experimental hypothesis: "A patient who takes drug A will be cured." Second, he or she rephrases the statement, introducing the concept of chance: "Patients who take drug A have the same chance to get well as those who do not take drug A." Third, the researcher formulates the null hypothesis with reference to specific populations: "Patients who take drug A still belong to the same population as patients who do not take drug A"; i.e., any difference observed between those who took the drug and those who did not is due to chance. The experimental hypothesis has now been translated into the null hypothesis, which can be tested by statistical inference.

Where the research hypothesis states that a difference will be found, the null hypothesis states that no difference will be found. Where an effect is expected, the null hypothesis states that no effect will be found. Where the researcher looks for correlation, the null hypothesis states that no correlation will be found—and so on.

Once the null hypothesis is formulated, the next step is to specify the alpha level of significance involved in rejecting the null hypothesis.

Step Three: Specify the Level of Significance and Related Concepts.
The *level of significance* is the probability of rejecting the null hypothesis
when it is true. The level of significance, however, means different things
depending upon whether *one tail* or *two tails* of the sampling-distribution
curve are to be used to test the null hypothesis. The *region of rejection*
is likewise related to the level of significance, since the *regions* consist of
the sample values (which are located in one or both tails), whose combined
probability is equal to the level of significance.

The *level of significance* is the probability that an observed relationship or value could be attributed to the sampling error—the tendency for
the sample statistic to fluctuate from one sample to the other as well as
from the population. The level of significance is often defined as the
probability of rejecting the null hypothesis when it is true, since the
selection of the level of significance determines whether or not a null
hypothesis will be rejected. The researcher may make an error when he
or she makes a decision to reject the null hypothesis—the null hypothesis
may be true. The researcher can estimate how often he or she is likely
to make such an error. This kind of error is called a Type I error and is
intimately tied to the level of significance set by the researcher. The level
of significance (set at .05, .01, .001, etc.) is set by the researcher as the
maximum risk or error that he or she is willing to run when rejecting
the null hypothesis. The researcher uses the level of significance to evaluate the probability that the sample statistic was obtained due to chance.
Statistical tests reported to be significant at the .05 or .01 level indicate
that the findings would occur by chance only five times in 100 (.05), or
one time in 100 (.01). If the result is likely to occur by chance and the
researcher rejects the null hypothesis, he or she is betting that the findings are not one of the 5 in 100. However, 5 percent of the time, the
researcher will probably be wrong. The level of significance is set at what
the researcher believes to be an appropriate level, given the nature of
the study and its consequences; but another researcher may set the level
of significance at a different level, thereby arriving at a different decision
to reject the null hypothesis. Studies that deal with vital issues of human
health and welfare usually require that the researcher set the level of
significance high (.01, .001, or higher). Less concern about the consequences of rejecting the null hypothesis allows the researcher to set the
level of significance lower; for example, .05 is often employed in sociological research. It should be clear that the level of significance has nothing
to do with the importance or meaning of the research, only with the
probability of chance occurrences. Moreover, rejection of the null hypothesis does not indicate what the nonchance factor is. It is the research
hypothesis that specifies alternatives to the null hypothesis.

Step Four: Complete all steps in the Planning Phase of the research
project.

Step Five: Draw the Sample. Reliance on a sample is the factor that makes the data and inferences probabilistic. Studies that do not employ random sampling, both in the selection of subjects from the population and in the assignment of subjects to the experimental and control groups, should not use tests of significance designated as parametric tests. Therefore, the sample must be drawn by one of the several methods of random sampling. Such sampling is not only scientific but may yield more valid data than those collected by other methods.

Sampling size is also important. The larger the size (N) of the sample, the smaller the probability of making a Type II error—of accepting the null hypothesis when it is actually false. However, it is important to distinguish between an error of sampling and an error of measurement that is caused by a defective instrument. Whether measuring blood pressure or attitudes, a defective instrument will not be corrected by increasing the number of observations. Such errors, called *systematic errors*, are corrected only by selecting a valid and reliable instrument.

Step Six: Collect and Summarize the Numerical Data. Data may be collected in many ways, including observation, questioning, and measurement. Data summaries are obtained by the use of descriptive statistics that calculate frequency, percentages, ratios, central tendencies, and variance.

Step Seven: Use Appropriate Statistical Tests. Statistical tests are classified as either nonparametric or parametric tests of statistical significance. *Nonparametric tests*, such as the Mann-Whitney U test, median test, or the chi-square test, are not as rigorous as parametric tests and are used when the measurement scale has been nominal or ordinal, when the sample size is small, and when a normal distribution of data cannot be assumed. Nonparametric tests require only that random sampling has been used to select the study sample and that the measurements are independent. *Parametric tests*, such a the t-test and the analysis of variance (ANOVA), require random sampling, measurement on a quantitative scale (such as an interval or ratio scale), and a normal distribution of data.

Step Eight: Make a Decision to Accept or Reject the Null Hypothesis. It is not possible to say, without question, that the null hypothesis is true or false. The researcher makes a decision to accept or reject the null hypothesis based upon judgment—how probable it is that observed differences were due to chance, rather than to factors proposed by the research hypothesis. Since the entire population was not examined but only a sample randomly selected from that population, the estimations are based on incomplete information and may not be accurate.

PARAMETRIC AND NONPARAMETRIC STATISTICAL TESTS

Parametric and nonparametric tests are two types of inferential statistics. They are alike in requiring that the study units be selected by random sampling. They differ in several ways: (1) in the size of the sample required; (2) in whether the variables under study are normally distributed; and (3) in the level of measurement that is required.

Parametric Tests

Parametric statistical tests are used with large, homogeneous samples whose variables are normally distributed—i.e., show a bell-shaped distribution curve—and whose measurements have been on at least an interval scale. They are appropriate statistical procedures for testing hypotheses. In fact, the first step in hypothesis testing is that of selecting the appropriate statistic. Parametric tests are powerful, *power* being defined as the ability of the inferential procedure to reject a null hypothesis when it should be rejected. Inferential parametric tests include the t-test, the analysis of variance, and the Pearson Product-Moment Correlation.

The t-test is used to test the significance of differences between means for independent samples and dependent, paired samples. *Independent samples* are those that involve two different groups that are independent; for example, the experimental group and the control group. *Dependent, paired samples* are included in a single group; for example, a single group that is tested before and after an experiment.

Analysis of variance (ANOVA) is used to test the significance of differences between means of three or more groups. It breaks down the total variability of a set of data into the data that result from the independent variable and the data that result from other variabilities. *One-way analysis of variance* deals with the effect of one independent variable on a dependent variable, while *multifactor analysis of variance* deals with the effect of two or more independent variables on a dependent variable.

Pearson's Product-Moment Correlation (r), the most frequently used correlational procedure, is both descriptive and inferential. As a descriptive variable, it is used when the relationship between two continuous variables is such that a change of a certain magnitude in one is consistently accompanied by a corresponding change in the other. As an inferential statistic, it is used to test hypotheses concerning population correlations.

When working with the computer and a software package, such as the Statistical Package for the Social Sciences (SPSS), once the researcher determines the test statistic to be used, the computer does the calculation and prints out the correlation.

Nonparametric Tests

Nonparametric statistical tests, like parametric tests, require that the researcher choose the study units by random sampling. Unlike the parametric statistical tests, nonparametric tests may be used when the data are on the nominal or ordinal level, when the sample is small, and when a normal distribution of variables is not assumed. Nonparametric tests include: the chi-square, used with the nominal scale; the Spearman rank-order correlation test, Kendall's tau, and the Mann-Whitney U test, all used with the ordinal scale; and the Pearson Product-Moment, used with the interval scale.

Chi-Square. The nonparametric correlation test most frequently used with both variables at the nominal level (i.e., homogeneous data) is the chi-square test (X^2). The chi-square test is used to test the differences in proportions, percentages, or frequencies between two or more groups. The test compares categories of data in order to look for associations between the variables. Like all nonparametric tests, it is not concerned with parameters of a population. It is an overall test of the significance of difference in the total pattern of data in the contingency table. The chi-square test seeks to answer the following questions: Have the research findings occurred as a result of chance? Is each variable independent of the other, or are they correlated with one another?

To find an answer to these questions, the researcher compares the research data, called the *observed frequencies* and designated by the symbol Fo, with a group of expected frequencies designated by the symbol Fe. The researcher has the observed frequencies in hand, but must determine what the expected frequencies are from one of the following: (1) a prior performance; for example, previous scores on a test may stand for expected frequency (Fe) for a researcher who wishes to determine if there is any relationship between a teaching program and the grades on a test after teaching; (2) empirical distribution; for example, the number of cases of depression found in health statistics may be used as expected data to compare with the number of cases of depression found in males and females in the observed data; (3) expectations that *no* relationship exists between the variables; i.e., that each variable is independent of the other. (To do this, the researcher states a null hypothesis, which predicts that an equal number of observations will fall in each of the categories.)

For example, a researcher may hypothetically conduct a survey to see if two nominal variables, level of education and compliance with a prescribed diabetic diet, are related. The observed data, which are hypothetical, are shown below:

Level of Compliance	Level of Education		Totals
	High (College)	Low (Grade School)	
High	40	10	50
Low	10	40	50
Totals	50	50	100

In comparing the figures, it seems clear that a person's education makes a difference when predicting compliance with a diabetic diet. Eighty per-cent of those with a college education had a high level of compliance. Thus, education and compliance seem to be correlated. To determine whether the correlation is statistically significant, a table of expected values (using the above totals) may be constructed to show no rela-tionship:

Level of Compliance	Level of Education		Totals
	High (College)	Low (Grade School)	
High	25	25	50
Low	25	25	50
Total	50	50	100

To determine whether the observed data found are significantly different from expected data in which there is no relationship (i.e., the variables are independent of one another), the researcher compares the two using the chi-square formula:

$$X^2 = \Sigma \frac{(Fo - Fe)^2}{Fe}$$

where:

X^2 = chi-square
Fo = observed frequency for a cell
Fe = expected frequency for a cell
Σ = sum of (Fo − Fe) square and divided by Fe for all cells.

$$X = \frac{(40 - 25)^2}{25} + \frac{(10 - 25)^2}{25} + \frac{(10 - 25)^2}{25} + \frac{(40 - 25)^2}{25}$$

$$= \frac{225}{25} + \frac{225}{25} + \frac{225}{25} + \frac{225}{25} = \frac{900}{25} = 36$$

To interpret what 36 means, a chi-square table must be consulted. This table is found in the back of most books on statistics (see Appendix C, p.

423). The researcher must also know the number of degrees of freedom (d.f.) in the table that he or she has constructed. "Degrees of freedom" is computed using the formula $(R - 1) \times (C - 1)$, where R stands for the number of rows in the table and C stands for the number of columns. In the 2×2 table used above, the number of rows is two, and the number of columns is two; therefore, d.f. $= (2 - 1) \times (2 - 1)$, or 1. Looking at a chi-square table, the researcher sees that, for 1 d.f., a chi-square value of 3.84 is significant at the .05 level (meaning that, if the researcher rejects the null hypothesis of independence, he or she will be wrong only 5 times out of 100). The value of 36 (above) exceeds 3.84 considerably; therefore, the researcher can conclude that the relationship between education and compliance with a diabetic diet is statistically significant at the p $=$ .05 level.

Ordinal Scale. Nonparametric correlational tests used with the ordinal scale include: (1) the Spearman rank-order correlation test, used to test correlation of ranks; (2) the Kendall's tau, used to test correlation of ranks; (3) the Mann-Whitney U test, based on rank order.

The *Spearman's rho* is used with: (1) homogeneous data (i.e., measurements obtained in the same form and at the same level); (2) at the ordinal level of measurement; and (3) with two sets of discrete data, obtained by ranking discrete variables. The Spearman's rho is one of the most frequently used correlation procedures for use with homogeneous data. This test is used to determine whether one sample has significantly higher ranks than the other sample, indicating whether the two samples were drawn from different populations or from the same population (with the observed differences due merely to chance).

Kendall's tau, like the Spearman rho, is used with homogeneous data, at the ordinal level of measurement, with two sets of discrete data obtained through ranking discrete variables. The purpose for using Kendall's tau is to provide an estimate of how the two ranks are associated. Some authors suggest using Kendall's tau when the number of study subjects is less than 10.

The *Mann-Whitney U test* is based on rank order. When data from two samples are in the form of ranks (such as occurs with the use of the ordinal scale) or in relative position (in terms of magnitude), the Mann-Whitney U test is used to determine whether one sample has significantly higher ranks than the other sample.

Interval Scale. Nonparametric correlational tests, to be used with the interval scale with homogeneous data, include the *Pearson Product-Moment Correlation*. This is the only test that demonstrates the relationships between two nondichotomous variables; i.e., that provides continuous data.

SUMMARY

Statistical inference is a combination of mathematical processes and logical principles that allows the researcher to test inferences and statistical or null hypotheses against actual data. Statistical inference is used both to estimate the probability that data found in a randomly drawn sample accurately reflect the target population and to test null hypotheses formulated from research hypotheses.

Descriptive statistics differ from inferential statistics, in that descriptive statistics summarize data from a sample, while inferential statistics infer characteristics of the population from which the sample was randomly drawn. Inferential statistics test statistical hypotheses as well. The major difference between the two is related to the use of randomization in inferential statistics, which allow the researcher to generalize from the sample to the target population; descriptive statistics summarize data from a sample and cannot be generalized beyond that sample.

A sample is any subset of a population, while a population is any set of persons, things, or measurements having an observable characteristic in common. Chance factors are the residual, unknown factors that affect events after the factors that determine the events have been isolated. The laws of probability upon which inferential statistics are based provide the basic ingredients necessary to calculate the chances that the researcher will take upon inferring from sample to population.

The standard error of the mean is the standard deviation of a theoretical distribution of sample means, used to construct the normal curve as a model for inference.

A population parameter is estimated from randomly drawn samples. However, the researcher needs to determine how close the mean of the sample is to the mean of the population, which may be unknown. Population means may be calculated through the use of sampling distributions, which calculate the mean of many sample means. The estimation of a population parameter begins after the data are collected.

The testing of a statistical hypothesis begins before the data are collected, when the researcher formulates the statistical hypothesis from the research hypothesis. The research hypothesis is tested by observing the specified variables both before and after an independent variable has been introduced. The researcher does not know whether the findings are the result of the manipulation of the independent variable or whether they occurred by chance. The statistical hypothesis is formulated to test statistically the probability that findings are due to chance alone. If the research hypothesis states that a difference will be found in the experimental and control groups, the statistical hypothesis states that no difference will be found. After testing, the researcher must make a decision to accept or reject the null hypothesis. If the null hypothesis is rejected when it is true, the researcher commits a Type I error. If the null hypothesis is accepted when it is false, the researcher makes a Type II error.

Parametric and nonparametric tests are two types of inferential statistics. They differ with respect to the size of the sample, assumptions of normal distribution, and level of measurement required. Parametric tests are used with large, homogeneous samples whose variables are normally distributed and whose measurements have been on at least an interval scale. Nonparametric tests are used when the data have been measured on the nominal or ordinal level, when the sample is small, and when a normal distribution of variables is not assumed.

EXAMPLES FROM NURSING RESEARCH

Data Analysis

Examples of the use of the chi-square test are numerous in nursing research. Recent reports include those of Flaskerud (1984), Miles (1985), and Lia-Hoagberg (1985).

Flaskerud compared perceptions of problematic behavior by six minority groups and a group of mental-health professionals from California. The minority ethnic or racial groups included: (1) Appalachians from a county in Pennsylvania; (2) black Fundamentalists who were resident members of a church in Louisiana; (3) Native Americans from the area around Detroit, representing several Indian tribes; (4) Chinese-Americans from Chinatown in Los Angeles; (5) Filipinos from a Filipino neighborhood in Los Angeles; and (6) Mexican-Americans born in Mexico and residing in east Los Angeles. She used the chi-square test to demonstrate significant differences in a number of characteristics, including education, marital status, and religion. Chi-square tests demonstrated significant educational differences between the group of mental-health professionals and the various ethnic or racial groups, as well as other differences (including religious differences) between the black Fundamentalists and the professionals from California. The internal characteristics of various groups were broken down by percentages, and measures of central tendency were used to calculate the mode, mean, and median.

Miles compared the emotional symptoms and physical health of groups of parents whose children had died by accident or chronic disease. She used the chi-square to explore group differences on characteristics of the two groups, such as hospital admissions, appetite changes, or an increased use of drugs. Lia-Hoagberg compared professional activities of nurse doctorates with those of academic women doctorates in other disciplines. She used chi-square statistics to test for differences between those who responded to the questionnaire that she mailed and those who did not.

STUDY QUESTIONS _____

1. Why is it important for nurses in research to understand what the term statistical inference means?

2. Can statistical inference allow the researcher to make completely accurate tests or estimates? Why or why not?
3. What is the basis for inference in research?
4. If a nurse has made a descriptive study, is it possible to use inference?
5. What is a statistic? What are descriptive statistics? Can a nurse who has data from a sample that was not drawn by random sampling use descriptive statistics? Why or why not?
6. What is random assignment? Can a nurse infer from one sample?
7. What is a population or universe? What is a population parameter?
8. What is the difference between a finite and an infinite population?
9. What is a sample?
10. What is chance? Why is it important for the nurse researcher to understand this concept?
11. What is the difference between a sampling distribution and the distribution of cases (frequency distribution)?
12. What is a null (statistical) hypothesis?
13. What is the difference between inferring from a sample to a population and testing a statistical (null) hypothesis?
14. Discuss the relationship between the research hypothesis and the null hypothesis.
15. Use the research hypothesis, "Patients who take drug A will be cured of cancer," and state a null hypothesis.
16. Distinguish between a Type I error and a Type II error.
17. Compare parametric and nonparametric statistical tests.

REFERENCES AND SUGGESTED READINGS

Bullough, V. (1981): Is the nurse practitioner role a source of increased work satisfaction? In Fox, D. and Lesser, I. (eds.), Readings on the Research Process in Nursing. New York: Appleton-Century-Crofts, pp. 221–223. *Chi-square.*

Byrne, T., and Edeani, D. (1984): Knowledge of medical terminology among hospital patients. Nursing Research, *33*, 178–181. *Percentages, mean, standard deviation, Pearson correlation.*

Chase, C. (1976): Elementary Statistical Procedures. New York: McGraw-Hill. *Chap. 8, probability and statistical inference.*

Cowan, M. and Murphy, S. (1985): Identification of postdisaster bereavement risk predictors. Nursing Research, *34*, 71–75. *Pearson correlation.*

Dixon, W. and Massey, F. (1957): Introduction to Statistical Analysis. New York: McGraw-Hill. *Chap. 4 and Chap. 7, universe, sample, statistical inference.*

Duncan, R., Knapp, R., and Miller, M. (1977): Introductory Biostatistics for Health Sciences. New York: Wiley. *Chap. 3, populations, samples, normal distribution.*

Flaskerud, J. (1984): A comparison of perceptions of problematic behavior by six minority groups and mental health professionals. Nursing Research, *33*, 190–197. *Chi-square, percentages, mode, median, mean.*

Fox, D. (1982): Fundamentals of Research in Nursing. Norwalk, Conn.: Appleton-Century-Crofts. *Chap. 22, inferential statistical concepts, procedures.*

Fox, R. and Ventura, M. (1984): Internal psychometric characteristics of the patient care quality scale. Nursing Research, *33*, 112–117. *Factor analysis.*

Gerber, R. and Van Ort, S. (1979): Topical application of insulin in decubitus ulcers. Nursing Research, *28*, 16–19. *Pearson product moment correlation coefficients, analysis of variance, frequency distribution, central tendency.*

Harris, R. and Hyman, R. (1984): Clean vs. sterile tracheotomy care and level of pulmonary infection. Nursing Research, *33*, 80–85. *Percentages, means, standard deviation, analysis of variance.*

Hasselmeyer, E. (1961): Behavior Patterns of Premature Infants. U.S. Public Health Service Publication No. 840. Washington, D.C.: Government Printing Office.

Hubbard, P., Muhlenkamp, A., and Brown, N. (1984): The relationship between social support and self-care practices. Nursing Research, *33*, 266–270. *Mean, standard deviation, range.*

Lia-Hoagberg, B. (1985): Comparison of professional activities of nurse doctorates and other women academics. Nursing Research, *34*, 1–19. *Chi-square, t-test, percentages.*

Lin, N. (1976): Foundations of Social Research. New York: McGraw-Hill. *Chap. 7, an introduction to statistical inference.*

Maxwell, A. (1961): Analyzing Qualitative Data. New York: Barnes & Noble. *Entire book on the chi-square and contingency table.*

Miles, M. (1985): Emotional symptoms and physical health in bereaved parents. Nursing Research, *34*, 76–81. *Percentages, reliability coefficient (Cronbach's alpha), mean, analysis of variance, analysis of covariance, chi-square.*

Mueller, J., Schuessler, K., and Costner, H. (1970): Statistical Reasoning in Sociology. New York: Houghton Mifflin. *Chap. 13, estimating parameters.*

Newman, M. and Gaudiano, J. (1984): Depression as an explanation of decreased subjective time in the elderly. *Pearson product moment correlation statistic, mean, standard deviation.*

Penckoffer, S. and Holm, D. (1984): Early appraisal of coronary revascularization on quality of life. Nursing Research, *33*, 60–63. *Percentage, mean, standard deviation, two-way ANOVA.*

Phillips, J. and Thompson, R. (1967): Statistics for Nurses. New York: Macmillan. *Inferences, using frequency and ranked data, means and variances.*

Rodgers, J. (1977): Relationship between sociability and personal space preference at two different times of day. In Downs, F. and Newman, M. (eds.), A Source Book of Nursing Research (2nd ed.). Philadelphia: F. A. Davis, pp. 171–177. *Means, standard deviations, and F values; Pearson product moment correlation coefficients.*

Rottkamp, B. (1981): A behavior modification approach to nursing therapeutics in body positioning of spinal cord injured patients. In Fox, D. and Lesser, I. (eds.), Readings on the Research Process in Nursing. New York: Appleton-Century-Crofts, pp. 107–114. *Mann-Whitney U test.*

Simon, J. (1978): Basic Research Methods in Social Science (2nd ed.). New York: Random House. *Chap. 27, "Inferential statistics: Introduction."*

Walizer, M. and Wienir, P. (1978): Research Methods and Analysis (2nd ed.). New York: Harper & Row, Chap. 16, p. 466.

Woods, N. (1985): Relationship of socialization and stress to perimenstrual symptoms, disability, and menstrual attitudes. Nursing Research, *34*, 145–149.

21

The Computer in Research

A *computer* is an electronic device that adds, subtracts, multiplies, and divides at tremendous speeds, thereby revolutionizing data analysis. The researcher who uses a computer with a word-processing program can also create documents or papers that look as if they came from a typesetter, can make changes within the paper, and can mix text with graphics (such as tables, graphs, and charts). The researcher can use a computer at all of the four different phases of the research process.

In the planning phase, the researcher can use a microcomputer at home, school, or office to cut down on the mass of paper normally used in this phase. With a word-processing program, the computer can store pages of data on small, thin compact disks about 3½ inches square (for the Apple Macintosh) to: (1) create and store bibliographies for immediate printing or easy updating later; (2) store or print summaries of articles and books on the small disks, which can be called up for viewing at a moment's notice; and (3) produce first and last drafts of paper-and-pencil instruments, such as questionnaires or interview schedules.

In the second phase, the collection of data, the researcher can use the word-processing program to type in and store all narrative data from unstructured interviews, observations, and field notes. In the third phase, the researcher can use a computer program already created for that purpose to analyze data with great speed and efficiency. In the fourth phase, the researcher can use a computer with a word-processing program to type drafts and the final research article and can instruct the printer to print a quality product with speed.

What the computer cannot do is take the place of the human observer and thinker, although it can be programmed to scan, survey, and monitor in places where the human observer cannot. The computer cannot think—it must rely completely on what the human thinker and programmer tells it to do. It cannot read narratives and select the one definition of a concept that the researcher wants. It cannot make judgments or inferences. But it is far superior to the human being with regard to the speed and accuracy with which it is able to calculate.

Upon completion of this chapter, the student should be able to: (1) identify different types of computers; (2) discuss types of computers; (3) describe, in simple terms, how a computer works; (4) discuss what a computer can and cannot do; (5) identify components and functions of a computer system; and (6) describe a mainframe computer or a mini-computer.

TYPES OF COMPUTERS

Computers vary from the large mainframe models centrally located in universities and businesses (sometimes in different cities), to the small, personal microcomputer, which may be portable. The researcher may not need to see the large computer, using (instead) the small, familiar console, or terminal (comprised of a keyboard and cathode-ray tube linked to the main computer), and the printer (which types out the results of the computer's calculations). One central processing unit can serve hundreds of terminals, due to its large storage, or memory, capacity. However, computer time must often be bought, whether by the individual researcher or by the college department for the student. Nevertheless, this is a bargain when it comes to data analysis, since the computer can perform in 1 minute calculations that it would take a person many hours to complete.

Families of computers include the digital computer and the analog computer. Digital computers, such as the computerized bank teller, require data represented by distinct numbers. Functions include counting and making comparisons. Activities include arithmetic processes, such as addition, subtraction, multiplication, and division. This is the type of computer used in nursing research. Analog computers, such as those that monitor patients in the ICU, provide continuous measurements that vary over time. They process data that represent physical qualities and provide a model analogous to the system that is simulated.

The Microcomputer

The microcomputer, or personal computer, began to appear on the market about 1978, and it immediately began to change the world's view of computers. Persons unable to gain access to larger machines now had the availability of the new, relatively portable, relatively inexpensive machines. Hassett (1985) predicts that, in a few years (by 1990), microcomputers will be in common use by nurses. In education, students will use a notebook-sized microcomputer for access to entire courses or for processing their own information. In nursing practice, nurses will use applications for direct patient care. Andreoli and Musser (1985) write that the microprocessor will soon take over more of the routine mental work that supports the judgments of health professionals.

Bertrand (1985) reports the expanding use of the microcomputer by health teams in developing countries. For example, a research team conducting a health survey in rural Bolivia used an IBM portable microcomputer and a word-processing program, Word Star, to produce, modify, and rework a questionnaire six times during a five-day period. A nine-page questionnaire and a seven-page field guide for interviewers were produced in one day. He notes that this experience was repeated in Zaire and Columbia. The newest technical innovation is the production of a completely portable, battery-powered disk drive that will increase mass storage capacity in the field.

In terms of statistical analysis and presentation of results, Bertrand writes that professional statisticians can be divided into two groups— those who are enthusiastic about the potential of microcomputers and those who insist that true statistics can only be worked on mainframe machines. However, most of the major statistical packages, such as the widely used SPSS (Statistical Package for the Social Sciences), are currently available for enhanced microcomputers, such as the IBM-compatible microcomputers.

Bellinger and Laden (1985) discuss the use by nurses of general-purpose microcomputer software programs. The authors give examples of possible applications, such as scheduling, report writing, unit budget planning, documentation of procedures, individualized care plans, research, performance evaluations, continuing education, clinical support modules (such as drug dosage interaction programs), and inservice tracking systems. The authors give the generic names of the programs to purchase, including the following:

1. *Spreadsheet Program* to simulate an accountant's spreadsheet, with rows and columns of interrelated numbers. The job function for this program includes planning, budgeting, and creating statistical reports such as a nurse-manager or unit coordinator would need.
2. *Database Program* for a nurse-manager, ward clerk, or secretary to maintain an index card system or to search and sort statistical records. This allows data to be selected, sorted, extracted, printed, or displayed in almost any format.
3. *Word-Processing Program* to create and maintain procedure manuals, forms, and mailing lists, as well as correspondence and report writing.
4. The *Integrated Package* to function in all of the ways described.

In addition, other functions (such as graphics and communication over telephone lines) may be available within the program.

The authors note that many different brand names, such as VisiCalc, Lotus 1–2–3, dBase II and III, Word Star, Word, Symphony, and Framework, are used by the manufacturers who produce these programs. More than 100 computer-software companies offer programs in one or more of these categories. The majority of available general-purpose programs is compatible with nearly all major brands of microcomputers.

HOW A COMPUTER WORKS

To understand how a digital computer works, it is helpful to compare its operation with that of a student with only a hand calculator. To analyze the data, the student using a hand calculator would use four kinds of equipment: (1) the calculator, to solve individual arithmetic problems; (2) a worksheet to write down the order in which the individual calculations were performed, as well as the intermediate and final totals; (3) mathematical tables, for reference; and (4) the student's mind, which would control the entire operation.

The corresponding parts of the computer include: (1) a high-speed arithmetic unit that can execute millions of operations in one second (this corresponds to the desk calculator; (2) a storage (or memory) unit, which corresponds to both the worksheet and the mathematical tables; and (3) a control unit, which corresponds to the mind of the human operator and which causes the computer to take the proper steps in their proper order.

The storage, or memory, unit of the computer includes the instructions for the problem to be solved, the numbers needed, and the intermediate results. The storage unit may be internal or external. External storage media are separate from the central processing unit and include: (1) paper products, such as punched cards, punched paper tape, and marked paper documents; and (2) magnetically treated products, such as tapes, disks, cards, a drum, or a core. Magnetic core memories, the most widely used type, are so fast that any part of the stored information can be selected and consulted in less than 10 one-millionths of a second.

Computer arithmetic is binary arithmetic—a numbering system that uses two digits, 0 and 1. Combinations of 0 and 1 can represent any number, letter, or symbol to be used by the computer. Each of the thousands of individual circuits is like an electric light switch that can be turned on or off.

To solve a problem on the computer, the researcher gives the computer a set of instructions, called a *program*. Numerous programs made by experts are available to the researcher. The computer center at a university has both a professional staff for consultation and a set of computer programs that can deal with the kind of data analysis that most researchers need. To use a microcomputer, the researcher obtains the program needed, whether a word-processing program or a program to analyze data.

What the Computer Can and Cannot Do

What the computer can do is perform more arithmetic in 1 second than the student could do in many months. In addition, the computer is accurate and never gets tired, overworked, or bored. Computers with word-processing programs can "shuffle" words around—they can create documents with many different type styles, such as the *italic*, the underline, the 𝐬𝐡𝐚𝐝𝐨𝐰 or the outline. Different sizes include the very small or the very large. The writer can move letters, words, sentences, and paragraphs around on the display screen with very simple, easily learned techniques. When the document is correct, a simple maneuver transfers it to the printer, where it is typed out.

However, computers do break down and, when they do, it takes an expert to repair them. A burned-out wire or an electrical surge may shut the computer down for hours. Most of all, the computer is limited by its inability to think, reason, or infer. The instructions programmed must be used in detail and one step at a time. However, programming is the task of computer experts, and it is big business. Students can rely on the consultants at the computer center or on computer statisticians to recommend the proper program for the research data. Programs for microcomputers are available at numerous computer centers in any medium-sized town. Most of the stores will instruct the potential purchaser in the use of the program and will allow practice on one of the store's computers. In addition, microcomputers come with step-by-step instructions that can be mastered in a fairly short time.

Components and Functions of Computer Systems

The components of a computer system (Fig. 21–1) include both the machines (hardware) and the programs (software) that specify what the computer is to do. The *hardware* for large computers consists of a number of machines, such as the keypunch, card reader, central processing unit, control panel (or console), card punch printer, and tape unit. Not all systems use all of the hardware available; some are basic.

The typical microcomputer, such as the Apple Macintosh or the IBM PC, consists of: (1) the main unit, which looks like a TV screen on the front (weighing about 16½ pounds); (2) the separate keyboard, which looks like a typewriter keyboard (weighing about 2½ pounds); (3) the "mouse" (in the Macintosh), a small box (weighing seven ounces), which

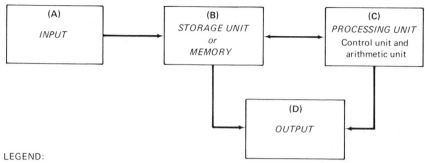

LEGEND:

(A) The program — a set of complete instructions to solve problems — is fed into computer. The raw data is fed into the computer. Program and data comprise the *INPUT.*

(B) The information is stored in the *MEMORY UNIT:* each cell can store either one instruction or one numerical value. The memory unit can store large amounts of information and allow rapid access to any portion of that information.

(C) Instructions stored in the memory are sent to the control unit, which interprets instructions, determines sequence of operations, and controls the processing of information. The control unit, together with the arithmetic unit (which does the arithmetic calculation), form the *DATA PROCESSING UNIT.*

(D) Information that results from the calculations of the computer comes out in an understandable form such as a printout — a verbal and numerical description of the findings — the *OUTPUT.*

Figure 21-1. Input, memory, processing, and output.

the operator moves about on a smooth surface to interact with the computer (the IBM PC uses the modem for interaction); and (4) a separate printer, which looks like the printing part of a typewriter and which rapidly types out all of the data put into the computer on command by the operator. An external disk drive may be purchased to hold more data. All of the parts fit on the top of an ordinary office desk. The programs, or software, are on small, thin, 3½-inch square disks, which are inserted into a slot in the front of the computer (or external disk drive) and which can be ejected from the computer when not in use and easily stored.

The receiving unit, or input, receives information in the form of the program and the data. In the case of the word-processing program, the data are inserted into the computer (after the program is inserted) by typing the information on the keyboard. The information immediately appears on the screen. The researcher can interact with the computer to move words, phrases, or paragraphs around; to correct spelling; or to delete or insert words, phrases, and paragraphs. The operator interacts with the main unit via the "mouse" to cause an arrow or a flashing bar on the screen to point to the place where a change or insertion is wished or to give instructions to the computer from preprinted lists, which appear at the top of the screen. The receiving unit consists of the storage media and reading devices. Microcomputers also have the means, via the phone connections, to hook onto the mainframe of a university computer.

The output unit receives the information from the computer and reproduces it in readable form. The information may be transferred from the computer by means of magnetic tape, disk drive, or high-speed printer to disks, magnetic tapes, punched cards, or printed documents. In the case of the microcomputer, the information is typed out on the printer, which is slow compared with the high-speed printers (which can print out paper documents as fast as 20,000 lines per minute) but which is fast compared with the ordinary typewriter.

STEPS TO TAKE IN USING THE COMPUTER

To use a mainframe computer to analyze data, the student begins early to take the first of several steps. Each will be examined briefly.

1. *Define what you wish the computer to analyze.* This information comes directly from the research proposal. The variables identify exactly what is to be studied and analyzed. For example, a nursing problem may be concerned with the number of persons in a community who have elevated blood pressure. The research proposal is to document, by interview and instrumentation, the blood pressure of a randomly selected sample of 100 adults in a specified community in order to discover how many blacks and how many whites have elevated blood pressures. The variables to be analyzed are blood pressure and race. The researcher can develop the interview schedule and blood-pressure records to indicate that race will be put in column one—*1* for black and *2* for white. Columns 2 through 8 can denote blood pressure.

2. *Consult a professional at the computer center.* The second step is to find an appropriate person to advise you throughout the project. The student, in particular, needs to know what program should be used. Canned programs, such as the Statistical Program for the Social Sciences (SPSS), are usually readily available in most university centers. Fortunately, it is not necessary for the student to learn either computer language or how to program the computer. Expert advice is usually forthcoming from those at the computer center, provided that the student has contacted a person early in the research process and has located the funds to pay for computer time.

3. *Transform the raw data into a medium that the computer can read.* The third step occurs after the data are collected. The student must now transform the data from the interview schedule and accompanying records to a medium that the computer can "read."

4. It is clear from these instructions how the computer must do its task. If the computer operation is to go forward accurately (or, indeed, at all), no step can be skipped.

5. *Examine the output of the computer.* The fifth step is to examine the analyzed data carefully for errors. Once errors are cleared up, the researcher must plan to store the data so that analysis is simple and access to the contents easy.

SUMMARY

The computer is an electronic device that has revolutionized the research process, because it can add, subtract, multiply, and divide at tremendous rates of speed. With assistance in the planning and analysis phases of a research project, the student can use the computer in her or his work: the researcher does not need to understand the inner workings of the computer in order to use it, but she or he must understand what the computer has the capability of doing.

Computers can be used at every phase of the research process, if a word-processing program and a statistical program are available. Computers vary in size from the large mainframe models, with large storage (or memory) capacity, to the small, personal microcomputer. The digital computer, used in research, functions to count; to make comparisons; to add, subtract, multiply, and divide; and to analyze data. Analog computers process data that represent physical qualities.

The microcomputer, appearing on the market about 1978, has revolutionized the use of the computer. Writers predict that microcomputers will soon be in common use in nursing education, practice, and research. Microcomputers are presently being used in field research. In remote areas without electricity, battery-operated microcomputers are coming into use. Such computers utilize software programs both for writing the research and for analyzing the data statistically.

Generic names for microcomputer programs useful in nursing include the "Spreadsheet Program," the "Database Program," the "Word-Processing Program," and the "Integrated Package."

The computer needs input—a program and raw data—to begin its operations. The memory (or storage) unit includes the instructions for the problem to be solved, the numbers or data needed, and the intermediate results. From the memory unit, information goes to the processing unit, which is (in turn) comprised of the control unit and the arithmetic unit. The control unit interprets the instructions, determines the sequence of operations, and controls the processing of information. The arithmetic unit does the arithmetic calculations. The control unit and the arithmetic unit form the data-processing unit. Information, or output, comes out of the computer in an understandable form, such as a printout. Data-processing terminology uses many common words to stand for particular computer operations. Many terms formerly referred to the data computer cards; now, magnetic tapes and disks are in common use.

The computer system is comprised of both hardware—the various machines that process data—and software—the programs that specify what the computer is to do and how.

In planning and executing a research project that includes the use of a computer, the student must be acquainted with several important steps. The student must define what the computer is to analyze; must consult a professional early in the planning stages; must transform raw data into a medium that the computer can read; must inform the computer how the data are set up; must carefully examine the output of the computer for errors; and must plan for the permanent storage of the data.

EXAMPLE FROM LITERATURE

Computer Use

Bertrand, William (1985): Microcomputer applications in health, population surveys: Experience and potential in developing countries. World Health Statistics, 38, 91–97.

Bertrand writes about the effect of the microcomputer, or personal computer, on researchers who had been unable to gain access to the larger machines. The new, portable, relatively inexpensive machines have caused an explosion in the last two years. These new products, along with relatively powerful database managers developed for large data sets, have become the first important tools for researchers in the health field. Software packages such as dBase II, Super Calc, or Lotus 1–2–3, combined with personal word-processing capability, have made the microcomputer an important tool.

Development is proceeding rapidly; differences between hand-held, highly portable microcomputers and the larger, desktop machines have virtually disappeared, with the exception of disk storage. The computer is essential in research in both developed and underdeveloped countries. (A survey carried out by a United States agency in Nepal in 1982 used over 40 microcomputers.)

The microcomputer is used in research in the following ways: First, the researcher may make initial drafts of study instruments and questionnaires, using portable microcomputers and a word-processing program. As larger disk-storage space becomes available, field revision of instruments can accelerate.

Second, sample selection, and retrospective and prospective sampling procedures, can be facilitated by the microcomputer. For example, a small program designed to generate random samples can assist even the least-sophisticated interviewer in choosing random houses and individuals as study units. In a large urban area, stratification and key parameters were tabulated, making the selection of a sample possible in a very short time. In the longitudinal design, so many data are generated that it is necessary to use the microcomputer to classify and record information. The most immediate innovation is the portable, battery-powered 3½ inch disk drive, which increases storage capacity.

Third, statistical analysis is being enhanced as microcomputers become more powerful. Most of the major statistical packages (such as the SPSS) are currently available for IBM-compatible microcomputers but not, as yet, for the truly portable machines. Analyses, such as frequency distribution, cross tabulations, simple univariate and bivariate statistics, and regression, are now feasible on small microcomputers.

Fourth, presentation of results associated with word processing appears at the end of the research. Bertrand closes by writing that the future looks bright for the use of microcomputers with a full range of statistical capabilities in the field.

STUDY QUESTIONS

1. What is a computer? Compare the operations of a computer with those of the researcher who uses a desk calculator to analyze data.
2. What are the advantages and disadvantages of using a computer?
3. What hardware is the student apt to use in computer operations?
4. What software is available?
5. If you were to use the computer in a research project of your own planning, what steps would you take?
6. What are the relationships among input, memory, processing, and output?
7. Locate the nearest computer center. Call to find the cost of using the computer for 5 minutes. Are there grants available that would enable you to use the computer?
8. What does the microcomputer revolution mean to nursing research and publication?

REFERENCES AND SUGGESTED READINGS

Andreoli, K. and Musser, L. (1985): Computers in nursing care: The state of the art. Nursing Outlook, *33*, 16–21.

Bellinger, K. and Laden, J. (1985): Nurse use of general-purpose microcomputer software. Nursing Outlook, *33*, 22–25.

Bertrand, W. (1985): Microcomputer application in health, population surveys: Experience and potential in developing countries. World Health Statistics, *38*, 91–97.

Billings, D. (1984): Evaluating computer-assisted instruction. Nursing Outlook, *32*, 50–53.

Hassett, M. (1985): Computers and nursing education in the 1980s. Nursing Outlook, *32*, 34–36.

McCormick, K. (1983): Preparing nurses for the technologic future. Nursing & Health Care, *4*, 379–382.

Nie, N. et al. (1975): Statistical Package for the Social Sciences. New York: McGraw-Hill.

Rieder, D. and Norton, D. (1984): An integrated nursing information system —a planning model. Computers in Nursing, *2*, 73–79.

Romano, C. (1984): A computerized approach to discharge care planning. Nursing Outlook, *32*, 23–25.

Worthley, J. (1982): Understanding computer technology. In Worthley, J. (ed.), Managing Computers in Health Care: A Guide for Professionals. Ann Arbor, Mich.: Health Administration Press, pp. 163–172.

Zielstorff, R. (ed.) (1980): Computers in Nursing. Wakefield, Mass.: Nursing Resources.

PART VII

The Research Report

22

The Research Report:
Organization and Self-Evaluation

A *research report* is a written or spoken communication that informs a selected audience about a research project. The objective of the report is to present what the audience wants or needs to know as clearly and succinctly as possible. The researchers extract the relevant material from their working papers, organize the content in logical order, and document each step with care, taking into consideration the needs of the audience.

Upon completion of this chapter, the student should be able to: (1) identify various audiences who read or hear nursing research reports; (2) state how to organize the content of the research report in a logical manner; (3) ask and answer questions that help self-critique the student's report; (4) identify various media in which reports may appear; and (5) identify sources helpful in developing styles of writing suitable for reports.

THE AUDIENCE

Effective communication of the research findings begins with the identification of the audience. The first audience reached by the student-researcher is usually composed of the researcher's supervising professors and classmates. The student should also plan to submit the paper, with the approval of the supervising professor, to professional meetings and suitable journals, in order to receive a wider review. The first meeting of professionals may be members of the faculty, who hear brief oral reports of the completed research. In addition, many nursing organizations have sections for student papers in their meetings, in order to encourage research among the rising generation of professionals. If such sections do not exist, it may be possible to initiate them. The supervising professor may join with the student to prepare the paper for submission to a professional meeting or journal.

The audience at professional meetings, or for nursing journals, may be diverse, including nursing researchers, practitioners, policy makers, sponsors of research, or interested members of the general public. Each of these may look for different information in a research report. Nurses engaged in basic or applied research may look for information that contributes to the body of nursing knowledge or to the practice of nursing. Practitioners may seek information helpful in the assessment, intervention, or evaluation of nursing care. Policymakers in nursing may look for information that could improve or change existing policies or administrative structures. Nursing professors may examine, in particular, the theories, concepts, and methods of data collection and analysis used in the study. Students must carefully consider the primary audience that they intend to reach, although secondary audiences also may be kept in mind.

To evaluate this element of his or her report, the student must answer the following questions: What is the primary audience that I am trying to reach? What is it that they want or need to know?

ORGANIZATION OF THE CONTENT OF THE REPORT

The organization of the research report varies from one scholar to another. Usually, the report follows the outline of activity pursued by the students as they planned and carried out the research activity: (1) introduction; (2) research statement (drawn from the research proposal); (3) review of the literature; (4) research design; (5) method of sampling; (6) research methods; (7) description of the pilot study, if any; (8) presentation, analysis, and interpretation of data; (9) conclusions; (10) bibliography and appendices; and (11) abstract (Table 22–1).

The main heading of the research report often follows rather faithfully the major steps of research depicted in Chapter 6. Each main head of the research report will be examined briefly, with accompanying questions for self-evaluation. The student may also wish to review the section on how to criticize a research report.

Introduction to the Report

The introduction to the report is not always easy to write. Sometimes the final version of the introduction is written after other parts of the report are complete. It is often helpful to examine how other researchers have introduced the general and specific problems in their report. For example,

TABLE 22–1. SUGGESTED OUTLINE FOR A RESEARCH REPORT

I. Introduction

  A. Importance of the general problem to nursing
  B. Specific problem

II. Research statement

  A. Statement of what the researcher studied and how
  B. Definitions of concepts/variables
  C. Hypotheses, if any
  D. Objectives of the study; purpose
  E. Ethical implications of the research

III. Review of the literature

  A. Review of related and competing theories
  B. Review of relevant research
  C. Specification of theory and research used in study
  D. Review of observations to formulate theory, if applicable

IV. Research design

  A. Description of the particular design used
  B. Description of control used, if any
  C. Discussion of the validity and reliability of the design

V. Sampling

  A. Description of the target population
  B. Discussion of how the sample was drawn, sample size, response rate.
  C. Discussion of bias, if any

VI. A. Description of the method of data collection used

  B. Descriptions of categories, instruments, scales, operational definitions
  C. Discussion of the reliability and validity of methods, instruments

VII. Pilot study

  A. Description of findings
  B. Subsequent revisions

VIII. Analysis and interpretation of data

  A. Description of statistics used and how the data were analyzed
  B. Summary of data in graphs and tables, with narrative explanation
  C. Interpretation of findings

IX. Conclusion

  A. Implication of findings for nursing
  B. Recommendations, suggestions for future research

X. Bibliography and appendices

XI. Abstract

McCorkle (1974) began her report on the effect of touch on seriously ill patients by noting the importance of verbal interaction in meeting the emotional needs of patients. Hays and Larson's *Interacting with Patients* (1963) was cited as a reference. Nonverbal communication was introduced in the next sentence as a second mode by which nurses can respond to patients' emotional needs. In the third sentence, the specific kind of nonverbal communication—touch—was introduced. In the fourth sentence,

McCorkle cited a reference, Clark's (1968) article on loneliness and nursing intervention, in order to establish the importance of touch in communicating with the patient. Therefore, in the space of four sentences, McCorkle introduced the reader to the general problem, the specific problem, its importance to nursing, and studies reported in the literature that establish the problem's significance to nursing. Upon completion of the introductory paragraph(s), the student should ask: Have I stated the general problem and the specific problem in terms of their importance to nursing? Are one or two references cited to establish this? Do the major concepts stand out? After reading the introduction, does the reader know precisely what was studied? Is the introduction clear, yet concise?

The Research Statement

The *research statement* is drawn from the research proposal. The proposal is forward-looking, defining what will be studied. The research proposal is converted into the research statement, which informs the audience precisely what was studied and how. Having informed the audience of the general and specific problems to be studied, the student now communicates, in summary form, all of the elements of the research: how the sample was drawn, how the data were collected, the time and site of the study, and any other pertinent information that sets the stage for the information that follows. The audience should not have to go searching through the report to discover whether or not the research design was experimental or a survey, or whether or not the sample was randomly selected. The following research statement summarizes what was studied, who was studied, and how:

> This study investigated the relationship between stressful environmental conditions in pregnancy and the subsequent pathology seen in the newborn. The data were collected by interview and by record review from 100 subjects. The subjects were selected by systematic sampling from a target population of pregnant women who attended prenatal clinics in Central City during the months of September and October. Those who gave informed consent were included in the study sample.

After writing the research statement, the student may go in one of two directions. If the researcher conducted an exploratory or descriptive study that did not use hypotheses, the report may next include definitions of concepts and objectives of the study. If the researchers did use hypotheses, these may be stated, followed by definitions of variables and, if desired, objectives.

The *definition of concepts*, a subheading of the research statement, informs the audience exactly what the researcher means by a particular term. Since a clear consensus does not exist on definitions of concepts, this is necessary. The student should both define the concept and give the source in the literature from which the definition was drawn. Next, the student gives the objectives that were set—what was planned to be accomplished by the research.

If hypotheses are used, they should be stated as a subhead of the research statement, followed by operational definitions of the variables used. Like definitions of all major concepts, operational definitions should be accompanied by references to the literature from which they were drawn.

Upon completion of the research statement, students should ask: Does the audience now know *what* I studied, *how* I collected the data, *who* the study subjects were, *how* I collected the sample from the population, and *when* and *where* the study took place? Have I noted here, or will I note later, the ethical implications of the study? Have I disguised the name and place of the study to ensure anonymity of agencies and subjects? Are concepts defined with reference to the nursing literature? Are the concepts observable and measurable, or have I referred the audience to an instrument, such as an operational definition, that makes the concept observable and measurable? Are the hypotheses clear and succinct? Is the source, or are the sources, of the hypotheses clearly stated, with reference to the theoretical literature? Does an operational definition of each variable follow each hypothesis so as to clarify how I observed and measured the variables? Have I clearly stated the objectives or intentions with which I began the study? Have I explained why I chose such objectives?

The Review of the Literature

The *review of the literature* informs the audience of several factors: (1) the extent to which the student researcher is familiar with current and classic publications; (2) the competing theories in the literature that propose to explain the phenomena under study; (3) the research that supports or refutes these theories; and (4) the theoretical viewpoint or assumptions (from which the research proceeded deductively) that best explains what has been observed.

A brief, critical review of the literature is preferable to a long, rambling description. However, the entire report may be a review of the literature; in such a case, the organization of the content should reflect this.

When the review of the literature has been written, the student should ask these questions: Does the review include primary, rather than secondary, sources? Does the review relate to the problem studied? Does the review include the most recent works, as well as the classics? Does the review contain a succinct report of different theories, as well as the research designed to test hypotheses formulated from them? Has the researcher made it clear which theory was used? Is the review written in such a way that the researcher can use it to interpret data? Are concepts that are identified in the literature clearly indicated? Are instruments that are located in the literature and used in research clearly documented? Are all citations included in the reference or bibliography? If the research is designed to formulate theory, are the observations of others clearly developed and reported?

The Research Design

The *research design* informs the audience about the plan of research—it describes the design (experimental, survey, historical/documentary, etc.) and the controls used, and notes any problems with validity or reliability. The researcher may want to inform the audience why this design was used rather than another, noting ethical implications or design problems that were experienced. Questions to be answered include the following: If an experimental design was used, has the method for sampling been clearly explained? Has the method of assigning subjects to the control or experimental groups been explained? Have the independent variable and the dependent variable been designated? Is it clearly explained how the researcher manipulated the variables? Is the control of extraneous variables explained? If a survey was used, does the report explain all elements of the research design? Is it clear whether a questionnaire or an interview was used? Are variations on these designs explained? Is it clear what the design intends to accomplish? If an historical design was used, does the researcher explain what records were used, how access was obtained, how the researcher determined whether the records were complete and accurate? In each of these cases, are the validity and reliability of the research design assessed and explained?

The Sampling Process

If the researcher has not reported about the sampling process, this should be next. The sampling process is one of the most crucial areas in the research process. The audience will want a clear description of exactly how the target population was identified and precisely how a sample was selected from the population. Subsequent analysis of data is dependent upon the account; therefore, the audience will scrutinize the sampling process closely. The researcher should make it clear exactly how the subjects were selected, as well as any problems that arose. This part of the report must be carefully examined to answer the following questions: What was the nature of the population: was it homogeneous or heterogeneous? Were members of the population accessible, or was it necessary to identify a population from which study subjects could be drawn? Did the researcher take the subjects as they arrived in the hospital or clinic? Was random sampling replaced with random assignment only? What was the size of the sample? Was it large enough to reflect the characteristics of a heterogeneous population? If probability sampling was not used, did the researcher identify possible biases? How many of the potential study subjects declined to take part in the research? What was the response rate to the questionnaire? Were any randomly selected patients' charts or other documents unavailable? Since subsequent data are dependent upon sampling, the student should scrutinize this part of the report.

Research Methods

The researcher must tell the audience exactly how he or she collected the data from the sample—whether by observation, questioning, measurement, or a combination of these. If observation was used, the researcher must explain the means used to observe: the operational definitions, the systems of classification and categorization, the instruments, as well as the reliability and validity of each. The researcher must explain to the audience the kind of observation used—participant or nonparticipant— and describe how many observers took part in the study and how they were trained. The audience must be informed of all behaviors observed and of how all observers were able to observe the same behavior.

If an interview was used, the interview schedule should be described or attached to the report in the appendix. The researcher should also describe how interviewers were selected and trained. In cases where an unstructured interview was used, the researcher must explain how data were recorded.

The use of a questionnaire requires that the researcher describe and/ or attach the questionnaire, together with the covering letter, to the research report. The source of the questions on the questionnaire may need explanation, and the researcher should describe how the questionnaire was formulated or obtained.

Upon completion of this portion of the report, the researcher should make certain that the following questions were answered: Is the method of data collection clearly described? Are all instruments, scales, and measures reported, together with the reliability and validity of each? If used, is the observational process carefully explained, including any steps to protect the subjects? If interviews were used, was the interview schedule well-developed and tested? Was a proper place for the interview arranged, in order to protect the privacy and confidentiality of the respondent? Does the report describe whether or not the interview was highly structured, or the degree of probing that may have occurred in an unstructured interview? Is the length of the interview reported?

The Pilot Study

The researcher reports the development of the pilot study in as much detail as space allows. The audience should be informed who was in the sample, what the findings were, how the instruments performed, what problems emerged, and how the researcher coped with these. Any elements of the research design that were revised as a result of the pilot study should be recorded.

Analysis of Data:
Presentation of Data:
The Results and Analysis of the Findings

The research design, methods, measurement level, and statistical procedures employed by the researcher all influence how the results of the study are presented. In general, the researcher plans to present the research data in the most clear, concise, and unambiguous format possible. The use of appropriate tables and graphs is essential to summarize material, but these must be accompanied by a narrative that explains them. The presentation must be completely objective, indicating what *was found* rather than what the researcher thought ought to be found.

If statistical procedures were used, the researcher must explain why he or she chose these and must give a statistical interpretation of the data. However, it is important to remember that the use of statistics is only the use of a helpful tool. The most sophisticated statistical analysis of data is of no use if the researcher has used an inappropriate research design or method of observing, questioning, measuring, and sampling.

Interpretation of Data

Interpretation is one of the most difficult tasks of the researcher, since the researcher must now make sense of the data. The difficulty of this task depends upon what the researcher found in the review of the literature—whether similar studies existed that were based upon similar assumptions, theory, designs, and methods. If so, the researcher can now compare and contrast his or her findings with those of others and can determine whether theories, hypotheses, assumptions or the data of others have been supported by the researcher's own findings.

If no sources were found in the literature, interpretation of data must be based on the researcher's own experience and preparation, the objectives of the study, the research design and method, the measurement level, and the use or invention of various instruments. If the study began with observations, the researcher should report whether these relate to known concepts or whether new concepts must be invented to stand for the observations. If possible, the researcher should attempt to integrate the findings or suggest tentative relationships among them. Upon completion of this part of the report, the student should ask the following questions: Have I discussed the objectives that I set at the beginning of the study? Have I met these objectives? Have I organized and interpreted the data in the best possible fashion? Have I worked in an unbiased way, reporting what was found rather than what I had hoped would be found?

Conclusions

The researcher's conclusion pulls the entire study together. For example, the conclusion may discuss the study's problems: its limitations in interpreting data due to sample size, the difficulty of establishing internal or external validity, and the subjective dilemmas (such as reading too much into data). In addition, the researcher may evaluate the study, noting its weaknesses and strengths. The purpose and objectives of the study may be reviewed in order to determine whether these were met or, if not, why not. The researcher may reach a conclusion concerning how the results of the study fit into the previous body of nursing knowledge and the implications of the study for nursing theory and practice. Finally, the researcher may recommend fruitful areas for future nursing research.

The Bibliography and Appendices

The researcher must review the manuscript and bibliography in order to determine whether there is a complete entry for all cited references and whether all of the entries are of the same acceptable bibliographic style. A review of the appendices must indicate that these are well-organized, complete, used effectively to present lengthy or supplementary materials, and referred to in the body of the manuscript.

Abstract

The researcher must write and criticize his or her own abstract in order to determine whether it includes a succinct description of the research question, design, method, sample, findings, and conclusion. Questions to answer include the following: Is the abstract too long or too short? Is it too vague or too detailed? Does it include what or who was studied, when, and how, and does it summarize the findings and conclusions?

Writing Style

The student who seeks to present a paper at a conference or submit it to a journal for publication should study the rules that govern participation or publications. A careful examination of the format used in research reports in a current journal may also be helpful.

Students wishing to improve their writing styles will benefit from an examination of a number of publications devoted to this purpose. Barzun and Graff (1970) include six chapters on writing: how to organize paragraphs, chapters, and parts; the use of plain words; how to write clear sentences; the art of quoting; the rules of citing; and how to revise for printer and public. Cordasco and Gatner published the brief *Research and Report Writing* (1963), which includes techniques of composition and specimen papers. Strunk and White's second edition of *The Elements of Style* (1972) includes elementary rules of usage, principles of composition, and an approach to style that is often recommended. The *Manual of Style* published by the University of Chicago Press includes an extensive section on style. Another popular book is Turabian's *A Manual for Writers of Term Papers, Theses, and Dissertations* (1973). In addition to these aids, the most valuable assistance is from the supervising professor or colleague who reads the paper and suggests areas that need improvement.

The Media

Oral presentations are common in the classroom; in local, state, or national professional meetings; and in nonprofessional clubs and associations that use health personnel as speakers.

Research reports may appear in nursing journals or in journals of allied disciplines. Technical reports are often printed within the school or university and, at times, professors use reports to accompany other teaching aids. Once the report appears in one medium, opportunities may arise to include it in edited books, conferences, or workshops. The student may also use a good report as a proposal for a grant, in job applications, or in application to graduate school.

SUMMARY

The research report is a written or spoken communication that informs an audience about the research findings and procedures. The researcher draws relevant material from the work, which he or she relays to an audience, beginning with a problem and ending with conclusions and recommendations.

The audience who is to hear the report or read the paper influences both the form and the content. Specific audiences will expect to hear selected portions of the research findings.

To write the report, the student begins with an organization of the data. The most helpful form of organization is an outline, which may be as informal or as formal as is desired. A carefully developed formal outline greatly assists in writing the report. The main heads and the subheads of the report lead both the writer and the reader into a logical discussion of the research process. Beginning with the introduction, the student may develop the report by following much the same organization proposed in the research design. A researchable problem is identified, and the research proposal records what the researcher studied and how it was studied. The identification and definition of significant concepts then follows, after which the hypothesis and the objects of the study are stated. Ethical implications of the study may be reported here or in conjunction with the research design. In either case, the third part of the report includes the review of the literature, or a summary of relevant theoretical and research reports. The research design, main heading number four, describes the plan of the research and what design was used—experimental, survey, or historical. The sampling process is then described in detail, followed by the research methods. Most readers scrutinize the research methods closely, so it behooves the researcher to write a careful and accurate account. The researcher follows this report with an account of the pilot study, if one was undertaken. The analysis and interpretation of the data are the heart of the research report. In this section, the researcher informs the reader how the data were analyzed and summarized and what the results of the study were.

The researcher uses the findings to draw implications for nursing practice. The research may suggest action in the assessment, intervention, or evaluation of nursing practice, or the researcher may recommend further refinement of the instruments or scales, in order to assure more valid findings.

The media in which the research report may appear include nursing conferences, workshops, meetings, journals, or books. The writing style in each of these may vary according to the nature of the audience.

STUDY QUESTIONS

1. Identify an audience for a research report that you are writing or would like to write.
2. Formulate an outline that is helpful in writing your own report or that can be a guide for future reports.
3. Write a one-paragraph introduction to your research report and evaluate it.
4. What is the value to the audience of the research statement?
5. Write a research statement for your own project.
6. What are the major criteria necessary in defining concepts or formulating hypotheses?
7. Discuss how a review of the literature is helpful to both the audience and the researcher.
8. In the section of the report entitled "research design," what elements of research does the student inform the audience about?
9. Discuss the crucial elements to document in the sampling process.
10. Discuss the questions that the student should ask to evaluate the research methods.
11. Describe what should be included in the report concerning the pilot project.
12. Why is the analysis and interpretation of data often called the heart of the research report?
13. Locate at least one source that is helpful in improving the writing style of a research report.
14. Identify one medium that you could use to present your report.

REFERENCES AND SUGGESTED READINGS

Barzun, J. and Graff, H. (1970): The Modern Researcher (rev. ed.). New York: Harcourt, Brace, & World, Part III.

Clark, E. (1968): Aspects of loneliness: Toward a framework of nursing intervention. In Zderad, L. (ed.), Developing Behavioral Concepts in Nursing. Atlanta, Ga.: Southern Regional Education Board, pp. 33–40. *Communication and loneliness.*

Cordasco, F. and Gatner, E. (1963): Research and Report Writing. New York: Barnes & Noble. *A College Outline primarily for college undergraduates, but generally useful. Includes specimen papers.*

Fox, D. (1976): Fundamentals of Research in Nursing (3rd ed.). New York: Appleton-Century-Crofts. *Chap. 13, "Critically Evaluating the Written Research Report."*

Goode, W. and Hatt, P. Methods in Social Research. New York: McGraw-Hill. *Chap. 21, "Preparing the Report."*

Hays, J. and Larson, K. (1963): Interacting with Patients. New York: Macmillan. *Communication with patients.*

The Chicago Manual of Style (13th ed.) (1982): Chicago: University of Chicago Press. *Part 2, "Style."*

McCorkle, R. (1974): Effects of touch on seriously ill patients. Nursing Research, *23,* 125–133. *Example of good introduction to research report.*

Polit, D. and Hungler, B. (1978): Nursing Research. Philadelphia: J. B. Lippincott, Chaps. 28 and 29.

Strunk, W. and White, E. (1972): The Elements of Style (2nd ed.). New York: Macmillan. *Short book of 78 pages, with helpful information.*

Turabian, K. (1973): A Manual for Writers of Term Papers, Theses and Dissertations. Chicago: University of Chicago Press. *Useful throughout.*

Webster's Dictionary of Synonyms (1951). Springfield, Mass.: G. & C. Merriam. *Helpful in finding a particular word.*

Appendix A

Observation Aids

INSTRUCTIONS TO OBSERVERS

1. Check the Observer's Schedule daily to confirm hours of work.
2. Observations should cover 2-hour periods (except for the night shift, which has fewer activities).
3. Every 10 (or 15) minutes, walk through the entire unit and record what each person (nursing personnel) in the unit is doing.
4. Whenever possible, observations of activities should be recorded in verb form. Example:
   a. Giving bath; not "bath"
   b. Taking TPR; not "TPR"
   c. Talking on telephone
   d. Is "off unit"
   e. Sitting; doing nothing
5. Activities of personnel need not be recorded in the order first observed. (The first person encountered may be a nursing student, and the second the head nurse; at the next observation, the first person encountered may be staff nurse no. 1.)
6. A code for persons observed is suggested to include:

   SU   —   Supervisor
   HN   —   Head nurse
   SN   —   Staff nurse
   NST   —   Nursing student
   PN   —   Practical nurse
   CI   —   Clinical instructor
   PN-I   —   Practical-nurse instructor
   NA   —   Nurse aide
   O   —   Orderly

OBSERVATION RECORDING SHEET

Nursing Activity Study

Observer _____ Date _____ Unit _____ Page _____ of _____ pages

TIME	PERSONNEL OBSERVED	ACTIVITY	LEVEL	AREA

WEEKLY SCHEDULE FOR OBSERVER

Observer's Schedule*

DATES

UNIT

Hours of Observation	Mon.	Tues.	Wed.	Thurs.	Fri.
7:00–9:00 A.M.					
9:00–11:00 A.M.	name				
11:00 A.M.–1:00 P.M.					
1:00–3:00 P.M.	name				
3:00–5:00 P.M.	name				
5:00–7:00 P.M.	name				
7:00–9:00 P.M.	name				
9:00–11:00 P.M.	name				
11:00 P.M.–1:00 A.M.					
1:00–3:00 A.M.					
3:00–5:00 A.M.					
5:00–7:00 A.M.					

*Areas blocked out have been eliminated by means of random selection of periods of observation.

7. If a person is away from the unit at observation time, ask the person later where she or he was and record the response.
8. Record the time of observation, personnel, and activity for each time period (10 or 15 minutes).

STUDY CODE

Classification of Activities by Level of Skill

Code

A = ADMINISTRATION ACTIVITIES (All coded as A in "Level Column")
Administration includes activities requiring nursing judgment. These involve responsibility for planning and providing effective patient care, for developing unit personnel, and for managing and operating the nursing unit.
  1. Patient care activities include:
  Assigning personnel to meet the individual needs of patients
  Planning and participating in unit education programs to ensure safe and effective nursing care
  Assisting the physician in the plan for patient care by directing the execution of orders and reporting to the physician the patient's symptoms, reactions, and progress
  Supervising and evaluating the effectiveness of patient care
  Giving nursing care for the purpose of observing a patient, establishing rapport with a patient, or teaching a member or members of the nursing staff
  Promoting, supervising, and evaluating the education and rehabilitation program for the patient and his or her family
  Making nursing rounds to assess the patient's condition, progress, and immediate environment
  2. Development of unit personnel includes:
  Planning for the participation of nursing personnel in continuous learning experiences
  Promoting personal growth and development of unit personnel
  Conducting written and oral evaluations of the performances of staff members
  3. Unit management activities include:
  Planning for and maintaining an environment conducive to the well-being of patients and personnel
  Promoting good interpersonal relationships
  Assisting in the development and implementation of nursing objectives and policies.

N = NURSING ACTIVITIES (all coded as N in "Level Column")
Nursing activities include those involved directly and indirectly in

giving nursing care to patients:

Preparation of a nursing care plan for direct patient care

Carrying out orders prescribed by the physician for individual patients

Observing and reporting on a patient's symptoms, reactions, and progress

Making out Rx sheet for direct patient care

Recording intake and output.

C = CLERICAL ACTIVITIES (all coded as C in "Level Column")
Clerical activities are those concerned with counting, copying, ordering, recording:

Assembling chart forms for new patients

Checking charts after discharge of patients

Copying records, such as time sheets

Transcribing orders, counting supplies or drugs

Checking drugs from pharmacy

Charting TPR on graph sheet

D = DIETARY ACTIVITIES (all coded as D in "Level Column")
Dietary activities are those concerned with the routine serving of fluids, food, and nourishment:

Caring for unit diet kitchen

Carrying or picking up trays

Cleaning water glasses and pitchers, and distributing fresh water and ice

Preparing and serving nourishment between meals

Setting up trays

H = HOUSEKEEPING ACTIVITIES (all coded as H in "Level Column")
Housekeeping activities are those concerned with the appearance of the unit environment and the care of supplies and equipment:

Making unoccupied beds

Cleaning floors, windows, bathrooms, and service rooms

Cleaning room after discharge of patient, including cleaning and making up the bed

Routine checking of the unit to maintain furnishings in good order

Dusting furniture, emptying wastebaskets, general cleaning of the nursing station

Distributing and collecting linens

M = MESSENGER ACTIVITIES (all coded as M in "Level Column")
Messenger activities are those requiring absence from the unit for transport services, escort service, and errands, such as:

Accompanying patients to other parts of the hospital

TABLE A–1. OBSERVATION OF ACTIVITY CHECKLIST GUIDE

Time	Personnel Observed	Area	Level	Activity
10:00 A.M.	RN_1	2.1	U	Reading new pamphlet on diabetes.
10:30 A.M.	RN_2	0.1	U	Drinking chocolate milk. .
11:00 A.M.	RN_3	0.2	U	Waiting to assist physician with a dressing.
11:30 A.M.	RN_4	0.1	U	Checking hour book for days off.

TABLE A–2

HN	1.4C	Copying medical order from order sheet to medicine tickets.
SN	1.4C	
NS	1.4C	
CI	1.4C	
HN	1.4A	Checking on orders as copied (by clerk).
SN	1.4A	
HN	2.1A	Showing nurse aide how to give a sitz bath.
SN	2.1A	
PN	2.1A	
SN	1.2A	Explaining intercom system to a new patient.
NA	1.2A	
HN	1.1N	Giving medicine to patient.
SN	1.1N	
PN	1.1N	
NST	1.1N	

Delivering requisitioned orders, both routine and emergency
Picking up drug and supply orders, both routine and emergency

U = UNCLASSIFIED ACTIVITIES (all coded as U in "Level Column")
Unclassified activities are those that, by definition, are eliminated from any of the preceding codes. Code U is used to identify those activities that refer to the person as an individual (see Table A–1).

The activity, not the person observed, is coded. The activity is classified or coded in two dimensions—area and level—simultaneously. This means that each activity, as entered on the Observation Recording Sheet, will be coded in the same manner, regardless of who performs it, whether a nurse, clerk, or nurse aide (see Table A–2).

Classification of Activities by Area of Nursing

Code   Subcode

1   PATIENT-CENTERED ACTIVITIES

These activities may occur in the patient's presence or away from the patient.

Code **Subcode**

1.1   *Direct Care*

Activities occurring in the presence of the patient that involve giving care, including:
> Carrying out nursing procedures
> Assisting doctors with treatments or procedures
> Giving or assisting patients with personal hygiene

1.2   *Other Patient Activities Relating to Direct Care*

Conversing or exchanging pleasantries with the patients (talking with patients)
> Evaluating the patients' need for care
> Escorting patients
> Interpreting procedures and practices to patients
> Observing the physical condition and behavior of patients
> Teaching patients
> Making unoccupied beds with patients at bedsides

1.3   *Exchange of Information Concerning Patients*

This is mainly oral communication. These activities include:
> Discussing an assignment of patient care
> Reading Kardex (nursing care plan)
> Examining reports on the patient with other members of the unit or hospital staff, physicians, the patient's family and friends, or other interested persons or agencies
> Holding or attending demonstrations for teaching staff members individually or collectively
> Giving or receiving planned or impromptu instruction
> Observing and evaluating the quality of work performed
> Orienting new unit staff members
> Reading or questioning to gain more information about a drug, treatment, etc.
> Listening to or giving the morning, afternoon, or evening report
> Ordering specific drugs, diet, supplies, or equipment by telephone for a particular patient or for a few patients, but not unit supplies

Code   *Subcode*

1.3   *Exchange of Information Concerning Patients* (cont.)

Participating in doctor's rounds
Receiving or giving an assignment related to patient care

1.4   *Indirect Care*

All patient centered activities not classified under Code Numbers 1.1, 1.2, 1.3, including:
Maintaining patient's records
Charting care given
Checking physician's orders
Completing form on patient's condition
Making out written requisition for specific drugs, diet, supplies, or equipment for a particular patient
Preparing medication and treatment trays
Setting up and performing immediate aftercare of equipment
Obtaining information from Kardex

2   PERSONNEL-CENTERED ACTIVITIES

These activities are primarily concerned with professional growth and development of nursing service personnel and with personnel management.

2.1   *Professional Development of Staff*

Participation in all activities conducive to improved nursing service, as well as planned and unplanned events that increase the knowledge and skill of the staff.

2.2   *Personnel:* Other

Activities having to do with personnel management (personnel centered activities), including:
Attending staff meetings
Participating in individual conferences on personal matters related to work
Maintaining personnel records and conferring on personnel matters
Obtaining physical examination on self by physician

Code   Subcode

2.3   *Professional Nursing Student Program* *

These activities include:
Discussing the nursing students' program with unit personnel, physicians, clinical instructors, and others
Observing and evaluating the quality of work performed by nursing students
Planning and selecting experience for nursing students
Giving nursing students impromptu or planned instruction

2.4   *Practical Nursing Student Program*

Activities concerned with the educational program or with experience for practical nursing students.

3   UNIT-CENTERED ACTIVITIES

These activities are concerned primarily with the patient's environment and with equipment and supplies for the unit.

3.1   *Environment*

Cleaning and maintenance activities for the order and safety of the unit, including:
Cleaning patient's unit (patient not at bedside)
Making unoccupied bed (patient not at bedside)
Caring for unit after patient's discharge
Cleaning of nurses' station, utility room, etc.

3.2   *Supplies and Equipment*

Activities concerned with obtaining, dispensing, or maintaining material for the unit, including:
Obtaining drug and linen supplies
Checking drugs delivered by pharmacy
Obtaining required supplies and equipment and conducting all discussions on this matter
Obtaining and serving all foods and fluids

---

*Activities in which nursing students are involved must be weighed carefully in terms of whether they are patient-centered or personnel-centered. If an activity is personnel-centered, a determination must be made as to whether it is for the student or for the unit staff of which the student is considered a part.

Code   Subcode

3.2   *Supplies and Equipment* (cont.)

Caring for supplies and equipment
Maintaining the Kardex

3.3   *Other Unit Activities*

These include:
Performing work related to the activity analysis study
Holding conversations to maintain rapport and good interpersonal relationships with unit and hospital staff, visitors, etc.
Delivering mail to patients
Holding discussions, compiling data, etc., in connection with any other studies
Running errands on behalf of unit personnel
Giving or receiving an interpretation of hospital policy as it affects the unit staff
Maintaining unit records, such as time sheets, leave records, daily reports
Reporting on or off duty
Serving on committees for the purpose of discussing, revising, or formulating hospital and nursing policy and procedure

0   OTHER-CENTERED ACTIVITIES

0.1   *Personal*

These activities include all activities of a personal nature; e.g., coffee breaks, conversations about personal affairs.

0.2   *Standby Time*

Time spent waiting for the arrival of a person or thing prior to the start of an activity, including:
Waiting for a doctor to arrive, in order to assist with a spinal puncture
Waiting for a sterile dressing tray to arrive, in order to change a patient's dressing

Appendix B

Sample Questionnaire And Interview Forms

SAMPLE QUESTIONNAIRE FORMAT

Directions

1. Please answer every question with a check mark ($\checkmark$) or short response.
2. It should take approximately 45 minutes to complete the questionnaire.
3. Your signature is optional. You will not be identified individually, and your response will be treated in confidence.
4. Please return the completed questionnaire to _____ .
5. Thank you for your cooperation.

I. Background Information   *Code*

1. Please check your age in the appropriate space.
   - a. 20 years or less   a. ____
   - b. 21–25 years   b. ____
   - c. 26–30 years   c. ____
   - d. 31–35 years   d. ____
   - e. 36–40 years   e. ____
   - f. 41–45 years   f. ____
   - g. 46–50 years   g. ____
   - h. 51–55 years   h. ____
   - i. More than 55 years   i. ____
2. From what type of basic educational program did you graduate? (Please check appropriate answer).
   - a. General nursing   a. ____

b. Mental nursing   b. ____

c. Other; specify _____ c. ____

3. What is your present position? (Please check appropriate answer.)
   a. Matron   a. ____
   b. Assistant matron   b. ____
   c. Departmental sister   c. ____
   d. Ward sister (Head nurse)   d. ____
   e. Staff nurse   e. ____
   f. Tutor (Instructor)   f. ____
   g. Other; specify _____ g. ____

4. How long have you worked in your present position? (Please check appropriate answer.)
   a. Less than 1 year   a. ____
   b. 1–3 years   b. ____
   c. 4–6 years   c. ____
   d. 7–9 years   d. ____
   e. 10–12 years   e. ____
   f. More than 12 years   f. ____

II. Patient Preference

1. What type of patients do you prefer to care for?

   _____

2. Please give the reason for your answer. ____

   _____

   _____

SAMPLE INTERVIEW SCHEDULE

1. a. Is this your first visit to the clinic?   Yes ____ No ____

   b. If the answer is "No," when was the last time you visited the clinic? _____

   c. Approximately how many times have you visited the clinic? _____

2. For what reason did you come to the clinic today?

   a. Complaint of pain _____
   b. Complaint of other symptoms _____
   c. Wanted to see doctor _____
   d. Wanted laboratory test _____
   e. Wanted an examination _____
   f. Other reason; specify _____

_____
_____
_____
_____

3. How are you feeling now?

   a. Sick (ill) _____
   b. Not sick but uncomfortable . _____
   c. Healthy _____
   d. Other; specify _____

_____
_____

TABULATION SHEET FOR RECORD REVIEW

CLINIC REGISTER NUMBER	CLINIC VISIT NUMBER	SEX	RACE	AGE	MARITAL STATUS	HEIGHT	DIET	MEDICAL DIAGNOSIS	SIGNS AND SYMPTOMS	REMARKS

DUMMY TABLE: INITIAL ANALYSIS FOR IDENTIFYING PATTERNS OF SIMILARITY OR DIFFERENCE

| LENGTH OF NURSING EXPERIENCE | TYPE OF PATIENT PREFERENCE | | | | | | | | | | TOTAL |
| | Medical | | Surgical | | Pediatric | | Geriatric | | |
	Acute	Chronic	Acute	Chronic	Acute	Chronic	Acute	Chronic	
Less than 6 months									
7 months to 5 years									
6–10 years									
11–15 years									
16–20 years									
21–25 years									
More than 25 years									
Total									

Appendix C

Distribution of Chi-Square Probability

DISTRIBUTION OF x^2 (CHI-SQUARE) PROBABILITY

df = (R−1)(c−1)	.05	.02	.01	.001
1	3 · 841	5 · 412	6 · 635	10 · 827
2	5 · 991	7 · 824	9 · 210	13 · 815
3	7 · 815	9 · 837	11 · 345	16 · 268
4	9 · 488	11 · 668	13 · 277	18 · 465
5	11 · 070	13 · 388	15 · 086	20 · 517
6	12 · 592	15 · 033	16 · 812	22 · 457
7	14 · 067	16 · 622	18 · 475	24 · 322
8	15 · 507	18 · 168	20 · 090	26 · 125
9	16 · 919	19 · 679	21 · 666	27 · 877
10	18 · 307	21 · 161	23 · 209	29 · 588
11	19 · 675	22 · 618	24 · 725	31 · 264
12	21 · 026	24 · 054	26 · 217	32 · 909
13	22 · 362	25 · 472	27 · 688	34 · 528
14	23 · 685	26 · 873	29 · 141	36 · 123
15	24 · 996	28 · 259	30 · 578	37 · 697
16	26 · 296	29 · 633	32 · 000	39 · 252
17	27 · 587	30 · 995	33 · 409	40 · 790
18	28 · 869	32 · 346	34 · 805	42 · 312
19	30 · 144	33 · 687	36 · 191	43 · 820
20	31 · 410	35 · 020	37 · 566	45 · 315
21	32 · 671	36 · 343	38 · 932	46 · 797
22	33 · 924	37 · 659	40 · 289	48 · 268
23	35 · 172	38 · 968	41 · 638	49 · 728
24	36 · 415	40 · 270	42 · 980	51 · 179
25	37 · 652	41 · 566	44 · 314	52 · 620
26	38 · 885	42 · 856	45 · 642	54 · 052
27	40 · 113	44 · 140	46 · 963	55 · 476
28	41 · 337	45 · 419	48 · 278	56 · 893
29	42 · 557	46 · 693	49 · 588	58 · 302
30	43 · 773	47 · 962	50 · 892	59 · 703

Glossary

Abstract: a short statement that gives the main ideas of an article or book.

Analysis: an examination of data to identify parts and their relationships to the whole; separation of a whole into its constituent parts.

   Analysis of data: the process by which the researcher summarizes and analyzes the collected data.

      Analysis of qualitative data, i.e., data whose characteristics must be abstracted before analysis:

         Content analysis: the systematic and objective procedure used to identify and analyze significant written, verbal, or visual data.

         Cross-cultural analysis: use of data from one or more cultures as a basis for comparative analysis.

         Frequency: the count of the number of subjects or objects under study.

         Index number: an average that indicates change between sets of data over time.

         Mode: the category, such as sex distribution, with the largest number of observations.

         Nominal scale: exhaustive and mutually exclusive named categories, such as female or male.

         Proportion: the relation in size of one thing compared to another.

         Percent: parts per 100.

         Rate: a quantity measured in proportion to something else, such as a norm or standard of reference.

         Ratio: the frequency of A, one category of observations, divided by the frequency of B, another category of observations.

Analysis of quantitative data, i.e., data that can be directly analyzed (treated as a number):

Analysis of covariance (ANCOVA): a procedure for controlling extraneous variables; adjusts data to equalize the groups studied after the independent variable has acted on the dependent variable; combines analysis of variance and regression analysis.

Analysis of variance (ANOVA): a statistical technique designed to test the significance of differences between the means of several groups; concerned with variance of the population, which can be estimated from the variances of several samples; tests the premise that the groups being compared do not differ, since they are all samples from the same population; treats data from experimental designs.

Analysis using descriptive summary measures: the measure of central tendency (mean, median, and mode); the measure of variance (range and standard deviation); and correlation coefficients (an index that summarizes the extent of the relationship between two variables). Used to summarize univariate and bivariate sets of data.

Analysis using statistical inference: a combination of mathematical processes and logical principles that allows the researcher to test estimations and statistical hypotheses against actual data in order to estimate the probability that the sample accurately reflects the target population from which it was drawn. The sample must have been drawn by random sampling from the population.

Computer analysis: the use of computers to process data and perform statistical operations.

Secondary analysis: the use of large-scale data sets in one's own research.

Applied research: a process in which the researcher scientifically collects data to be used in the clinical, administrative, or instructional area, in order to find solutions to nursing problems; evaluate nursing practices, procedures, policies, or curricula; assess the needs of patients, staff, or students; and/or make decisions to change or continue various nursing processes.

Array: a list of observations in which data are ranked from lowest to highest.

Art: a skill or craft; nursing art is the ability to apply nursing knowledge in a practical manner and with proficiency and expertise.

Assumption: a basic principle often documented and assumed to be true but not proven.

Basic research: a process in which data are scientifically collected in order to advance knowledge without particular reference to its immediate or practical use.

Bias: to prejudice, slant, influence, or improperly affect research data.
  Experimenter bias: expectancies of the researcher that may affect outcomes.
  Hawthorne effect: knowledge of being included in a study may change the behavior of study subjects.
  Interviewer bias: the tendency of the interviewer to influence the respondent's reply.
  Measurement bias: the use of inappropriate, invalid, or unreliable instruments to measure data.
  Observer bias: the tendency of the observer to see, hear, and remember only what he or she wants to see, hear, and remember.
    Halo effect: the observer is influenced by characteristics not related to the variable under study.
  Rater bias: the rater may be influenced by the halo effect, or may rate too positively or too harshly.
  Record bias: distortions introduced due to selective deposit, retrieval, survival, and recording of data.
  Respondent bias: the tendency of the respondent to distort verbal self-report because of unwillingness or inability to answer correctly.
  Response-set bias: factors that interfere with measurement of attitudes or answers to questions, such as the wish to project a favorable self-image.
  Sampling bias: the use of study subjects that are not representative of the target of population; loss of study subjects during research; nonresponse of study subjects to questionnaires or queries.

Bibliography: an alphabetical list of writings related to topic under study; includes dates of printing, editions, author, title, etc.
  Annotated bibliography: a bibliography with notes added to comment or explain.

Bivariate descriptive statistics: those derived from the analysis of two variables (an independent and a dependent) simultaneously.

Case study: a research design involving the in-depth study of an individual, group, community, institution, whole society, incident, or situation. The case study may be descriptive or analytical. It may examine changes that have occurred in a social unit after nature has introduced a stimulus. A case study that seeks to explain change, rather than describe characteristics, has been called a *pre-experimental design* by Campbell and Stanley (1963).

Category: a class or division for the purpose of organizing observations.

Causation: a process in which an event or phenomenon, called the *causative agent*, precedes, leads to, produces, or results in a change in another factor.

Cell: in a table, the intersection of a row and a column.

Central tendency: a statistical summary measure that is representative of a series of measures; includes the mean (average) score, the median (middle) score, and the mode (most frequent) score.

Chi-square test (χ^2): a nonparametric statistical test used to determine whether observed values differ from expected values; compares groups in terms of qualitative variables.

Class interval: a subdivision of the total range of a quantitative variable, divided into intervals of equal size.

Classification studies: studies that place observations into named categories.

Coding: transforming research data into the symbols used in computer analysis.

Coefficient of correlation: an index that summarizes the extent of the relationship between two or more variables from -1 to 0 to $+1$. Minus one is a perfect negative relationship, 0 is no relationship, and $+1$ is a perfect positive relationship.

Cohort: study objects who are grouped together on the basis of a common characteristic, such as age.

Comparative studies: studies of more than one group so as to compare and contrast data.

Computer: an electronic device that adds, subtracts, multiplies, divides, and performs other operations at tremendous speeds.
  Computer software: instructions for performing computer operations from a set of instructions, called a program.
  Computer hardware: input device, memory, control unit, arithmetic–logic unit, output device.

Concept: complex observations or symbols that the mind organizes into a single word or idea.

Concept-formulation studies: studies that organize the researcher's observations and experiences into a meaningful whole, expressed by a word or concept.

Conceptual framework: interrelationships among the concepts that underlie the research proposal or theory.

Conceptualization: a process by which data are arranged according to concepts.

Concomitant variation: the consistent and persistent manner in which phenomena vary or change together, either because a causal connection exists between the two or because both are caused by a common factor.

Confidence interval: a range within which the true value of the population parameter is estimated to lie at a stated level of probability.

Confidentiality: an element of ethical research, it is the researcher's ability to keep data sources protected by using numbers instead of names and by using locked records that reveal code names/numbers.

Consent: a free decision to participate in an action.
Informed consent: subjects have full knowledge and understanding about the research project in which they are being asked to participate.

Constructs: concepts.

Contingency table: a table that summarizes descriptive data and provides a cross-tabulation of data; may be used to depict nominal data from qualitative studies, for analysis using the chi-square test, and with data from ordinal scales that contain few ranks.

Control: to rule, regulate, restrain, check, correct, or limit error or distortion of knowledge.
Experimental control: a process of randomization, manipulation, and/ or modification of experimental conditions by the researcher.

Control group: a group of study subjects who are similar or equivalent to the experimental group in every way possible, except that the control group is not exposed to the experimental variable.

Correlation coefficient: an index that summarizes the extent of a relationship from -1 to 0 to $+1$.

Correlational studies: studies of how variables change in terms of one another; an increase in the magnitude of one is associated with a change (either increase or decrease) in the other.

Cronbach's alpha: a reliability index; estimates the homogeneity of a measure; also called coefficient alpha.

Cross-sectional study: the collection and analysis of data from one point in time.

Data: units of information.

Data analysis: a summary of completed observations designed to answer the research question; a study of the relationships between the parts and the whole.

Data tabulation: the process of arranging data in a concise and logical order, such as in tables.

Deductive reasoning: logical thought that moves from theory to fact by means of propositions stated as hypotheses.

Delphi technique: a research technique in which successive waves of questionnaires elicit responses from a panel.

Demography: the study of population variables, such as fertility, mortality, age, sex, and migration.

Descriptive research: research designed to recount, characterize, narrate, describe, or classify observations.

Dispersion of scores: the range and standard deviation that summarize how scores are spread out.

Documentary-historical design: a plan to collect research data by using documents, records, and/or oral history.

Ecology: the reciprocal relationship between humankind and its total environment.

Edge coding: the use of the margin of data sources, such as questionnaires, to write a code that is a symbol for the answer; for example, *1* for female, *2* for male, etc.

Effect: an event that follows the action of a causal agent; the response to the action of an independent variable, as manifested in the dependent variable.

Empirical: data obtained from using the human senses.

Empirical generalization: a statement of the observed relationships between concepts.

Error: a mistake or inaccuracy.
    Alpha, or Type I, error: rejection of a true null hypothesis.
    Beta, or Type II, error: acceptance of a false null hypothesis.
    Measurement error: an inaccuracy that arises from the measurement process.
    Observer error: a mistake that the observer makes due to inadequate training or psychological bias.
    Response error: an inaccurate or incomplete answer given by a respondent.
    Sampling error: the tendency for statistics from different samples drawn from the same population to fluctuate.

Ethics: the study and evaluation of human conduct.
    Applied ethics: actual human conduct in real situations, such as in research.

Evaluation research: research designed to judge the characteristics (good or poor) of an entity, such as nursing practices or policies.

Ex-post-facto research: research conducted from "after the fact"—after nature or life has introduced the stimulus whose effect the researcher wishes to study.

Experiment: research designed to examine cause and effect or correlations.

Experimental design: a plan of research that includes randomization, manipulation, and/or control.

    Solomon four-group experimental design: a combination of the "true," or "classic," design and the two-after-group control design.

    True, or classic, experimental design: a four-cell design in which study subjects or objects are randomly selected from the total population, randomly assigned to either the experimental or the control group, and measured both before and after the researcher manipulates the independent variable by introducing it into the experimental group and by withholding it from the control group.

    Two-after-group control design: a two-cell design in which a randomly selected group of study subjects is randomly divided into an experimental group and a control group, neither of which is measured or tested before the researcher introduces the independent variable into the experimental group.

Experimental group: the group of study subjects or objects into which the researcher introduces the independent variable.

Explanatory design: a plan of research that seeks to explain and predict.

Exploratory design: a form of descriptive research that is specifically focused.

External criticism: an examination of the validity of historical data.

External validity: the extent to which data from a sample can be generalized to the population from which they were drawn.

Fact: an empirically verifiable observation that the mind orders into a concept.

Factor analysis: a statistical technique that attempts to find unitary traits or common characteristics in a number of correlated variables. Rather than analyze the interrelationships among several variables, it analyzes the structure of the interrelationship in order to determine the number and kinds of variables needed to explain it.

Field study: research that uses a natural site for study, such as a community.

Frequency distribution: the summarization of research data by enumeration.

Generalization: the application of findings from the study sample to the broader population from which the sample was drawn; the application of the findings to a broader situation.

Halo effect: a generalization of one characteristic of a subject or object to other characteristics that may influence the observer or rater.

Hawthorne effect: the response of subjects who know they are being watched or studied, which tends to influence their behavior.

Heterogeneous: a mixture of unlike subjects, objects, or elements of research.

Histogram: a frequency distribution graph.

Homogeneous: a category or grouping of like characteristics, subjects, or objects.

Hypothesis: a proposition that states the expected relationships to be found.
> **Null hypothesis:** a statement predicting that the differences to be obtained in the values between the groups being compared could have occurred by chance alone.
> **Research hypothesis:** a proposition that states what the expected relationships among variables will be upon observation.
> **Working hypothesis:** a prediction that lies close to observed data.

Index: an alphabetical listing of references, often by both subject and author.

Inductive reasoning: a process in which the researcher begins with observations and facts and moves toward generalizations.

Inference: an estimation or judgment based on data other than direct observation; a generalization from a sample to the population from which the sample was drawn.

Inferential statistics: a theory and method of analyzing quantitative data that allows the researcher to attach probability estimates to the generalizations drawn from data.

Informed consent: an ethical approach to research in which the study subjects are given full knowledge about the research project in which they are being asked to participate.

Instrumentation: the construction and use of instruments by the researcher in order to observe, measure, and analyze data.

Internal consistency: the extent to which the parts of an instrument, such as a questionnaire or test, measure the same characteristic. A form of reliability.

Interpretation of data: the researcher's reasoning that gives meaning to the data.

Interrator reliability: the extent to which two independent raters agree.

Intervention: the manipulation of the independent variable (the treatment) by the experimenter so as to study its effect on the dependent variable.

Interview: an interaction between researcher and respondent in which questioning elicits verbal data.

> **Partially structured interview:** the use of an interview schedule that also allows the interviewer the latitude to move in interesting and productive directions.
>
> **Clinical interview:** the use of an interview schedule that combines observation with free questioning.
>
> **Focused interview:** the use of an interview schedule that focuses on questions and topics to be covered during the interview but that allows the researcher the freedom to deviate from the schedule.
>
> **Structured interview:** the use of a standardized interview schedule by an interviewer who asks the same questions, with the same wording, in the same order, using procedures identical to those of all other interviewers in the research project.
>
> **Telephone interview:** questioning by telephone.
>
> **Unstructured interview:** a general approach in which the interviewer encourages the respondent to broach and explore topics as long as he or she wishes; includes projective techniques.

Interview schedule: a series of questions that the interviewer asks.

Level of significance: a probability level that states the risk of rejecting the null hypothesis when it is true.

Literature review: a search and summary of research on a particular topic in order to identify theories utilized, research that does or does not support theory, definitions of concepts, instruments used, suggestions for further research, and research that needs replication or clarification.

Manipulation: a process by which the researcher treats or manages the independent variable, in order to study its effect on the dependent variable.

Matching: utilization of identical characteristics in a pair of study subjects so as to enhance control over extraneous variables.

Measure of central tendency:

> **Mean:** a descriptive measure computed by summing all values or scores and dividing by the number of scores (the average value).
>
> **Median:** a descriptive measure computed by identifying the value in the exact middle of a distribution of values (the value that exactly divides a distribution of values into two parts).
>
> **Mode:** a descriptive measure computed by identifying the value that occurs most frequently in a distribution of values.

Measurement: a procedure whereby rules assign symbols or numerals to objects or events, in order to determine relationships, such as quantities, degrees, or extent of observations; including counting, comparing, and ranking.

MEDLARS (Medical Literature Analysis and Retrieval System): a computer-based literature retrieval system available at libraries; it retrieves specialized bibliographical information from the National Library at Bethesda, Md.

Methods of research: how the researcher collects data: by observation, questioning, measuring, or a combination of these methods.

Model: the symbolic or physical representation of an idea; an analogy of the actual phenomenon.

Methodological design: a plan to develop or evaluate tools for research.

Multivariate methods: correlational procedures for three or more variables.

Multiple regression: a correlational procedure that analyzes the effects of two or more independent variables on a dependent variable, measured on an interval or ratio scale.

Nominal data: observations and facts that can only be separated into mutually exclusive categories.

Normal curve: a bell-shaped curve in which the mean (average), median (middle), and mode (most frequent) scores are clustered about the curve's center, with few values or measurements at either extreme end.

Nursing: a profession based on the art and science of caring for persons in sickness and health.

Nursing research: a scientific process designed to collect observable, verifiable data, in order to describe, explain, or predict nursing phenomena.

Nursing science: both the body of knowledge and the scientific method of approach to the empirical world of nursing.

Observation: a method of collecting data in which the researcher scientifically watches and records pertinent information.
  Nonparticipant observation: the observer watches and records but does not participate as a member of the group of study subjects being observed.
  Participant observation: the observer watches, collects, and records data while interacting with the group of study subjects as a member of the group.
  Unobtrusive observation: the simple observation—of exterior signs, expressive movements, physical positioning, language, or time usage —in which the researcher does not intrude.

Observation method: a means of observation devised before the researcher begins to observe, including systems of classification, operational definitions, instrumentation, scaling, and measurements.

Operational definition: a set of directions or procedures that designate precisely how to observe, measure, and record the phenomena to be observed.

Parameter: data such as the mean and standard deviation, obtained from all sampling units in the population under study, which summarize the characteristics of that population.
>   **Population parameter:** a hypothetical true value for a population; any measurable characteristic of the population, such as the population mean or variance.

Phenomenon: an observed datum.

Pilot study: a study carried out at the end of the planning phase of research, in order to explore and test the research elements.

Population: the total category of persons or objects that meets the criteria for study established by the researcher; any set of persons, objects, or measurements having an observable characteristic in common; a universe.
>   **Accessible population:** that category of persons or objects available to the researcher.
>   **Target population:** the total category of persons or objects from which the study sample was drawn and about which the researcher wishes to generalize.

Probability theory: an explanation of the possibility that events occurred by chance.

Proposition: a statement of the interrelationships observed among concepts (empirical generalization) or predicted between variables (hypothesis).

Prospective design: a plan of research beginning with the collection of data and proceeding forward in time.

Purpose: the end or aim; the purposes of nursing research are to observe in order to know; to know in order to predict; to predict in order to control, practice, and prescribe in a professional manner.

Q-sort: a method of collecting data in which the subject sorts cards with written words, phrases, or messages, in terms of a particular characteristic, such as approve–disapprove; or high priority–low priority.

Questionnaire: a technique of collecting data by means of written questions that subjects answer in writing, with little (if any) help from the researcher.

Random sampling: a method of sampling that allows every member of the population an equal chance of being selected for the study sample.

Random start: selecting numbers or names from a list by closing the eyes and touching the list blindly in order to choose a random starting point.

Randomization: a process that affords each member of the target population an equal chance of being chosen for the study sample or for assignment to either the experimental or the control group.

Reasoning:
   Deductive reasoning: reasoning that begins with theory or assumptions; develops propositions (such as hypotheses) that predict what will be found upon observations.
   Inductive reasoning: reasoning that begins with observation, develops a proposition (the empirical generalization) that summarizes the observed relationship between two concepts, and moves toward theory.

Reliability: the extent to which data are consistent, accurate, and precise; the extent to which procedures, such as measurement, yield consistent data; stability, equivalence, and internal homogeneity of instruments.

Research: the systematic, careful collection, analysis, and interpretation of data in order to obtain new knowledge, add to existing knowledge, or solve problems.
   Applied nursing research: a process whereby the researcher collects data to be used in the clinical, administrative, or instructional areas. Designed to find solutions to nursing problems; evaluate nursing practices, procedures, policies, or curricula; assess needs of patients, staff, students; and/or make decisions to change or continue aspects of nursing.
   Basic nursing research: a process whereby the researcher collects data so as to advance nursing knowledge, whether or not this knowledge is immediately usable in nursing.
   Scientific research: a process in which observable, verifiable data are systematically collected from the empirical world we know through our senses, in order to describe, explain, or predict events.

Research design: a plan or structure that guides the research process. Includes descriptive-exploratory designs; experimental, quasi-experimental, and pre-experimental designs; surveys; documentary-historical designs; methodological designs; ex-post-facto designs; correlational designs; and various mixtures and modifications of these.
   Correlational design: one that looks for patterns of variation between two or more phenomena.
   Descriptive and Exploratory designs: one that proposes to observe, describe, explore, and assemble new knowledge. Includes the case study, the comparative-descriptive study, the classificatory study, and the concept-formulation study.
   Evaluation design: one that enables the researcher to judge the success of a practice, policy, or program.

Experimental design: one that includes randomization, manipulation, and control; the researcher has maximum control over the independent variable and over the selection and assignment of subjects or objects to different experimental conditions.

Ex-post-facto design: one that researches the effect of an event that happened in the past.

Historical/Documentary design: one that collects and interprets data by examining material that already exists.

Methodological design: one that studies the methods and instruments used in research.

Needs assessment design: one that determines what needs a category of persons requires of services and policies.

Prospective design: a plan of research that begins with the collection of data in the present and proceeds forward in time.

Qualitative design: one in which the researcher plans to observe, discover, describe, compare, and analyze the characteristic attributes, themes, and underlying dimensions of a particular unit.

Quantitative design: one that measures the magnitude, size, or extent of a phenomenon.

Quasi-experimental design: one in which full experimental control, usually randomization, is not possible.

Retrospective design: one that links the effect of a dependent variable seen in the present with a presumed cause that occurred in the past.

Secondary analysis of data design: one that uses large sets of data already collected for a re-analysis from a new perspective.

Research methods: ways and means by which the researcher collects data; primarily observation, questioning, and measurement.

Research model: a symbolic or physical representation of the research plan; may represent steps to take in a temporal framework.

Research problem: a question or dilemma that the researcher wishes to investigate.

Research proposal: a written statement that summarizes what the researcher plans to do, how, and why it is important to nursing.

Review of the literature: an extensive, exhaustive, and systematic examination of publications relevant to a research project.

Critical review: a process by which the strengths and weaknesses of publications are assessed.

Sample: a portion of a larger population of subjects or objects.

Sampling: a process of selecting a portion of a target population for study.

Accidental sampling: a process in which study subjects are chosen solely by convenience.

Cluster sampling: a process in which the target population is first divided into categories or clusters, often geographic; then, the unit for study is selected from each cluster by random sampling.

Nonprobability sampling: a process in which subjects or objects are selected for study by other than probability sampling.

Probability sampling: a process in which each element of the population is given an equal chance of being included in the study sample.

Purposive sampling: a process in which study subjects are chosen that are judged to be typical of the population.

Quota sampling: a process in which study subjects are chosen to reflect the characteristics of the population being studied.

Simple random sampling: a basic probability design that gives each element in the population an equal chance of being chosen.

Systematic sampling: a process in which every *nth* element is drawn from a list of the entire target population.

Stratified random sampling: a process in which, prior to sampling, units of a population are grouped, with respect to a significant characteristic, into homogeneous strata; then, a sample is drawn by simple, systematic, or cluster sampling.

Scale: a device for measuring quantitative or qualitative variables.

Interval scale: a quantitative scale with equal intervals and an arbitrary zero point; for example, the Fahrenheit scale.

Nominal scale: a qualitative scale that enables the researcher to place variables in discrete, mutually exclusive and exhaustive, named categories; for example, sex, race, diagnosis.

Ordinal scale: a qualitative scale in which categories may be ranked; for example, Likert-type scales.

Graphic rating scale: a paper-and-pencil attitude scale in which the respondent ranks variables, constructed along a continuum, from highest to lowest or from most to least.

Guttman scale: measures attitudes by using a set of cumulative statements with which respondents are asked to agree or disagree.

Likert scale: a series of statements designed to measure attitude; respondents are asked to read prepared statements and then select one of several categories, such as Strongly Agree . . . Strongly Disagree, that most clearly expresses their view.

Semantic differential scale: a method for measuring the meaning of concepts and emotional-evaluative components of attitudes.

Ratio scale: a quantitative scale with equal intervals and an absolute zero point; for example, Kelvin temperature scale, length, weight, etc.

Science: a way of thinking and method of studying the empirical world.

Statistics: *singular:* the science of classifying relative numbers of occurrences as a ground for induction; *plural:* classified facts that can be expressed in numbers.

Descriptive statistics: a process of summarizing and synthesizing data from a sample.

Inferential statistics: a process that uses data from randomly drawn samples from which to infer characteristics of the population from which the sample was drawn and to test statistical hypotheses.

Statistic: a summary value calculated from a sample of observations and an estimator of some population value (parameter).

Summary measures: mode, median, means, range, standard deviation, percentages, and similar summations computed from measurements of sample units.

Survey: a collection of data by questionnaire or interview.

Theory: a statement that explains the interrelationships among propositions, concepts, or observations; summarizes what is known from past work and predicts what will be found on future observation.

Adaptation theory: seeks to explain the interrelationships among adjustment of organisms to a particular environment in order to function, survive, and leave offspring.

Stress theory: seeks to explain the interrelationships among tension, change in the physical and social environment, and health and illness.

Homeostasis theory: seeks to explain the regulation of a system by negative feedback.

Culture theory: seeks to explain the learned traditional way of life of a people.

Cultural ecology: seeks to explain the interrelationships of a culture and its total environment, including technology, social structure, and ideology.

Cultural relativity: a value-free explanation of the interrelationships among the system of values and the internal cultural system of a people.

Transcultural nursing theory: seeks to explain the interrelationship among a set of cross-cultural nursing concepts and hypotheses that take into account the caring behaviors, values, and beliefs of individuals and groups.

Value orientation: explains the distinctive profile of a particular culture in terms of the interrelationships among human nature, nature, time orientation, and values of being or doing.

Demographic theory: seeks to explain the interrelationships among birth rates, death rates, mortality rates, and migration rates of human populations.

Developmental theory: seeks to explain the changes that occur through time in the physical, mental, psychological, and social structure.

Learning theory: seeks to explain the process in which past experience results in a lasting change in behavior, motivation, or perception.

Behaviorism (operant conditioning): the interrelationships among learning, stimulus, response, and reinforcement.

Conditioning: the interrelationships between imposed learning and innate reflexes, between stimulus (external or internal event that brings about an alteration in behavior) and response (the alteration in behavior).

Gestalt and Cognitive learning: explains the interrelationships among knowing, learning, and thinking—problem solving, insight, and cognitive structure.

Social learning: the interrelationships among social elements, such as imitation and identification, in the learning process.

Social-network theory: seeks to explain the interrelationships between an individual or group, the web of social relations built between the individual and others over time, and social support—the extent to which an individual or group can depend on primary or secondary groups in times of need.

Social stratification theory: an explanation for the interrelationships among ranking and property, power, and prestige.

Symbolic interaction theory: explains the interrelationships among meanings, roles, symbols, and their interaction.

Systems theory: an explanation for the interrelationships among the parts of an organization such that a change in one part brings about a change in all parts.

Johnson's behavioral system: an explanation for the interrelationships among seven subsystems of human behavior.

Neuman's health-care system: an explanation for the interrelationships among the total person (as an open system) and tension-producing stimuli that may cause disequilibrium, crisis, or stress.

Time factors: research that occurs in different time frameworks.

Cross-sectional studies: collecting data at one point in time.

Longitudinal studies: collecting data over a period of time so as to study population changes or changes in the characteristics of study subjects.

Panel studies: interviewing the same subjects at two or more points in time.

Trend studies: repeatedly asking the same questions of equivalent samples of different individuals.

Validity: the extent to which a component of research—such as method, scale, instrument, or measure—reflects the theory, concept, or variable that the researcher intends it should. A valid instrument measures what it purports to measure.

Concurrent validity: the extent to which an instrument or design measures present observable behavior.

Construct validity: the extent to which a research tool measures the concept or variable that the researcher wants it to measure, whether or not the subject possesses the characteristic presumed to be reflected by the scale or test.

Content validity: concerned with sampling adequacy; it judges whether the content of the questionnaire, interview schedule, or checklist is

representative of all possible questions or observations; a panel of judges in the content area is helpful to review the adequacy of the instrument.
External validity: the extent to which the researcher is able to generalize from the study sample to the larger population from which the sample was drawn.
Face validity: the extent to which the instrument is judged appropriate by an experienced researcher.
Internal validity: the judgment of measures or designs within the study sample; for example, whether or not the independent variable actually made a difference to the research findings of an experimental study.
Predictive validity: sometimes called *empirical validity*; the ability of the instrument, such as an I.Q. test, to measure and predict performance accurately.

Values: ideas and evaluations that members of a group share about what is important; the standards by which means and ends are judged.

Variable: a concept defined by operational definition in such a way that changes or variations can be observed and measured.
Attribute variable: a pre-existing characteristic of study subjects, such as age, income, occupation.
Dependent variable: also called the *effect, response,* or *criterion measure*; a behavior or outcome that the researcher wishes to predict, study, or explain. It is observed to determine the effect of the independent variable upon it.
Extraneous variables: those variables present in large numbers in the research environment—especially in research involving human subjects—that may interfere with the research findings by acting as unwanted independent variables, thereby confusing the results of the research.
Independent variable: also called the *cause, stimulus, experimental variable,* or *treatment*; the variable that is manipulated by the researcher, in order to study its effect upon the dependent variable.

Bibliography

Aamodt, A. (1972): The child's view of health and healing. In Batey, M. (ed.), Communicating Nursing Research. Boulder, Colo.: WICHE, pp. 38–56.

Abbey, J. (1980): FANCAP: What is it? In Riehl, J. and Roy, C. (eds.), Conceptual Models for Nursing Practice (2nd ed.). New York: Appleton-Century-Crofts.

Abdellah, F. et al (1960): Patient-Centered Approaches to Nursing. New York: Macmillan.

Abdellah, F. and Levine, E. (1965): Better Patient Care Through Nursing Research. New York: Macmillan.

Abdellah, F. (1967): Approaches to protecting the rights of human subjects. Nursing Research, 16, 316–320.

Abdellah, F. (1971): Forward. In Murphy, F. (ed.), Theoretical Issues in Professional Nursing. New York: Appleton-Century-Crofts.

Abdellah, F. and Levine, E. (1979): Better Patient Care Through Nursing Research (2nd ed.). New York: Macmillan.

Adorno, T. et al (1950): The Authoritarian Personality. New York: Harper and Row.

Ailinger, R. (1982): Hypertension knowledge in a Hispanic community. Nursing Research, 31, 207–213.

Akutagawa, D. (1965): A Study in Construct Validity of the Psychoanalytic Concept of Latent Anxiety and a Test of Projection Distance Hypothesis. Unpublished Ph.D. dissertation, Univ. of Pittsburgh.

Alderson, M. (1974): Effects of increased body temperature on the perception of time. Nursing Research, 23, 43–49.

Alexy, B. (1985): Goal setting and health risk reduction. Nursing Research, 34, 283–288.

Amborn, S. (1976): Clinical signs associated with the amount of tracheobronchial secretions. Nursing Research, 25, 121–126.

American Nurses' Association (1968): The nurse in research: ANA guidelines on ethical values. In Nursing Research, 17, 104–107. (1975): Human Rights Guidelines for Nurses in Clinical and Other Research. Code No. D–465M. Kansas City: The Association. (1976): Preparation of Nurses for Participation in Research. Code No. D–54 2500. Kansas City: The Association. (1976): Research in Nursing. Kansas City: The Association.

Ammon, K. (1969): The effects of music on children in respiratory distress. In ANA Clinical Sessions. New York: Appleton-Century-Crofts, 127–133.

Andreoli, K. and Musser, L. (1985): Computers in nursing care: The state of the art. Nursing Outlook, *33*, 16–21.

Annas, G. et al (1977): The Subject's Dilemma. Cambridge: Ballinger.

Arminger, B. (1977): Ethics of nursing research: profile, principles, perspective. Nursing Research, *26*, 330–336.

Armstrong, F. (1981): Parametric statistics and ordinal data: A pervasive misconception. Nursing Research, *30*, 60–62.

Auger, J. (1976): Behavioral Systems and Nursing. Englewood Cliffs, N.J.: Prentice-Hall.

Austin, A. (1957): History of Nursing Source Book. New York: G. P. Putnam's Sons.

Austin, A. (1958): The historical method in nursing. Nursing Research, *7*, 4–10.

Babbie, E. (1975): The Practice of Social Research. Belmont, Calif.: Wadsworth.

Backstrom, C. and Hursh, G. (1980): Survey Research (2nd ed.). Evanston, Ill.: Northwestern University Press.

Baer, E. (1985): Nursing's divided house—An historical view. Nursing Research, *34*, 32–35.

Barnard, K. (1973): The effect of stimulation on the sleep behavior of the premature infant. In Batey, M. (ed.), Communicating Nursing Research. Boulder, Colo.: WICHE, pp. 12–33.

Barnard, K. and Neal, M. (1977): Maternal-child nursing research: review of the past and strategies for the future. Nursing Research, *26*, 193–200.

Barzun, J. and Graff, H. (1970): The Modern Researcher (rev.). New York: Harcourt, Brace, & World.

Batey, M. (ed.) (1968–1978): Communicating Nursing Research. Boulder, Colo.: WICHE. Eleven volumes.

Baziak, A. and Denton, R. (1965): The language of the hospital and its effect on the patient. In Skipper, J. and Leonard, R. (eds.), Social Interaction and Patient Care. Philadelphia: J. B. Lippincott.

Beard, M. and Scott, P. (1975): The efficacy of group therapy by nurses for hospitalized patients. Nursing Research, *24*, 120–124.

Bell, J. (1977): Stressful life events and coping methods in mental-illness-and-wellness behavior. In Nursing Research, *26*, 136–141.

Bellinger, K. and Laden, J. (1985): Nurse use of general-purpose microcomputer software. Nursing Outlook, 33, 22–25.

Benne, D. and Bennis, W. (1959): The role of the professional nurse. American Journal of Nursing, May, 837–882.

Benoliel, J. (1975): Research related to death and the dying patient. In Verhonick, P. (ed.), Nursing Research I. Boston: Little, Brown, pp. 189–227.

Bensberg, G. et al (1965): Teaching the profoundly retarded self-help activities by behavior shaping techniques. American Journal of Mental Deficiency, *69*, 674–679.

Bertrand, W. (1985): Microcomputer application in health, population surveys: Experience and potential in developing countries. World Health Statistics, *38*, 91–97.

Besch, L. (1979): Informed consent: A patient's right. Nursing Outlook, *27,* 32–35.

Blake, M. (1980): The Peplau development model for nursing practice. In Riehl, J. and Roy, C. (eds.), Conceptual Models for Nursing Practice (2nd ed.). New York: Appleton-Century-Crofts.

Bloch, D. (1974): Some crucial terms in nursing: what do they really mean? Nursing Outlook, *22,* 689–694.

Billings, D. (1984): Evaluating computer assisted instruction. Nursing Outlook, *32,* 50–53.

Bogdan, R. and Biklen, S. (1982): Qualitative Research for Education: An Introduction to Theory and Method. Boston: Allyn & Bacon.

Boggardus, E. (1959): Social Distance. Yellow Springs, Ohio: Antioch Press.

Bonjean, C., et al (1967): Sociological Measurement: An Inventory of Scales and Indices. San Francisco: Chandler.

Borg, W. and Gall, M. (1971): Educational Research. New York: David McKay.

Borkovec, T. et al (1976): Assessment of anxiety. In Ciminero, A., Calhoun, K., and Adams, H. (eds.), Handbook of Behavioral Assessment. New York: Wiley.

Boruck, R. (ed.) (1978): Secondary Analysis. San Francisco: Jossey Bass.

Bott, E. (1957): Family and Social Network. London: Tavistock.

Bowlby, J. (1956): Maternal-child separation. In Soddy, K. (ed.), Mental Health and Infant Development. New York: Basic Books.

Branch, H. (1979): Women in pain. In Kjervik, D. and Martinson, I. (eds.), Women in Stress: A Nursing Perspective. New York: Appleton-Century-Crofts, pp. 237–255.

Brill, E. and Kilts, D. (1980): Foundations for Nursing. New York: Appleton-Century-Crofts.

Brink, P. (1984): Value orientation as an assessment tool in cultural diversity. Nursing Research, *33,* 198–203.

Brink, P. and Wood, M. (1978, 1983): Basic Steps in Planning Nursing Research. Monterey, Calif.: Wadsworth.

Brown, E. (1948): Nursing for the Future. New York: Russell Sage. (1961): Newer Dimensions of Patient Care I. New York: Russell Sage. (1962): Newer Dimensions of Patient Care II. New York: Russell Sage.

Brown, J. et al (1984): Nursing's search for scientific knowledge. Nursing Research, *33,* 26–32.

Brown, M. et al (1977): Drug–drug interactions among residents in homes for the elderly. Nursing Research, *26,* 47–52.

Brown, M. and Grunfel, C. (1980): Taste preferences of infants for sweetened or unsweetened food. Research in Nursing and Health, *3,* 11–17.

Buckley, W. (1967): Sociology and Modern Systems Theory. Englewood Cliffs, N.J.: Prentice-Hall.

Bullough, B. (1974): Is the nurse practitioner role a source of increased work satisfaction? Nursing Research, *23,* 14–19. (1980): Factors contributing to role expansion for registered nurses. In Bullough, B. (ed.), Law and the Expanding Nursing Role (2nd ed.). New York: Appleton-Century-Crofts.

Bullough, B. (ed.) (1980): The Law and the Expanding Nursing Role (2nd ed.). New York: Appleton-Century-Crofts.

Bullough, V. (1981): Is the nurse practitioner role a source of increased work satisfaction? In Fox, D. and Lesser, I. (eds.), Readings on the Research Process in Nursing. New York: Appleton-Century-Crofts, 221–223.

Burkhart, C. (1985): The impact of arthritis on quality of life. Nursing Research, *34*, 11–16.

Burnside, J. (1973): Caring for the aged: touching is talking. American Journal of Nursing, *73*, 2060–2063.

Buros, O. (ed.) (1978): The Eighth Mental Measurement Yearbook. Highland Park, N.J.: Gryphon Press.

Byrne, T. and Edeani, D. (1984): Knowledge of medical terminology among hospital patients. Nursing Research, *33*, 178–181.

Cahell, J. and Warburton, F. (1967): Objective Personality and Motivation Tests. Chicago: University of Chicago Press.

Caldwell, R. et al (1983): Sex differences in separation and divorce. Issues in Mental Health Nursing, *5*, 103–120.

Calley, J. et al (1980): The Orem self-care nursing model. In Riehl, J. and Roy, C. (eds.), Conceptual Models for Nursing Practice (2nd ed.). New York: Appleton-Century-Crofts, pp. 53–59.

Campbell, D. and Stanley, J. (1963): Experimental and Quasi-Experimental Designs for Research. Chicago: Rand McNally.

Cannon, W. (1939): Wisdom of the Body (2nd ed. rev.). New York: W. W. Norton.

Caplow, T. (1971): Elementary Sociology. Englewood Cliffs, N.J.: Prentice-Hall.

Capron, A. (1973): Legal considerations affecting clinical pharmacological studies in children. Clinical Research, *21*, 141–150.

Carlson, C. (ed.) (1970): Behavioral Concepts and Nursing Intervention. Philadelphia: J. B. Lippincott.

Carr-Saunders, A. and Wilson, P. (1933): Professions. In Seligman, E. (ed.), Encyclopaedia of the Social Sciences. New York: Macmillan.

Cassidy, C. (1976): The relationship between daily life changes, physical symptoms, and body temperature range: Temperature changes related to adjustments to life events. Image, *8*, 30–35.

Cattell, R. and Scheier, I. (1961): Neuroticism and Anxiety. New York: Ronald.

Caty, S., Ellerton, M., and Ritchie, J. (1984): Coping in hospitalized children: An analysis of published case studies. Nursing Research, *33*, 277–282.

Chapin, F. (1970): Social participation scale. In Miller, D. (ed.), Handbook of Research Design and Social Measurement (2nd ed.). New York: David McKay.

Chapman, J. (1977): Effects of different nursing approaches upon selected postoperative herniorrhaphy patients. In Downs, F. and Newman, M. (eds.), A Sourcebook of Nursing Research. Philadelphia: F. A. Davis, pp. 15–23.

Charter, S. (1975): Understanding Research in Nursing. Geneva: WHO Offset Pub. No. 14.

Chase, C. (1976): Elementary Statistical Procedures. New York: McGraw-Hill.

Chesney, M. and Tasto, D. (1975): The development of the menstrual symptom questionnaire. Behavior Research and Therapy, *13*, 237–244.

Chinn, P. (ed.) (1983): Advances in Nursing Theory Development. Rickville, Md.: Aspen Systems Corp.

Christensen, M. et al (1979): Professional development of nurse practitioners. Nursing Research, *28*, 51–56.

Christy, T. (1975): The methodology of historical research. Nursing Research, *24*, 189–192.

Chun, K. et al (1975): Measures of Psychological Assessment. Ann Arbor: Survey Research Center.

Chung, H. (1977): Understanding the Oriental maternity patient. Nursing Clinics of North America, *12*, 67–75.

Ciminero, A. et al (eds.) (1977): Handbook of Behavioral Assessment. New York: Wiley.

Clark, E. (1968): Aspects of loneliness: Toward a framework of nursing intervention. In Zderad, L. (ed.), Developing Behavioral Concepts in Nursing. Atlanta, Ga.: Southern Regional Education Board, pp. 33–40.

Cleland, V. (1977): Investigations in the clinical setting. In Verhonick, P. (ed.), Nursing Research II. Boston: Little, Brown, pp. 33–75.

Code for Nurses (1977): American Journal of Nursing, *77*, 876.

Coleman, L. (1980): Orem's self-care concept of nursing. In Riehl, J. and Roy, C. (eds.), Models for Nursing Practice (2nd ed.). New York: Appleton-Century-Crofts.

Conant, J. (1947): On Understanding Science. New Haven: Yale University Press.

Cook, T. and Reichardt, C. (eds.): Qualitative and Quantitative Methods in Evaluation Research. Beverly Hills, Calif.: Sage.

Cooley, C. (1902): Human Nature and the Social Order (rev. ed., 1922). New York: Scribner's.

Cordasco, F. and Gatner, E. (1963): Research and Report Writing. New York: Barnes & Noble.

Cornell, S. (1974): Development of an instrument for measurement of the quality of nursing care. Nursing Research, *23*, 108–117.

Cornell Medical College (1956): Cornell Medical Index Health Questionnaire (rev. ed.). Ithaca, N.Y.: The College.

Cortin, L. and Flaherty, M. (1982): Nursing Ethics: Theories and Pragmatics. Bowie, Md.: Brady.

Cowan, M. and Murphy, S. (1985): Identification of post-disaster bereavement risk predictors. Nursing Research, *34*, 71–75.

Cox, C. (1985): The Health Self-Determinism Index. Nursing Research, *34*, 177–183.

Craddock, R. and Stanhope, M. (1980): The Neuman health-care systems model: Recommended adaptation. In Riehl, J. and Roy, C. (eds.), Conceptual Models for Nursing Practice (2nd ed.). New York: Appleton-Century-Crofts.

Cronenwett, L. (1985): Network structure, social support, and psychological outcomes of pregnancy. Nursing Research, *34*, 93–99.

Dailey, A. (1985): Burnout test. American Journal of Nursing, *85*, 270–271.

Davis, A. (1985): Informed consent: How much information is enough? Nursing Outlook, *33*, 40–42.

Davis, A. (1979): Ethics rounds with intensive care nurses. Nursing Clinics of North America, *14*, 45–55.

Davis, A. and Aroskar, M. (1978): Ethical Dilemmas and Nursing Practice. New York: Appleton-Century-Crofts.

Davis, A. and Underwood, P. (1976): Role, function, and decision making in community mental health. Nursing Research, *25*, 256–259.

Deardorff, M., Denner, P., and Miller, C. (1976): Selected National League for Nursing achievement test scores as predictors of state board examination scores. Nursing Research, *25*.

Dee, F. et al (1965): Self-acceptance of nurses and acceptance of patients: an exploratory investigation. Nursing Research, *14*, 345–350.

Dempsey, P. and Dempsey, R. (1981): The Research Process in Nursing. New York: D. Van Nostrand.

Deridarian, A. and Clough, D. (1976): Patients' dependence and independence levels on a prehospitalization–postdischarge continuum. Nursing Research, *25*, 27–34.

De Walt, E. and Haines, A. (1977): The effects of specified stressors on healthy oral mucosa. In Downs, F. and Newman, M. (eds.), A Sourcebook of Nursing Research (2nd ed.). Philadelphia: F. A. Davis.

Dickoff, J., and James, P. (1968): A theory of theories—a position paper. Nursing Research, *17*, 197–203. Researching research's role in theory development. Nursing Research, *17*, 204–206.

Diers, D. (1979): Research in Nursing Practice. Philadelphia: J. B. Lippincott.

Dilorio, C. (1985): First trimester nausea in pregnant teenagers: Incidence, characteristics, intervention. Nursing Research, *34*, 372–374.

Dixon, J. (1984): Effect of nursing interventions on nutritional and performance status in cancer patients. Nursing Research, *33*, 330–335.

Dixon, W. and Massey, F. (1957): Introduction to Statistical Analysis. New York: McGraw-Hill.

Downs, F. (1967): Ethical inquiry in nursing research. Nursing Forum, *6*, 12–20. (1977): Maternal stress in primigravidas as a factor in the production of neonatal pathology. In Downs, F. and Newman, M. (eds.), A Sourcebook of Nursing Research (2nd ed.). Philadelphia: F. A. Davis.

Downs, F. (1984): Elements of a research critique. In Downs, F. (ed.), A Source Book of Nursing Research (3rd ed.). Philadelphia: F. A. Davis.

Downs, F. (1983): One dark and stormy night. Nursing Research, *32*, 259.

Downs, F. (1964): Maternal stress in primigravidas as a factor in the production of neonatal pathology. Nursing Science, *2*, 348–367.

Downs, F. (ed.) (1984): A Source Book of Nursing Research (3rd ed.). Philadelphia: F. A. Davis.

Downs, F. and Fleming, J. (eds.) (1979): Issues in Nursing Research. New York: Appleton-Century-Crofts.

Downs, F., and Fitzpatrick, J. (1976): Preliminary investigation of the reliability and validity of a tool for the assessment of body position and motor activity. Nursing Research, *25*, 404–408.

Downs, F. and Newman, M. (eds.) (1977): A Sourcebook of Nursing Research. Philadelphia: F. A. Davis.

Du Bois, C. (1944): The People of Alor. Minneapolis: University of Minnesota Press.

Dumas, R. and Leonard, R. (1963): The effect of nursing and the incidence of postoperative vomiting: a clinical experiment. Nursing Research, *12*, 12–15.

Dunbar, S. (1982): Critical care and the Neuman model. In Neuman, B. (ed.), The Neuman System Model. Norwalk, Conn.: Appleton-Century-Crofts, pp. 297–301.

Duncan, R. et al (1977): Introductory Biostatistics for the Health Sciences. New York: Wiley.

Dunn, O. (1967): Basic Statistics. New York: Wiley.

Durand, B. (1975): Failure to thrive in a child with Down's syndrome. Nursing Research, *24*, 272–286.

Durkheim, E. (1951): Suicide (trans. Spaulding and Simpson). Glencoe, Ill.: The Free Press.

Eckland, B. (1965): Academic ability, higher education and occupational mobility. American Council on Education.

Elder, R. (1976): Orientation of senior nursing students toward access to contraception. Nursing Research, *25*, 338–345.

Erikson, E. (1950): Childhood and Society. New York: Norton.

Evans, et al (1968): A new measure of effects of persuasive communications: a chemical indicator of tooth brushing behavior. Psychological Reports, *23*, 731 –736.

Evans, J. (1982): Invitation to Psychological Research. New York: Holt, Rinehart & Winston.

Farr, L., Keene, A., Samson, D., and Michel, A. (1984): Alterations in circadian excretion of urinary variables and physiological indicators of stress following surgery. Nursing Research, *33*, 140–146.

Felton, G. (1970): Effect of time cycle changes on blood pressure and temperature in young women. Nursing Research, *19*, 48–58.

Fessler, D. (1952): The development of a scale for measuring community solidarity. Rural Sociology, *17*, 144–152.

Festinger, L. (1957): A Theory of Cognitive Dissonance. Stanford, Calif.: Stanford University Press.

Field, S. (1975): A Summary of Integrated Nursing Theory (2nd ed.). New York: McGraw-Hill.

Fielo, S. (1975): A Summary of Integrated Nursing Theory (2nd ed.). New York: McGraw-Hill.

Fieve, R. et al (1971): A critical trial of methysergate and lithium in mania. In Kuper, D. (ed.), Lithium and Psychiatry Journal Articles. Medical Examination Pub.

Fink, A. and Kosecoff, J. (1980): An Evaluation Primer Workbook: Practical Exercises for Health Professionals. Beverly Hills: Sage.

Fitts, W. (1964): Tennessee Self-Concept Scale. Nashville: Counselor Recordings and Tests.

Flaskerud, J. (1979): Use of vignettes to elicit responses toward broad concepts. Nursing Research, *29*, 210–212.

Flaskerud, J. (1984): A comparison of perceptions of problematic behavior by six minority groups and mental health professionals. Nursing Research, *33*, 190–194.

Fleming, J. (1979): The future of nursing research. In Downs, F. and Fleming, J. (eds.), Issues in Nursing Research. New York: Appleton-Century-Crofts.

Fleming, J. and Hayter, J. (1974): Reading research reports critically. Nursing Outlook, *22*, 172–176.

Floyd, J. (1984): Interaction between personal sleep–wake rhythms and psychiatric hospital rest–activity schedules. Nursing Research, *33*, 255–259.

Flynn, B. (1984): An action research framework for primary health care. Nursing Outlook, *32*, 316–318.

Ford, V. (1973): Medicine among the Teton Dakota, Rosebud Indian Reservation, South Dakota. In Batey, M. (ed.), Communicating Nursing Research. Boulder, Colo.: WICHE.

Foster, G. and Anderson, B. (1978): Medical Anthropology. New York: Wiley.

Fox, D. (1976): Fundamentals of Research in Nursing (3rd ed.). New York: Appleton-Century-Crofts.

Fox, D. (1982): Fundamentals of Research in Nursing (4th ed.). Norwalk, Conn.: Appleton-Century-Crofts.

Fox, D. and Lesser, I. (1981): Readings on the Research Process in Nursing. New York: Appleton-Century-Crofts.

Fox, D. and Ventura, M. (1984): Internal psychometric characteristics of the quality patient care scale. Nursing Research, *33*, 112–117.

Franck, P. (1979): A survey of health needs of older adults in northeast Johnson County, Iowa. Nursing Research, *28*, 360–368.

Freihofer, P. and Felton, G. (1976): Nursing behaviors in bereavement. *Nursing Research, 25*, 332–337.

Freud, S. (1938): The Basic Writings of Sigmund Freud. New York: Random House.

Gebbie, K. (1976): Summary of the Second National Conference on Classification of Nursing Diagnoses. St. Louis: St. Louis University.

Geer, J. (1965): The development of a scale to measure fear. Behavior Research and Therapy, *3*, 45–53.

Gerber, R. and Van Ort, S. (1979): Topical application of insulin in decubitus ulcers. Nursing Research, *28*, 16–19.

Gesell, A. et al (1956): Youth: The Years from Ten to Sixteen. New York: Harper and Row.

Gibbs, et al (1974): Patterns of reproductive health care among the poor of San Antonio, Texas. American Journal of Public Health, *64*, 37–40.

Glaser, B. and Strauss, A. (1966): Awareness of Dying. Chicago: Aldine.

Glaser, B. and Strauss, A. (1967): The Discovery of Grounded Theory. Chicago: Aldine.

Glittenberg, J. (1978): Fertility patterns and child rearing of the Ladinos and Indians of Guatemala. In Leininger, M., Transcultural Nursing. New York: Wiley, pp. 417–432.

Goode, W. (1960): A theory of role strain. American Sociological Review, 25, 483–493.

Goode, W. and Hatt, P. (1952): Methods in Social Research. New York: McGraw-Hill.

Goodwin, L. and Goodwin, W. (1984): Qualitative vs. quantitative research or qualitative and quantitative research? Nursing Research, *33*, 378–379.

Gordon, M. (1979): The concept of nursing diagnosis. In The Nursing Clinics of North America. Philadelphia: W. B. Saunders.

Gorenberg, B. (1983): The research tradition of nursing: An emerging issue. Nursing Research, *32*, 347–349.

Gortner, S. (1975): Research for a practice profession. Nursing Research, *24*, 193–197.

Gortner, S. (1982): Ethics issues: The boundaries between practice and research. CNR (Council of Nurse Researchers) Newsletter, *10*, 2.

Gortner, S., Hydes, M., and Zyzanskik, S. (1984): Appraisal of values in the choice of treatment. Nursing Research, *33*, 319–324.

Goslin, D. (ed.) (1969): Handbook of Socialization Theory and Research. Chicago: Rand McNally.

Grant, E. (1971): Facial expression and gesture. Journal of Psychosomatic Research, *15*.

Gray, B. (1976): An assessment of institutional review committees in human experimentation. Nursing Digest, *4*.

Gray, B. (1976): Health needs of the elderly. Nursing Research, *25*, 433–438.

Griggs, V. (1977): A systems approach to the development and evaluation of a minicourse for nurses. Nursing Research, *26*, 34–41.

Grosieki, J. (1968): Effects of operant conditioning on modification of incontinence in neuropsychiatric geriatric patients. Nursing Research, *17*, 304–311.

Gunning, S. and Holmes, T. (1973): Dance therapy with psychotic children. Archives of General Psychiatry, *28*.

Habenstein, R. (ed.) (1970): Pathways to Data. Chicago: Aldine.

Hain, M. and Chen, S. (1976): Health needs of the elderly. Nursing Research, *25*, 433–439.

Hall, V. (1975): Statutory Regulation of the Scope of Nursing Practice—A Critical Survey. Chicago: National Joint Practice Commission.

Hallenbeck, W. (ed.): Psychology of Adults. Washington, D.C.: Adult Education of the USA.

Hamm, B. and Brodt, D. (1982): GUTS: Teaching assertiveness skills by simulation & gaming. Nursing Research, *31*, 246–247.

Hampe, S. (1974): Needs of the grieving spouse in the hospital setting. Nursing Research, *24*, 113–120.

Hanson, R. (1973): Effects of administering cold and warmed tube feedings. In Batey, M. (ed.), Communicating Nursing Research. Boulder, Colo.: WICHE.

Hardy, M. (ed.) (1975): Theoretical Foundations for Nursing. New York: MSS Information Corp.

Hardy, M. and Conway, M. (1978): Role Theory: Perspectives for Health Professionals. New York: Appleton-Century-Crofts.

Harrington, M. (1962): The Other America. New York: Macmillan.

Harris, R. and Hyman, R. (1984): Clean vs. sterile tracheotomy care and level of pulmonary infection. Nursing Research, *33*, 80–85.

Hash, V., Donlea, J., and Walljasper, D. (1985): The telephone survey: A procedure for assessing educational needs of nurses. Nursing Research, 126–128.

Hasselmeyer, E. (1961): Behavior Patterns of Premature Infants. Washington, D.C.: Government Printing Office.

Hassett, M. (1985): Computers and nursing education in the 1980s. Nursing Outlook, *32*, 34–36.

Havighurst, R. (1952): Developmental Tasks and Education. New York: Longmans, Green.

Hayden, M., Davies, L., and Clore, E. (1982): Facilitators and inhibitors of the emergency nurse practitioner role. Nursing Research, *31*, 294–299.

Hayter, J. (1979): Issues related to human subjects. In Downs, F. and Fleming, J. (eds.), Issues in Nursing Research. New York: Appleton-Century-Crofts.

Heineken, J. (1982): Disconfirmation in dysfunctional communication. Nursing Research, *31*, 211–213.

Henderson, V. and Nite, G. (1978): Principles and Practices of Nursing (6th ed.). New York: Macmillan.

Highriter, M. (1977): The status of community health nursing research. Nursing Research, *26*, 183–238.

Hilbert, G. (1985): Spouse support and myocardial infarction. Nursing Research, *34*, 218–220.

Hinsvark, I. (1974): Implications for action in the expanded role of the nurse. Nursing Clinics of North America.

Hodge, R. et al (1964): Occupational prestige in the United States 1925–1964. American Journal of Sociology, *70*, 286–302.

Hofling, C. et al (1967): Basic Psychiatric Concepts in Nursing (2nd ed.). Philadelphia: J. B. Lippincott.

Holaday, B. (1974): Achievement behavior in chronically ill children. Nursing Research, *23*, 25–30. (1980): Implementing the Johnson model for nursing practice. In Riehl, J. and Roy, C. (eds.), Conceptual Model for Nursing Practice. New York: Appleton-Century-Crofts.

Hollingshead, A. and Redlich, F. (1958): Social Class and Mental Illness. New York: Wiley.

Holsti, O. (1968): Content analysis. In Lindzey, G. and Aronson, E. (eds.), The Handbook of Social Psychology. Reading, Mass.: Addison-Wesley.

Horn, B. (1978): Transcultural nursing and child-rearing of the Muckleshoot people. In Leininger, M. (ed.), Transcultural Nursing. New York: Wiley, pp. 286–302.

Hubbard, P., Muhlenkamp, A., and Brown, N. (1984): The relationship between social support and self-care practices. Nursing Research, *33*, 266–270.

Huckaby, L. (1978): Cognitive and affective consequences on formative evaluation in graduate nursing students. Nursing Research, *7*.

Hughes, E. et al (1958): Twenty Thousand Nurses Tell Their Story. Philadelphia: J. B. Lippincott.

Hurwitz, F. and Eadie, F. (1977): Psychologic impact on nursing students of participation in abortion. Nursing Research, *26*, 112–120.

Iannik, G. and Orr, M. (1979): Toward a rapprochement of quantitative and qualitative methodologies. In Cook, T. and Reichardt, C. (eds.), Qualitative and Quantitative Methods in Evaluation Research. Beverly Hills: Sage, pp. 87–98.

Jacobson, G., Thiele, J., and McCune, J. (1985): Hand washing: Ring-wearing and number of microorganisms. Nursing Research, *34*, 186–187.

Jacobson, S. (1973): Ethical issues in experimentation with human subjects. Nursing Forum, *12*, 58–71.

Jacox, A. (1974): Theory construction in nursing: an overview. Nursing Research, *23*, 4–13.

Jacox, A. and Steward, M. (1973): Psychosocial Contingencies of the Pain Experience. Iowa City, Iowa: University of Iowa College of Nursing.

Jalowiec, A., Murphy, S., and Powers, M. (1984): Psychometric assessment of the Jalowiec coping scale. Nursing Research, *33*, 157–161.

Jerome, N., Kandel, R., and Pelto, G. (eds.): Nutritional Anthropology. Pleasantville, N.Y.: Redgrave.

Jerome, N., Pelto, G., and Kandel, R. (1980): An ecological approach to nutritional anthropology. In Jerome, N., Kandel, R., and Pelto, G. (eds.), Nutritional Anthropology. Pleasantville, N.Y.: Redgrave, pp. 13–45.

Johnson, A. (1977): Social Statistics Without Tears. New York: McGraw-Hill.

Johnson, D. (1959): The nature of a science of nursing. Nursing Outlook (1968): Theory in nursing: borrowed and unique. Nursing Research, *17*, 206. (1980): The behavioral system model for nursing. In Riehl, J. and Roy, C. (eds.), Conceptual Models for Nursing Practice. New York: Appleton-Century-Crofts.

Johnson, D. (1968): Theory in nursing: Borrowed and unique. Nursing Research, *17*.

Johnson, J. et al (1977): Altering children's distress behavior during orthopedic cast removal. In Downs, F. and Newman, M., A Sourcebook of Nursing Research (2nd ed.). Philadelphia: F. A. Davis, pp. 33–45.

Johnson, M. (1975): Outcome criteria to evaluate postoperative respiratory status. American Journal of Nursing, *75*, 1474–1475.

Johnston, M. (1977): Folk beliefs and ethnocultural behavior in pediatrics: Medicine or magic? Nursing Clinics of North America, *12*, 77–84.

Jordan-Marsh, M. (1985): Development of a tool for enhancing compliance. Nursing Research, *34*, 103–107.

Josten, L. (1979): Child abuse. In Jervik, D. and Martinson, I. (eds.), Women in Stress: A Nursing Perspective. New York: Appleton-Century-Crofts, pp. 218–236.

Kalish, B., Kalish, P., and Belcher, B. (1985): Forecasting for nursing policy: A news-based image approach. Nursing Research, *34*, 44–49.

Kane, F. (1959): Clothing worn by out-patients to interviews. In Psychiatric Communications.

Kassenbaum, G. (1970): Strategies for the sociological study of criminal correctional systems. In Habenstein, R. (ed.), Pathways to Data. Chicago: Aldine.

Kelly, K. and McClelland, E. (1979): Signed consent: Protection or constraint? Nursing Outlook, *27*, 40–42.

Kendall, K. (1978): Maternal and child nursing in an Iranian village. In Leininger, M. (ed.), Transcultural Nursing. New York: Wiley, pp. 399–416.

Kerlinger, F. (1974): Foundations of Behavioral Research (2nd ed.). New York: Holt, Rinehart, and Winston.

Kim, H. (1983): The Nature of Theoretical Thinking in Nursing. Norwalk, Conn.: Appleton-Century-Crofts.

King, I. (1971): Toward a Theory for Nursing. New York: Wiley.

King, I. (1981): A Theory for Nursing: Systems, Concepts, Process. New York: Wiley.

Kjervik, D. and Martinson, I. (eds.) (1979): Women in Stress: A Nursing Perspective. New York: Appleton-Century-Crofts.

Klein, R. et al (1972): Psychiatric staff: uniforms or street clothes? Archives of General Psychiatry, *26* (Jan.).

Klenow, D. (1981): Qualitative methodology: A neglected resource in nursing research. Research in Nursing and Health, *4*, 281–282.

Kluckhohn, C. and Murray, H. (eds.) (1971): Personality in Nature, Society, and Culture (2nd ed., revised). New York: Knopf.

Kluckhohn, F. (1971): Dominant and variant value orientations. In Kluckhohn, C. and Murray, H. (eds.), Personality in Nature, Society, and Culture (2nd ed., revised). New York: Knopf.

Knafl, D. and Howard, M. (1984): Interpreting and reporting qualitative research. Research in Nursing and Health, *7*, 17–24.

Knapp, R. (1978): Social Statistics Without Tears. New York: McGraw-Hill.

Knapp, T. (1985): Validity, reliability, and neither. Nursing Research, *34*, 189–192.

Kohlenberg, R. (1973): Operant conditioning of human anal sphincter pressure. In Journal of Applied Behavior Analysis, *6*, 201–208.

Kovacs, A. (1985): The Research Process: Essentials of Skills Development. Philadelphia: F. A. Davis.

Kuhn, T. (1962): The Structure of Scientific Revolutions. Chicago: University of

Chicago Press.

LaFleur, J. and Novotny, M. (1981): Study of human figure drawing by amputee children and verbalization of their general adjustment. In Krampitz, S. and Pavlovich, N. (eds.), Readings for Nursing Research. St. Louis: C. V. Mosby.

Lamontagne, L. (1984): Children's locus of control beliefs as predictors of preoperative coping behavior. Nursing Research, *33*, 76–79.

Lamontagne, L. et al (1985): Effects of relaxation on anxiety in children: Implications for coping with stress. Nursing Research, *34*, 289–292.

Langer, E. (1966): Human experimentation: New York verdict affirms human rights. Science, *151*, 663–666.

La Rocco, S. and Polit, D. (1980): Women's knowledge about the menopause. Nursing Research, *29*, 10–13.

Leavitt, M. (1975): The discharge crisis: the experience of families of psychiatric patients. Nursing Research, *24*, 33–40.

LeCompte, M. and Goetz, J. (1982): Problems of reliability and validity in ethnographic research. Review of Educational Research, *52*, 31–60.

Leininger, M. (1968): The research critique: nature, function and art. In Batey, M. (ed.), Communicating Nursing Research. Boulder, Colo.: WICHE. (1976): Doctoral programs for nurses: trends, questions and projected plans. Nursing Research, *24*, 434–441. (1978): Transcultural Nursing. New York: Wiley.

Leininger, M. (1978): Transcultural Nursing. New York: Wiley.

Lia-Hoagberg, B. (1985): Comparison of professional activities of nurse doctorates and other women academics. Nursing Research, *34*, 155–159.

Leipold, W. (1963): Psychological distance in a dyadic interview as a function of introversion, extraversion, anxiety, social desirability and stress. Unpublished dissertation, University of North Dakota.

Leonard, R. et al (1975): The application of behavioral science to patient care as illustrated by the etiology and control of stress in clinical settings. In Verhonick, P. (ed.), Nursing Research I. Boston: Little, Brown, pp. 93–112.

Levine, M. (1967): The four conservation principles of nursing. Nursing Forum, *6*, 45.

Lin, N. (1976): Foundations of Social Research. New York: McGraw-Hill.

Lindeman, C. (1975): Delphi survey of priorities in clinical nursing research. Nursing Research, *24*, 434–441.

Lindeman, C. and Van Aernam, B. (1977): Nursing intervention with the presurgical patient—the effects of structured and unstructured preoperative teaching. In Downs, F. and Newman, M. (eds.), A Sourcebook of Nursing Research. Philadelphia: F. A. Davis.

Lindzey, G. and Aronson, E. (eds.): The Handbook of Social Psychology. Reading, Mass.: Addison-Wesley.

Lofland, J. and Lofland, L. (1984): Analyzing Social Settings: A Guide to Qualitative Observation and Analysis (2nd ed.). Belmont, Calif.: Wadsworth.

Loomis, M. (1983): Emerging content in nursing: An analysis of dissertation abstracts and titles: 1976–1982. Nursing Research, *34*, 113–118.

Lowery, B. and DuCette, J. (1976): Disease-related learning and disease control in diabetes as a function of the locus-of-control. Nursing Research, *25*, 358–362.

Lubin, B. (1965): Adjective checklists for measurement of depression. Archives of General Psychiatry, *12*, 57–62.

Lynch, K. (1983): Qualitative and quantitative evaluation: Two terms in search of meaning. Educational Evaluation and Policy Analysis, 5, 461–464.

Mager, R. (1962): Preparing Instructional Objectives. Palo Alto, Calif.: Fearon.

Magilvy, J. (1985): Quality of life of hearing-impaired older women. Nursing Research, 34, 140–144.

Mahl, G. (1956): Disturbances and silences in the patient's speech in psychotherapy. Journal of Abnormal and Social Psychology, 53, 1–15.

Marshack, A. (1972): The Roots of Civilization. New York: McGraw-Hill.

Marshall, L. (1972): Patient reaction to sound in an intensive coronory care unit. In Batey, M. (ed.), Communicating Nursing Research. Boulder, Colo.: WICHE, pp. 81–97.

Mathwig, G. (1971): Nursing science—the theoretical core of nursing knowledge. Image, 4, 20–23.

Maxwell, A. (1961): Analysing Qualitative Data. New York: Barnes & Noble.

McCorkle, R. (1981): Effects of touch on seriously ill patients. In Fox, D. and Leeser, I. (eds.), Readings on the Research Process in Nursing. New York: Appleton-Century-Crofts.

McGillicuddy, M. (1977): A study of the relationship between mothers' rooming-in during their children's hospitalization and changes in selected areas of children's behavior. In Downs, F. and Newman, M. (eds.), A Sourcebook of Nursing Research (2nd ed.). Philadelphia: F. A. Davis.

Mead, G. (1934): Mind, Self and Society. Chicago: University of Chicago.

Merton, R. (1968): Social Theory and Social Structure. New York: The Free Press.

Messick, D. (1968): Mathematical Thinking in Behavioral Sciences. San Francisco: W. H. Freeman.

Mill, J. (1930): A System of Logic (8th ed.). New York: Longmans.

Miller, D. (ed.) (1970): Handbook of Research Design and Social Measurement (2nd ed.). New York: David McKay.

Mikaelian, H. (1972): A technique for measuring eye-foot coordination without visual guidance. Behavior Research Methods and Instrumentation, 4, 17–18.

Mitchell, P. (ed.) (1973): Concepts Basic to Nursing. New York: McGraw-Hill.

Moore-Nunnally, D. and Aguiar, M. (1981): Patients' evaluation of their prenatal and delivery care. In Fox, D. and Leeser, I. (eds.), Readings on the Research Process in Nursing. New York: Appleton-Century-Crofts.

Nakagawa, H. (1972): An epidemiological study of psychiatric symptom pattern change. In Batey, M. (ed.), Communicating Nursing Research. Boulder, Colo.: WICHE.

National Commission for the Study of Nursing and Nursing Education (1970): An Abstract for Action. New York: McGraw-Hill.

National Institute of Health (1974): Research projects involving human subjects.

National League for Nursing (1978): Characteristics of Baccalaureate Education in Nursing.

Nightingale, F. (1859): Notes on nursing (1970 ed.). London: Gerald Duckworth.

Neuman, G. (1980): The Betty Neuman health-care system model. In Riehl, J. and Roy, C. (eds.), Conceptual Models for Nursing Practice (2nd ed.). New York: Appleton-Century-Crofts.

Nolan, J. (1985): Work patterns of mid-life female nurses. Nursing Research, 34, 150–154.

Nordal, D. and Sato, A. (1980): Peplau's model applied to primary nursing in clinical practice. In Riehl, J. and Roy, C. (eds.), Conceptual Models for Nursing Practice. New York: Appleton-Century-Crofts.

Norris, C. (1975): Restlessness: A nursing phenomenon in search of meaning. Nursing Outlook, *23*, 103–107.

Notter, L. (1963): Nursing research is every nurse's business. Nursing Outlook, *11*, 49–51.

Notter, L. (1972): The case for historical research in nursing. Nursing Research, *21*, 483.

Nursing Theories Conference Group: Nursing Theories: The Base for Professional Nursing Practice. Englewood Cliffs, N.J.: Prentice-Hall.

O'Brien, M. (1980): Hemodialysis regimen compliance and social environment. Nursing Research, *29*, 250–255.

O'Connell, K. and Duffey, M. (1978): Research in nursing practice: Its present scope. In Chaska, N. (ed.), Images of Nursing Views Through the Mist. New York: McGraw-Hill.

Olade, R. (1984): Evaluation of the Denver developmental screening in test as applied to African children. Nursing Research, *33*, 204–207.

Olgas, M. (1974): Relationship between parent's health status and body image of their children. Nursing Research, *23*, 319–324.

O'Neil, S. (1972): The application and methodological implication of behavior modification in nursing research. In Batey, M. (ed.), Communicating Nursing Research. Boulder, Colo.: WICHE.

Orem, D. (1971): Nursing: Concepts of Practice. New York: McGraw-Hill.

Orlando, I. (1961): The Dynamic Nurse–Patient Relationship. New York: G. P. Putnam's Sons.

Osgood, C. et al (1957): The Measurement of Meaning. Urbana: University of Illinois Press.

O'Shea, H. (1982): Role orientation and role strain of clinical nurse faculty in baccalaureate programs. Nursing Research, *31*, 306–310.

Parten, M. (1950): Surveys, Polls and Samples. New York: Harper and Brothers.

Pavlov, I. (1928): Lectures on Conditioned Reflex (trans. W. H. Gantt). New York: International Pub.

Pelto, P. and Pelto, G. (1978): Anthropological Research: The Structure of Inquiry (2nd ed.). Cambridge: Cambridge University Press.

Pelto, G., Jerome, N., and Kandel, R. (1980): Methodological issues in nutritional anthropology. In Jerome, N., Kandel, R., and Pelto, G. (eds.) (1980), Nutritional Anthropology: Contemporary Approaches to Diet & Culture. Bedford Hills, N.Y.: Redgrave, pp. 48–59.

Penckofer, S. and Holm, K. (1984): Early appraisal of coronary revascularization on quality of life. Nursing Research, *33*, 60–63.

Peplau, H. (1952): Interpersonal Relations in Nursing. New York: G. P. Putnam's Sons.

Petrovich, D. et al (1968): Nursing apparel and psychiatric patients: a comparison of uniforms and street clothes. Journal of Psychiatric Nursing, *6*, 344.

Phillips, B. (1966): Social Research. New York: Macmillan.

Phillips, J. and Thompson, R. (1967): Statistics for Nurses. New York: Macmillan.

Phillips, L., and Rempusheski, V. (1985): A decision-making model for diagnosing and intervening in elder abuse and neglect. Nursing Research, *34*, 134–139.

Polit, P. and Hungler, B. (1978): Nursing Research. New York: J. B. Lippincott.

Polit, P. and Hungler, B. (1983): Nursing Research. Philadelphia: Lippincott.

Polit, P. and Hungler, B. (1985): Essentials of Nursing Research. New York: Lippincott.

Porter, C. (1974): Grade school children's perception of their internal body parts. Nursing Research, *23*, 384–391.

Primeaux, M. (1977): American Indian health care practices. Nursing Clinics of North America, *12*, 55–65.

Puttock, D. (1972): Dance therapy. Nursing Times, *68*, 960–961.

Quint, J. (1967): The Nurse and the Dying Patient. New York: Macmillan.

Rathus, S. (1973): A thirty item schedule for assessing assertive behavior. Behavior Therapy, *4*, 398–406.

Reeder, L. et al (1976): Handbook of Scales and Indices of Health Behavior. Pacific Palisade, Calif.: Goodyear Pub.

Resio, D. and Verhonick, P. (1973): On the measurement and analysis of clinical data in nursing. Nursing Research, *22*, 388–393.

Richardson, F. and Tasto, D. (1976): Development and factor analysis of a social anxiety inventory. Behavior Therapy, *7*, 453–462.

Rieder, D. and Norton, D. (1984): An integrated nursing information system —a planning mode. Computers in Nursing, *2*, 73–79.

Riehl, J. and Roy, C. (eds.) (1980): Conceptual Models for Nursing Practice. New York: Appleton-Century-Crofts.

Robb, S. (1985): Urinary incontinence verification in elderly men. Nursing Research, *34*, 278–280.

Robinson, J. and Shaver, P.: Measures of Psychological Attitude (rev.). Ann Arbor: University of Michigan.

Robinson, V. (1970): Humor in nursing. In Carlson, C. (ed.), Behavioral Concepts and Nursing Intervention. Philadelphia: Lippincott.

Robischon, P. (1971): Pica practice and other hand-mouth behavior and children's developmental level. Nursing Research, *20*, 4–16.

Rodgers, J. (1972): Relationship between sociability and personal space preference at two different times of day. Perceptual and Motor Skills, *35*, 519–526.

Rogers, M. (1970): An Introduction to the Theoretical Basis of Nursing. Philadelphia: F. A. Davis.

Romano, C. (1984): A computerized approach to discharge care planning. Nursing Outlook, *32*, 23–35.

Rose, A. (1980; orig. 1962): A systematic summary of symbolic interaction theory. In Riehl, J. and Roy, C. (eds.), Conceptual Models for Nursing Practice. New York: Appleton-Century-Crofts.

Rose, M. (1972): The effects of hospitalization on the coping behaviors of children. In Batey, M. (ed.), Communicating Nursing Research. Boulder, Colo.: WICHE.

Rotter, J. et al (1962): Internal versus external control of reinforcement: A major variable in behavior theory. In Washburn, N. (ed.), Decisions, Values and Groups. Elmsford, N.Y.: Pergamon Press.

Rotter, J. (1966): Genealized expectancies for internal versus external control of reinforcement. Psychology Monographs, *80*, 1–28.

Rottkamp, B. (1981): A behavior modification approach to nursing therapeutics in body positioning of spinal-cord-injured patients. In Fox, D. and Lesser, I. (eds.), Readings on the Research Process in Nursing. New York: Appleton-Century-Crofts.

Rottkamp, F. (1976): A behavior modification approach to nursing therapeutics in body positioning of spinal cord injured patients. Nursing Research, *2*, 181–

185; reprinted in Fox, D. and Lesser, I. (1981). New York: Appleton-Century-Crofts, pp. 107–114.

Roy, C. (1980): The Roy adaptation model. In Riehl, J. and Roy, C. (eds.), Conceptual Models for Nursing Practice. New York: Appleton-Century-Crofts, pp. 179–188.

Roy, S. and Roberts, S. (1981): Theory Construction in Nursing: An Adaptation Model. Englewood Cliffs, N.J.: Prentice-Hall.

Rugh, J. and Schwitzgebel, R. (1977): Instrumentation for behavioral assessment. In Ciminero et al (eds.), Handbook of Behavioral Assessment. New York: Wiley, pp. 79–113.

Samples, J. et al (1985): Circadian rhythms: Basis for screening for fever. Nursing Research, *34*, 278–280.

Santopietro, M. (1980): Effectiveness of a self-instructional module in human sexuality counseling. Nursing Research, *29*, 14–19.

Schlotfeldt, R. (1975): The need for a conceptual framework. In Verhonick, P. (ed.), Nursing Research II. Boston: Little, Brown.

Schmitt, F. and Wooldridge, P. (1981): Psychological preparation of surgical patients. In Fox, D. and Lesser, I. (eds.), Readings on the Research Process in Nursing. New York: Appleton-Century-Crofts.

Schoen, D. (1975): Comparing the body systems and conceptual approaches to nursing education. Nursing Research, *24*, 383–387.

Schulmann, J. and Reisman, J. (1959): An objective measurement of hyperactivity. American Journal of Mental Deficiency, *64*, 455–456.

Scott, D. et al (1984): Stress-coping response to genitourinary carcinoma in men. Nursing Research, *33*, 325–329.

Seaman, C. (1976): Elementary Research Methods. Charlottesville: University of Virginia Printing Press.

Selltiz, C. et al (1976): Research Methods in Social Relations. New York: Holt, Rinehart, and Winston.

Selye, H. (1965): The Stress of Life. New York: McGraw-Hill.

Shaw, E. (1958): Female circumcision. American Journal of Nursing '85, 685–687.

Shipley, R. and Harley, R. (1971): A device for estimating stability of stance in human subjects. Psychophysiology, *7*, 287–292.

Sieber, S. (1978): The integration of field work and survey methods. In N. Denzin (ed.), Sociological Methods: A Sourcebook (2nd ed.). New York: McGraw-Hill, pp. 358–380.

Simon, J. (1978): Basic Research Methods in Social Science (2nd ed.). New York: Random House.

Skinner, B. (1953): Science and Human Behavior. New York: Macmillan.

Skipper, J. and Leonard, R. (eds.) (1965): Social Interaction and Patient Care. Philadelphia: Lippincott.

Small, V. (1980): Nursing visually impaired children with Johnson's model as a conceptual framework. In Riehl, J. and Roy, C. (eds.), Conceptual Models for Nursing Practice (2nd ed.). New York: Appleton-Century-Crofts.

Sohier, R. (1978): Gaining awareness of cultural difference: A case study. Leininger, M. (ed.), Transcultural Nursing. New York: Wiley.

Spradley, J. (1980): Participant Observation. New York: Holt, Rinehart & Winston.

Steffen, M. and Francis, F. (1978): Transcultural nursing experience and care with migrant children. In Leininger, M. (ed.), Transcultural Nursing. New York: Wiley, pp. 283–297.

Stern, P. (1980): Grounded theory methodology: Its uses and abuses. Image, *12*, 20–23.

Stetler, C. and Marram, G. (1976): Evaluating research findings for applicability in practice. Nursing Outlook, *24*, 559–563.

Stevens, B. (1979): Nursing Theory. Boston: Little, Brown.

Stevens, S. (1959): Measurement, psychophysics, and utility. In Churchman, C. and Ratoosh, P. (eds.), Measurement: Definitions and Theories. New York: Wiley, 18–63.

Stevenson, J. (1982): Construction of a scale to measure load, power, and margin in life. Nursing Research, *31*, 222–225.

Stillman, M. (1977): Women's health beliefs about breast cancer and breast self-examination. Nursing Research, *26*, 121–127.

Stouffer, S. (1950): Some observations on study design. American Journal of Sociology, *55*, 356–359.

Strunk, W. and White, E. (1972): The Elements of Style (2nd ed.). New York: Macmillan.

Swanson, A. (1977): Fearfulness of children in relation to maternal anxiety, self-differentiation and accuracy of perception. In Downs, F. and Newman, M. (eds.), A Sourcebook of Nursing Research (2nd ed.). Philadelphia: F. A. Davis.

Swanson, J. and Chenitz, S. (1982): Why qualitative research in nursing? Nursing Outlook, *30*, 241–245.

Swider, S., McElmurry, B., and Yarling, R. (1985): Ethical decision making in a bureaucratic context by senior nursing students. Nursing Research, *34*, 108–112.

Taylor, A., Skelton, J., and Butcher, J. (1984): Duration of pain condition and physical pathology as determinants of nurses' assessments of patients in pain. Nursing Research, *33*, 4.ff.

Treece, E. and Treece, J. (1977): Elements of Research in Nursing (2nd ed.). St. Louis: C. V. Mosby.

Triplett, J. (1977): Characteristics and perceptions of low-income women and use of preventive health services: an exploratory study. In Downs, F. and Newman, M. (eds.), A Sourcebook of Nursing Research. Philadelphia: F. A. Davis.

Tripodi, T. et al (1969): The Assessment of Social Research. Itasca, Ill.: F. E. Peacock.

Tripp-Reimer, T. (1982): Barriers to health care: Variation in interpretation of Appalachia client behavior by Appalachian and Non-Appalachian health professionals. Western Journal of Nursing Research, *4*, 179–181.

Tripp-Reimer, T. and Friedl, M. (1977): Appalachians: A neglected minority. Nursing Clinics of North America, *12*, 41–54.

Turabian, K. (1973): A Manual for Writers of Term Papers, Theses, and Dissertations (4th ed.). Chicago: University of Chicago Press.

Trussell, P., Brandt, A., and Knapp, S. (1981): Using Nursing Research: Discovery, Analysis and Interpretation. Wakefield, Mass.: Nursing Resources, 123–130.

Updike, P., Accurson, F., and Jones, R. (1985): Physiologic circadian rhythmicity in preterm infants. Nursing Research, *34*, 160–163.

Valadez, A. and Anderson, E. (1972): Rehabilitation workshops: change in attitude of nurses. Nursing Research, *21*, 132–137.

Van Gennap, A. (1909, trans. 1960): The Rites of Passage. London: Routledge and Kegan Paul.

Van Ort, S. and Gerber, R. (1976): Topical application of insulin in the treatment of decubitus ulcers. Nursing Research, *25*, 9–12.

Veatch, R. and Branson, R. (eds.) (1976): Ethics and Health Policy. Cambridge: Ballinger.

Ventura, M., Fox, R., Corley, M., and Mercurio, S. (1982): A patient satisfaction measure as a criterion to evaluate primary nursing. Nursing Research, *31*, 226–230.

Verhonick, P. (ed.) (1975): Nursing Research I. Boston: Little, Brown. (1977): Nursing Research II. Boston: Little, Brown.

Verhonick, P. (1961): Decubitus Ulcer Observations Measured Objectively. Nursing Research, *10*, 211–214.

Verhonick, P. (ed.) (1977): Nursing Research II. Boston: Little, Brown.

Vietze, P., et al (1974): A portable system for studying head movement in infants in relation to contingent and noncontingent sensory stimulation. Behavior Research Methods and Instrumentation, *6*, 338–340.

Vincent, P. and Price, J. (1977): Evaluation of a VNA mental health project. Nursing Research, *26*, 361–367.

Volicer, B. and Bohannon, M. (1970): A hospital stress rating scale. Nursing Research, *24*, 32–39.

Wagner, T. (1985): Smoking behavior of nurses in western New York. Nursing Research, *34*, 58–60.

Wald, F. and Leonard, R. (1964): Toward development of nursing practice theory. Nursing Research, *13*, 309–313.

Walizer, M. and Wienir, P. (1978): Research Methods and Analysis. New York: Harper and Row.

Walk, R. (1956): Self-ratings of fear in a fear-invoking situation. Journal of Abnormal and Social Psychology, *52*, 171–178.

Walker, L. and Avant, K. (1983): Strategies for Theory Construction in Nursing. Norwalk, Conn.: Appleton-Century-Crofts.

Wallace, W. (1971): The Logic of Science in Sociology. Chicago: Aldine.

Warner, W. et al (1949): Social Class in America. Chicago: Science Research Associates.

Warner, W. (ed.) (1963): Yankee City. New Yaven, Conn.: Yale.

Watson, A. (1982): Informed consent of special subjects. Nursing Research, *31*, 43–47.

Webb, E. et al (1966): Unobtrusive Measures. Chicago: Rand McNally.

Webster's Dictionary of Synonyms (1951). Springfield, Mass.: Merriam.

Weiss, S. and Davis, P. (1985): Validity and reliability of the collaborative practice scales. Nursing Research, *34*, 299–304.

Wells, N. (1982): The effect of relaxation on postoperative muscle tension and pain. Nursing Research, *31*, 236–238.

White, C. and Maguire, M. (1973): Job satisfaction and dissatisfaction among hospital nursing supervisors. Nursing Research, *22*, 25–31.

Williams, A. (1972): Study of factors contributing to skin breakdown. Nursing Research, *21*, 238–243.

Williams, M. (1972): A comparative study of postsurgical convalescence among women of two ethnic groups: Anglo and Mexican-American. In Batey, M. (ed.),

Communicating Nursing Research (Vol. 5). Boulder: WICHE, 58–73.

Windwer, C. (1977): Relationship among prospective parents' locus of control, social desirability, and choice of psychoprophylaxis. Nursing Research, *26*, 96–99.

Winslow, E., Lane, L., and Gaffney, F. (1985): Oxygen uptake and cardiovascular responses in control adults and acute myocardial infarction patients during bathing. Nursing Research, *34*, 164–169.

Wolff, C. (1948): A psychology of gesture. London: Methuen.

Woods, N. (1985): Relationship of socialization and stress to perimenstrual symptoms, disability and menstrual attitudes. Nursing Research, *34*, 145–149.

Woods, N. (1984): Employment, family roles, and mental ill health in young married women. Nursing Research, *34*, 4–9.

Wooldridge, P. et al (1968): Behavioral Science, Social Practice, and the Nursing Profession. Cleveland: The Press of Case Western Reserve University.

Wooldridge, P., Leonard, R., and Skipper, J. (1976): Methods of Clinical Experimentation to Improve Patient Care. St. Louis: C. V. Mosby.

Worthley, J. (1982): Understanding computer technology. In Worthley, J. (ed.), Managing Computers in Health Care: A Guide for Professionals. Ann Arbor, Mich.: Health Administration Press.

Young, P. (1939): Scientific Social Surveys and Research. New York: Prentice Hall.

Zielstorff, R. (eds.) (1980): Computers in Nursing. Wakefield, Mass.: Nursing Resources.

Zif, J. (1976): Optional vs. fixed information systems in a simulation game. Simulation Games, *7*, 35–52.

Zuckerman, M. (1960): The development of an affective adjective checklist for the measurement of anxiety. Journal of Consulting and Clinical Psychology, *24*, 457–462.

Index

Page numbers followed by *f* indicate figures; followed by *t* indicate tables.

Brigitte Couture